S
OUT

Theory and Problems of
MATHEMATICS
FOR
NURSES

SCHAUM'S
OUTLINE OF

Theory and Problems of

MATHEMATICS FOR NURSES

Second Edition

EIZO NISHIURA, Ph.D.

Associate Professor of Mathematics
Queensborough Community College

LARRY J. STEPHENS, Ph.D.

Professor of Mathematics
University of Nebraska at Omaha

LANA C. STEPHENS, M.S.N., ARNP

Nurse Practitioner, Alegent Health
Omaha, Nebraska

Schaum's Outline Series

McGRAW-HILL
New York   Chicago   San Francisco   Lisbon
London   Madrid   Mexico City   Milan   New Delhi
San Juan   Seoul   Singapore   Sydney   Toronto

The **McGraw·Hill** Companies

EIZO NISHIURA is an Associate Professor of Mathematics at Queensborough Community College, where he has been a full-time faculty member since 1972. He received his B.A. from San Jose State College, an M.S. in mathematics from the University of Illinois, and a Ph.D. in mathematics from Wayne State University.

LARRY J. STEPHENS is a Professor of Mathematics at the University of Nebraska at Omaha, where he has been a full-time faculty member since 1974. He received his B.S. from Memphis State University, an M.A. in mathematics from the University of Arizona, and a Ph.D. in statistics from Oklahoma State University.

LANA C. STEPHENS is a Nurse Practitioner at Alegent Health, where she has been since 1998. She received her BSN from Creighton University in 1979, her MSN from University of Nebraska Medical Center in 1989, and her Family Nurse Practitioner Certification in 1997.

Schaum's Outline of Theory and Problems of
MATHEMATICS FOR NURSES

Copyright © 2003, 1986 by The McGraw-Hill Companies, Inc. All rights reserved. Printed in the united States of America. Except as permitted under the Copyright Act of 1976, no part of this publication may be reproduced or distributed in any form or by any means, or stored in a data base or retrieval system, without the prior written permission of the publisher.

Portions of MINITAB Statistical Software input and output contained in this publication/book are printed with permission of Minitab Inc.

1 2 3 4 5 6 7 8 9 10 11 12 13 14 15 16 17 18 19 20 VLP VLP 0 9 8 7 6 5 4 3 2

ISBN 0-07-140022-2

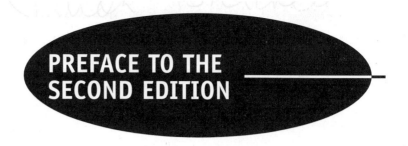

PREFACE TO THE SECOND EDITION

Much has changed in the field of nursing since 1986, when this book was first published. The apothecary system has practically disappeared and has been replaced by the metric system of measurement in the area of medicine dosages. Clark and Fried's rule have disappeared as a means of estimating a safe dosage for a child based on his or her weight and age. Mitchell J. Stoklosa and Howard Ansel, in the tenth edition of *Pharmaceutical Calculations*, state that "Today these rules are not, in general, used because age alone is no longer considered a singularly valid criterion in the determination of children's dosage, especially when calculated from the usual adult dose, which itself provides wide clinical variations in response." Because of this, we have dropped the section that includes Clark and Fried's rule. We have also replaced all problems that involve apothecary measurements of drugs. For historical reasons, we have left the part in Chapter 4 that relates apothecary measurements to other measurements.

Also, if drugs have disappeared from use we have left them out of the book. If a drug was mentioned in examples or problems but we could not find that drug in the *Nursing 2002 Drug Handbook* or in the *2002 Physicians, Desk Reference*, we replaced it with another drug that is in wide use. We have continued the emphasis on dimensional analysis in the working of problems and examples. We have replaced some problem statements by the labels that accompany the drug and ask for the computation given that the drug is available in the strength stated on the label.

We have added a chapter on statistics that is intended to help the nurse with the statistics course that she or he is required to take. We have incorporated into this chapter output from Microsoft Excel and Minitab that nurses may find integrated into their course. I have taught a course that all nurses who enter the graduate nursing program at the University of Nebraska are required to take. In this course, I integrate Excel and Minitab. I have found nearly all my students have Excel on their own home computers and are delighted to be introduced to it in their statistics course. The nursing student will be happy to find that I have been able to explain statistics with a minimum amount of mathematical formulas.

I wish to thank my wife, Lana Stephens, for her part in producing a book that is up to date and for helping me when I needed help, understanding some nursing concepts that I did not fully understand. She is a former nursing instructor and is currently an active Nurse Practitioner. She is well aware of the need that nurses have for mathematics and statistics. I wish to thank my good friend and long-time technical partner, Stanley Wileman. He was there when I needed to scan labels or pictures of syringes to incorporate into the book.

1. I also wish to thank Deidre Wall of Becton Dickinson and Company for the right to use their pictures of 3/10, 5/10, and 1-cc syringes.

2. I wish to thank Jamie Stoker at GlaxoSmithKline for her help in securing labels to be used in the book.

3. I wish to thank Karen McCann at Merck & Co, Inc., for her help in securing labels to be used in the book. The labels for the products Prinivil, Vioxx, and Zocor are reproduced with permission of Merck & Co, Inc., copyright owner.

4. I wish to thank Tiffany Trunko at Pfizer, Inc., for her help in securing labels to be used in the book. The labels are reproduced with permission of Pfizer, Inc.

5. I wish to thank Micaela Tanes of Eli Lilly, Inc., for her help in securing labels to be used in the book.

6. I wish to thank Minitab for permission to include output in the book. MINITAB™ is a trademark of Mintab, Inc., in the United States and other counties and is used herein with the owner's permission. Minitab may be reached at www.minitab.com or the following address:

Minitab Inc.
3081 Enterprise Drive
State College, PA 16801-3008

LARRY J. STEPHENS
LANA C. STEPHENS

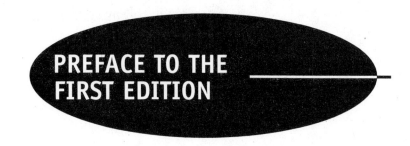

PREFACE TO THE FIRST EDITION

This book is an introduction to the mathematics needed by the nurse in modern clinical practice. It will be useful (1) as a self-review text for those preparing for nursing licensing examinations or (2) as a classroom or adjunct text for a course in nursing mathematics.

The book consists of two parts. The first part is a review of basic arithmetic, and the second discusses nursing applications.

A feature of this book is the use of a particularly easy approach to the solution of proportion problems, namely, dimensional analysis. Dimensional analysis is commonly used in the physical sciences and engineering for problems in conversion of a measurement from one unit to another. This is the same kind of problem which the nurse must master in order to convert a medication order to a form in which it can be administered to a patient.

The first three chapters comprise the arithmetic review. Those who have a good foundation in arithmetic can begin directly with the second part of the book which starts with Chapter 4 on systems of measurement and the method of dimensional analysis. A thorough grasp of this chapter is necessary to understand the remaining chapters on nursing applications.

A further feature of this book is the inclusion of material on the use of the hand-held electronic calculator to perform dosage calculations.

Each chapter contains examples to illustrate the material under discussion. In addition, each chapter contains a large collection of solved problems which are accompanied by detailed solutions to each problem, and a collection of supplementary problems, answers to all of which are supplied.

I would like to thank my wife, Ruth Nelson, R.N., for her support and professional advice during the writing of this book, Moriko Nishiura for proofreading the mathematics, and Melissa Scholz, R.N., for professional advice.

I would also like to express my appreciation for much help and valued advice to Professor E. J. Dickason of the Nursing Department of Queensborough Community College, and to my editors, Karl Weber and Jeff McCartney.

EIZO NISHIURA

CONTENTS

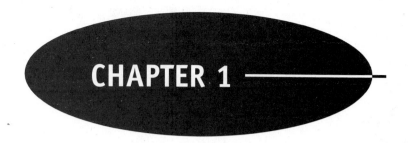

Whole Number Arithmetic

1.1 NUMBER

Counting is the process used to answer the question: How many? The numbers used for counting—"one, two, three, four, five," and so on—are called the *natural numbers*. The set of natural numbers, together with the number "zero," is called the set of *whole numbers*. Numbers may be represented either by words or by symbols called *numerals*. There are many systems of representing whole numbers by numerals, of which the most commonly used is the *base ten* system. In this system the whole numbers are written as 0, 1, 2, 3, 4, 5, 6, 7, 8, 9, 10, 11, 12, and so on.

1.2 THE BASE TEN SYSTEM

In the base ten system the first ten whole numbers—0, 1, 2, 3, 4, 5, 6, 7, 8, 9—are used as *digits*. All other whole numbers are written in terms of these digits. Numerals are classified according to how many digits they contain. Thus, the first ten numerals are called *single-digit* numerals. On the other hand, 63 is a *two-digit* numeral since it contains two digits; similarly, 504 is a *three-digit* numeral. Any numeral with more than one digit is called a *multiple-digit* numeral. Thus, 63 and 504 are multiple-digit numerals.

The digits in a base ten numeral tell how many "ones," "tens," "hundreds," and so on, the number contains. For example, the number of things in the collection on the left in Fig. 1-1 is represented by the numeral 26, since the collection can be separated into 2 groups of ten plus 6 ones, as on the right.

2 tens   +   6 ones = 26

Fig. 1-1

Similarly, the number of things in Fig. 1-2 is represented by the numeral 235 since it consists of 2 groups of a hundred, plus 3 groups of ten, plus 5 ones. As these two examples show, the digits of a numeral are assigned *place values* according to where they stand in the numeral by the following scheme:

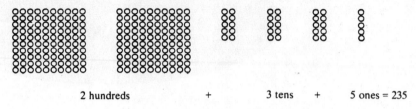

2 hundreds   +   3 tens   +   5 ones = 235

Fig. 1-2

1. The digit farthest to the right has *place value one*.
2. Proceeding to the left, the place value of each digit is ten times the place value of the digit immediately to the right.

Since the digit farthest to the right has place value one, the second digit from the right has place value ten (ten times one), the third digit from the right has place value a hundred (ten times ten), the fourth digit from the right has place value a thousand (ten times a hundred), and so on. Figure 1-3 illustrates these place values. The numeral 52,703 shown in the figure has 5 ten thousands, 2 thousands, 7 hundreds, 0 tens, and 3 ones.

Trillion	Hundred billion	Ten billion	Billion	Hundred million	Ten million	Million	Hundred thousand	Ten thousand	Thousand	Hundred	Ten	One
								5	2	7	0	3

Fig. 1-3   Place values of base ten digits.

EXAMPLE 1.1   Give the place values of each digit in the following numerals and tell how many ones, tens, hundreds, and so on the number contains: (*a*) 51; (*b*) 207; (*c*) 6000.

(*a*)   The 5 has place value ten and the 1 has place value one. Therefore 51 contains 5 tens and 1 one.

(*b*)   The 2 has place value a hundred, the 0 has place value ten, and the 7 has place value one. Therefore 207 contains 2 hundreds, 0 tens, and 7 ones (or simply 2 hundreds and 7 ones).

(*c*)   The 6 has place value a thousand, the first 0 has place value a hundred, the second 0 has place value ten, and the third 0 has place value one. Therefore 6000 contains 6 thousands, 0 hundreds, 0 tens, and 0 ones (or simply 6 thousands).

1.3   READING NUMERALS

Note that the place values in Fig. 1-3 are separated into groups of three. Starting from the right, the first group consists of the ones, tens, and hundreds; the second group consists of the thousands, ten thousands, and hundred thousands; the third group consists of the millions, ten millions, and hundred millions; and so on. In practice, the use of commas to separate digits in a numeral into groups of three aids in reading the number.

EXAMPLE 1.2   Read the numbers (*a*) 12,420; (*b*) 1,300,190; (*c*) 4,300,000,000. The commas make it easier to see what the place value of the leftmost digit is.

12,420

thousands

(a)   Read: twelve thousand, four hundred twenty

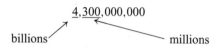

(b)   Read: one million, three hundred thousand, one hundred ninety

4,300,000,000

billions   millions

(c)   Read: four billion, three hundred million.

EXAMPLE 1.3   Write the following numbers as base ten numerals.

(a)   Five hundred seventy thousand
(b)   Fourteen million, six hundred thousand
(c)   Two billion, three hundred eighty million

  (a) 570,000; (b) 14,600,000; (c) 2,380,000,000.

1.4   EXPANDED FORM

When a number is written to show how many ones, tens, hundreds, and so on that it contains, it is said to be in *expanded form*. For example:

$$472 = 4 \text{ hundreds} + 7 \text{ tens} + 2 \text{ ones}$$

Since

$$4 \text{ hundred} = 400$$
$$7 \text{ tens} = 70$$
$$2 \text{ ones} = 2$$

the same number can also be written

$$472 = 400 + 70 + 2$$

This also is called expanded form.

EXAMPLE 1.4   Write the following numbers in expanded form in both ways: (a) 49; (b) 631; (c) 5714; (d) 12,605.

(a) $49 = 4 \text{ tens} + 9 \text{ ones}$
   $= 40 + 9$
(b) $631 = 6 \text{ hundreds} + 3 \text{ tens} + 1 \text{ one}$
    $= 600 + 30 + 1$
(c) $5714 = 5 \text{ thousands} + 7 \text{ hundreds} + 1 \text{ ten} + 4 \text{ ones}$
     $= 5000 + 700 + 10 + 4$
(d) $12,605 = 1 \text{ ten thousand} + 2 \text{ thousands} + 6 \text{ hundreds} + 5 \text{ ones}$
      $= 10,000 + 2000 + 600 + 5$

In the last case, note that the 0 tens was not written. Only nonzero digits need be expressed when a number is written in expanded form.

1.5   THE FUNDAMENTAL OPERATIONS

The four fundamental operations of arithmetic are addition ($+$), subtraction ($-$), multiplication ($\times$), and division ($\div$). Some of the properties of and procedures for performing these calculations will now be discussed.

1.6   ORDER OF OPERATIONS (FOR ADDITION AND MULTIPLICATION)

When a series of additions and/or multiplications is performed, the order in which these operations are carried out is as follows.

1. In a series of additions, the additions are performed in order from left to right. For example:

$$
\begin{aligned}
2 + 5 &+ 3 + 1 \\
= \quad 7 &+ 3 + 1 \qquad \text{(First add } 2 + 5 = 7) \\
= \quad 10 &+ 1 \qquad \text{(Then add } 7 + 3 = 10) \\
= \quad 11 & \qquad \text{(Finally add } 10 + 1 = 11)
\end{aligned}
$$

2. In a series of multiplications, the multiplications are performed in order from left to right. For example:

$$
\begin{aligned}
2 \times 5 &\times 4 \times 2 \\
= \quad 10 &\times 4 \times 2 \qquad \text{(First multiply } 2 \times 5 = 10) \\
= \quad 40 &\times 2 \qquad \text{(Then multiply } 10 \times 4 = 40) \\
= \quad 80 & \qquad \text{(Finally multiply } 40 \times 2 = 80)
\end{aligned}
$$

3. When multiplications are combined with additions, the multiplications are performed first. Then the results are added. For example:

$$
\begin{aligned}
3 \times 2 &+ 1 \times 4 \\
= \quad 6 &+ 4 \qquad \text{(First do the multiplications)} \\
= \quad 10 & \qquad \text{(Then do the addition)}
\end{aligned}
$$

4. Operations within parentheses are performed first. Then the resulting calculations are performed according to the previous rules. For example:

$$
\begin{aligned}
3 + (2 &+ 5) \\
= 3 + \quad 7 & \qquad \text{(First add } 2 + 5 \text{ within the parentheses)} \\
= \quad 10 & \qquad \text{(Then add the results } 3 + 7 = 10) \\
4 \times (3 &+ 2) \\
= 4 \times \quad 5 & \qquad \text{(First add } 3 + 2 = 5 \text{ within the parentheses)} \\
= \quad 20 & \qquad \text{(Then multiply the results } 4 \times 5 = 20)
\end{aligned}
$$

EXAMPLE 1.5   Perform the following calculations: (a) $6 + 2 \times 4$; (b) $(6 + 2) \times 4$; (c) $(5 + 3) \times (4 + 2)$.

(a) $6 + 2 \times 4$
$= 6 + \quad 8 \qquad$ (First do the multiplication)
$= \quad 14 \qquad$ (Then add the results)

(b) $(6 + 2) \times 4$
$= \quad 8 \quad \times 4 \qquad$ (First do the operation within the parentheses)
$= \quad 32 \qquad$ (Then multiply the results)

(c) $(5 + 3) \times (4 + 2)$
$= \quad 8 \quad \times \quad 6 \qquad$ (First do the operations within the parentheses)
$= \quad 48 \qquad$ (Then multiply the results)

1.7 ADDITION OF WHOLE NUMBERS

When a set of numbers is added, the numbers being added are called *addends*. The result of an addition is called a *sum*. Two important properties of addition are the following.

1. *The Commutative Property*. The sum of two numbers is not affected by the order of the addends. For example, $2 + 3 = 3 + 2$. Both sums are equal to 5.
2. *The Associative Property*. When adding three numbers, the third added to the sum of the first two is equal to the first added to the sum of the last two. For example, $(2 + 5) + 3 = 2 + (5 + 3)$, since

$$(2 + 5) + 3 = 7 + 3 = 10$$

and

$$2 + (5 + 3) = 2 + 8 = 10$$

A useful consequence of these properties is that *any set of numbers can be added in any order*. For example, $3 + 2 + 5 + 4 = 5 + 3 + 4 + 2$. Both sums are equal to 14.

The Addition Table. To perform additions of numbers with multiple digits, the sums of single-digit numbers must first be memorized. These sums are given in Table 1-1 (the Addition Table). The following example shows how to use this table. For the sum $6 + 9$, the first addend (6) is located at the left-hand side of the table, and the second addend (9) is located at the top of the table. The sum $6 + 9 = 15$ is found where the row containing the 6 crosses the column containing the 9.

Table 1-1   Addition Table

	0	1	2	3	4	5	6	7	8	9
0	0	1	2	3	4	5	6	7	8	9
1	1	2	3	4	5	6	7	8	9	10
2	2	3	4	5	6	7	8	9	10	11
3	3	4	5	6	7	8	9	10	11	12
4	4	5	6	7	8	9	10	11	12	13
5	5	6	7	8	9	10	11	12	13	14
6	6	7	8	9	10	11	12	13	14	15
7	7	8	9	10	11	12	13	14	15	16
8	8	9	10	11	12	13	14	15	16	17
9	9	10	11	12	13	14	15	16	17	18

Addition of Multiple-Digit Numbers. To add numbers with more than one digit, the addends are arranged vertically so that *digits with the same place value are aligned in the same vertical column*. There will then be a column for the ones digits, a column for the tens digits, a column for the hundreds, and so on. The process of *carrying* will be needed for some addition problems, and not for others. Both cases will be explained below.

Addition with No Carry Needed. After the addends have been arranged as described above, the columns are added in turn from right to left starting from the ones column. Each sum is written under its column to obtain the answer.

EXAMPLE 1.6   Calculate the sum $312 + 13 + 224$.

1. Write the addends so that digits with the same place value are in the same column.

```
 ┌─────── hundreds
 │ ┌───── tens
 │ │ ┌─── ones
312
 13
224
```

2. Starting with the ones column, add each column and place each sum under its column.

Step 1	Step 2	Step 3
$2 + 3 + 4 = 9$	$1 + 1 + 2 = 4$	$3 + 2 = 5$
312	312	312
13	13	13
224	224	224
9	49	549 Answer

The same procedure is also used when the final column added gives a two-digit sum.

EXAMPLE 1.7   Calculate the sum $653 + 9102 + 8024$.

1. Write the addends so that digits with the same place value are in the same column.

```
   653
  9102
  8024
 17,779
```

2. Add each column and place each sum under its column.

Addition with Carry Needed.   When the sum of a column is a two-digit number, only the ones digit of the answer is placed under the column. The tens digit is then *carried* to the top of the next column on the left, and is included in the addition of that column.

EXAMPLE 1.8   Calculate the sum $56 + 39$.

1. Arrange the addends vertically.

```
  56
 +39
```

2. Add the ones column $6 + 9 = 15$. The sum is a two-digit number; therefore, write down the 5 and carry the 1 to the next column.

```
  1  ← carry
  56
 +39
   5
```

3. Add the tens column (including the carry) and write the answer $1 + 5 + 3 = 9$.

```
  1
  56
 +39
  95        Answer
```

Understanding the Carry.   The process of carrying can be understood by performing the addition with the number written in expanded form.

1.   Write 56 and 39 in expanded form.

$$56 = 5 \text{ tens} + 6 \text{ ones}$$
$$39 = 3 \text{ tens} + 9 \text{ ones}$$

2.   Add the ones column, writing $15 = 1 \text{ ten} + 5 \text{ ones}$. The 1 ten is carried to the tens column.

$$\begin{array}{l} \overset{1 \text{ ten}}{5 \text{ tens}} + 6 \text{ ones} \\ \underline{3 \text{ tens} + 9 \text{ ones}} \\ \qquad\qquad 5 \text{ ones} \end{array}$$

3.   Add the tens column, including the 1 ten carried.

$$\begin{array}{l} \overset{1 \text{ ten}}{5 \text{ tens}} + 6 \text{ ones} \\ \underline{3 \text{ tens} + 9 \text{ ones}} \\ 9 \text{ tens} + 5 \text{ ones} = 95 \end{array}$$

EXAMPLE 1.9   Calculate the sum $567 + 15 + 338$.

1.   Arrange the addends vertically.

$$\begin{array}{r} 567 \\ 15 \\ \underline{338} \end{array}$$

2.   Add the ones column $7 + 5 + 8 = 20$. Write the 0 and carry the 2.

$$\begin{array}{r} \overset{2}{5}67 \\ 15 \\ \underline{338} \\ 0 \end{array}$$

3.   Add the tens column, including the carry, $2 + 6 + 1 + 3 = 12$. Write the 2 and carry the 1.

$$\begin{array}{r} \overset{12}{5}67 \\ 15 \\ \underline{338} \\ 20 \end{array}$$

4.   Add the hundreds column, including the carry, $1 + 5 + 3 = 9$.

$$\begin{array}{r} \overset{12}{5}67 \\ 15 \\ \underline{338} \\ 920 \end{array}$$ Answer

1.8   SUBTRACTION OF WHOLE NUMBERS

To *subtract* 5 from 9 means to find the number which, when added to 5, gives 9. The answer is 4 since $5 + 4 = 9$. Thus we write $9 - 5 = 4$. When one number is subtracted from another the result is called a *difference*. The number that is subtracted is called the *subtrahend* and the number from which it is subtracted is call the *minuend*. In the example above, 4 is the difference, 5 is the subtrahend, and 9 is the minuend. In subtraction of whole numbers the subtrahend must always be equal to or less than the minuend. For example, $5 - 9 = ?$ has no answer in whole numbers since there is no whole number which, when added to 9, gives 5.

Subtraction of Multiple-Digit Numbers.   To subtract two numbers with more than one digit, the numbers are first arranged vertically as for addition, with the subtrahend under the minuend. The subtraction is then carried out column by column, starting with the ones column. Each difference is written under its column. In some subtractions of multiple-digit numbers, *borrowing* is needed; in others, it is not. Both cases are explained below.

Subtraction with No Borrowing Needed

EXAMPLE 1.10   Calculate the difference $879 - 372$.

1. Arrange vertically with the subtrahend under the
    minuend.

$$\begin{array}{r} 879 \\ -372 \\ \hline \end{array}$$

2. Starting with the ones column, subtract each
    column and place each difference under its
    column.

Step 1	Step 2	Step 3
$9 - 2 = 7$	$7 - 7 = 0$	$8 - 3 = 5$
879	879	879
372	372	372
7	07	507

Subtraction When Borrowing Is Needed.   In the example above, each digit of the minuend was greater than or equal to the corresponding digit of the subtrahend. When this is not the case—that is, when a digit of the minuend is less than the corresponding digit of the subtrahend—then borrowing is needed.

EXAMPLE 1.11   Calculate the difference $64 - 39$.

1. Arrange vertically with the subtrahend under
    the minuend.

$$\begin{array}{r} 64 \\ -39 \\ \hline \end{array}$$

2. In the ones column the upper digit 4 is less than
    the lower digit 9. Therefore the digits cannot be
    subtracted in this form. Borrowing is needed.
    This is performed as follows: Take away 1 from
    6, which reduces it to 5. This 1 ten is added to
    4, which makes it 14.

$$\begin{array}{r} \overset{5}{\cancel{6}}{}^{1}4 \\ -3\ 9 \\ \hline \end{array}$$

3. The subtraction can now be carried out: Subtract
    9 from 14: $14 - 9 = 5$. Then subtract 3 from 5:
    $5 - 3 = 2$.

$$\begin{array}{r} \overset{5}{\cancel{6}}{}^{1}4 \\ -3\ 9 \\ \hline 2\ 5 \end{array}$$

Understanding Borrowing.   To understand the idea of borrowing, write the number 64 in expanded form.

$$64 = 6 \text{ tens} + 4 \text{ ones}$$

Since 6 tens $= 5$ tens $+ 1$ ten, this can also be written as

$$64 = 5 \text{ tens} + 1 \text{ ten} + 4 \text{ ones}$$

Since 1 ten $+ 4$ ones $= 14$ ones, this can be written as

$$64 = 5 \text{ tens} + 14 \text{ ones}$$

Thus the borrowing consists of expressing 6 tens $+ 4$ ones as 5 tens $+ 14$ ones.

EXAMPLE 1.12   Calculate the difference $534 - 178$.

1. Arrange vertically with the subtrahend under the
    minuend

$$\begin{array}{r} 534 \\ -178 \\ \hline \end{array}$$

2. Since 4 is less than 8, we must borrow 1 from 3,
    then subtract $14 - 8 = 6$.

$$\begin{array}{r} \overset{2}{5}\overset{}{\cancel{3}}{}^{1}4 \\ -17\ 8 \\ \hline 6 \end{array}$$

3. Since 2 is less than 7, we must borrow 1 from 5,
    then subtract $12 - 7 = 5$.

$$\begin{array}{r} \overset{4}{}\overset{1}{}\overset{2}{} \\ \cancel{5}\ \overset{}{\cancel{3}}{}^{1}4 \\ 17\ 8 \\ \hline 5\ 6 \end{array}$$

4. Subtract $4 - 1 = 3$.

$$\begin{array}{r} \overset{4}{}\overset{1}{}\overset{2}{} \\ \cancel{5}\ \overset{}{\cancel{3}}{}^{1}4 \\ 17\ 8 \\ \hline 3\ 5\ 6 \end{array}$$

Borrowing across Zeros.   When borrowing is needed and the next digit to the left is 0, the procedure for borrowing can be understood as follows. Consider, for example, the number 503. In expanded form,

$$503 = 5 \text{ hundreds} + 0 \text{ tens} + 3 \text{ ones}$$
$$= 4 \text{ hundreds} + 10 \text{ tens} + 3 \text{ ones} \qquad (\text{Borrow 1 hundred} = 10 \text{ tens from 5 hundreds})$$
$$= 4 \text{ hundreds} + 9 \text{ tens} + 13 \text{ ones} \qquad (\text{Borrow 1 ten from 10 tens})$$
$$= \overset{4}{\cancel{5}} \qquad \overset{9}{\cancel{0}} \qquad {}^{1}3$$

Thus 1 ten is *borrowed across the 0* by writing $\overset{4\,9}{\cancel{5}\cancel{0}}{}^{1}3$. The 5 becomes 4, the 0 becomes 9, and the 3 becomes 13.

EXAMPLE 1.13   Calculate the difference $503 - 168$.

Borrow across the zero, then subtract.

$$\begin{array}{r} \overset{4\ 9}{\cancel{5}\cancel{0}}{}^{1}3 \\ -16\ 8 \\ \hline 33\ 5 \end{array}$$

Borrowing across two or more zeros is performed similarly.

EXAMPLE 1.14   Calculate the difference $24{,}002 - 6{,}534$.

1. Borrow across the zeros, then subtract.

$$\begin{array}{r} \overset{3\ 9\ 9}{2\,4{,}\cancel{0}\cancel{0}}{}^{1}2 \\ -6\ 53\ 4 \\ \hline 46\ 8 \end{array}$$

2. Borrow from 2, then subtract.

$$\begin{array}{r} \overset{1}{\ }\overset{1}{}3\ 9\ 9 \\ \cancel{2}\,4{,}\cancel{0}\cancel{0}{}^{1}2 \\ -6\ 53\ 4 \\ \hline 1\,7{,}46\ 8 \end{array}$$

1.9   MULTIPLICATION OF WHOLE NUMBERS

When two or more whole numbers are multiplied, the result is called their *product*. The numbers multiplied are called *factors* of the product. Multiplication of whole numbers can be defined as repeated addition. For example, the product 3×4 means $4 + 4 + 4$. That is, "three times four" means "the sum of three fours." Similarly,

$$0 \times 3 = 0 \quad \text{(zero threes is zero)}$$
$$1 \times 3 = 3 \quad \text{(one three is three)}$$
$$2 \times 3 = 6 \quad \text{(two threes is six)}$$
$$3 \times 3 = 9 \quad \text{(three threes is nine)}$$

and so on. A *multiple* of a number is the product of that number and another whole number (except 0). For example, as is shown above, the numbers 3, 6, 9, and so on are multiples of 3. Similarly, the multiples of 2 are 2, 4, 6, 8, 10, 12, and so on, since $2 = 2 \times 1, 4 = 2 \times 2, 6 = 3 \times 2$, and so on. The multiples of 2 are called the *even numbers*. The numbers 1, 3, 5, 7, 9, and so on, which are *not* multiples of 2, are called the *odd numbers*.

The Multiplication Table. To perform multiplication of whole numbers, the multiplication table (Table 1-2) for single-digit numbers must be memorized. This table is read in the same way as Table 1-1. For example, to find the product of 6 and 8, read across the row with 6 at the left and down the column with 8 at the top.

Table 1-2   Multiplication Table

	0	1	2	3	4	5	6	7	8	9
0	0	0	0	0	0	0	0	0	0	0
1	0	1	2	3	4	5	6	7	8	9
2	0	2	4	6	8	10	12	14	16	18
3	0	3	6	9	12	15	18	21	24	27
4	0	4	8	12	16	20	24	28	32	36
5	0	5	10	15	20	25	30	35	40	45
6	0	6	12	18	24	30	36	42	48	54
7	0	7	14	21	28	35	42	49	56	63
8	0	8	16	24	32	40	48	56	64	72
9	0	9	18	27	36	45	54	63	72	81

Properties of Multiplication. Like addition, multiplication has the commutative and associative properties (see Sec. 1.7). From these properties follows the useful fact that *the multiplication of a set of numbers can be performed in any order.* Another important property of multiplication is the *distributive property*. The product of a number and the sum of two or more addends can be calculated by multiplying the number by each addend and then adding the results. For example, the product $3 \times (2 + 4)$ can be calculated as $3 \times 2 + 3 \times 4$. The results will be the same:

$$3 \times (2 + 4) = 3 \times 6 = 18$$
$$3 \times 2 + 3 \times 4 = 6 + 12 = 18$$

Multiplication of a Single-Digit Number by a Multiple-Digit Number.   To multiply a number with more than one digit by a single-digit number, write the single-digit factor under the ones digit of the other factor. The multiplication is carried out by multiplying each digit of the top factor by the bottom factor, starting from the right and proceeding to the left. In some cases carrying is needed; in others, it is not. Both cases are explained below.

Multiplication with No Carry Needed

EXAMPLE 1.15   Calculate the product 3×432.

1. Arrange the factors vertically with the single-digit
    factor below.

$$432$$
$$\times 3$$

2. Multiply the single-digit factor by each digit of
    the top factor, starting from the right and
    proceeding to the left.

Step 1	Step 2	Step 3	
$2 \times 3 = 6$	$3 \times 3 = 9$	$4 \times 3 = 12$	
432	432	432	
3	3	3	
6	96	1296	Answer

Understanding the Procedure.   The procedure outlined above can be understood by writing the number 432 in expanded form. The multiplication is carried out using the distributive property.

$$3 \times 432 = 3 \times (4 \text{ hundreds} + 3 \text{ tens} + 2 \text{ ones})$$
$$= 3 \times 4 \text{ hundreds} + 3 \times 3 \text{ tens} + 3 \times 2 \text{ ones}$$
$$= 12 \text{ hundreds} + 9 \text{ tens} + 6 \text{ ones}$$
$$= 1296$$

Multiplication with Carry Needed. When a multiplication of digits results in a two-digit answer, the ones digit of the answer is written down and the tens digit is carried mentally, to be added to the result of the next multiplication.

EXAMPLE 1.16   Calculate the product 4×57.

1. Arrange the factors vertically with the single-digit
    factor below.
2. Multiply the single-digit factor by each digit in
    the top factor.

Step 1.   Multiply $4 \times 7 = 28$. Write the 8 and
carry the 2.

$$57$$
$$\times 4$$
$$8$$ (Carry the 2 in your head)

Step 2.   Multiply $4 \times 5 = 20$, then add the
carry 2 to this answer, $20 + 2 = 22$.

$$57$$
$$\times 4$$
$$228$$ Answer

Understanding the Procedure.   The procedure of carrying outlined above can be understood by writing the number 57 in expanded form. The multiplication is carried out using the distributive property.

$$4 \times 57 = 4 \times (5 \text{ tens} + 7 \text{ ones})$$
$$= 4 \times 5 \text{ tens} + 4 \times 7 \text{ ones}$$
$$= 20 \text{ tens} + 28 \text{ ones}$$

Since 28 ones = 2 tens + 8 ones, the above can be written as

$$4 \times 57 = 20 \text{ tens} + 2 \text{ tens} + 8 \text{ ones} \qquad \text{(The 2 tens is the digit 2 that was carried mentally)}$$
$$= 22 \text{ tens} + 8 \text{ ones}$$
$$= 228$$

Multiplication by Multiples of the Place Values. The multiples of the place values ten, hundred, thousand, and so on, are:

Multiples of 10: 10, 20, 30, 40, 50, 60, ...

Multiples of 100: 100, 200, 300, 400, 500, 600, ...

Multiples of 1000: 1000, 2000, 3000, 4000, 5000, ...

and so on. Multiplication by such numbers can be performed by a shortcut method shown in Example 1.17.

EXAMPLE 1.17 Calculate the following products: (a) 2×300; (b) 40×200; (c) 200×500.

(a) Multiply $2 \times 3 = 6$, then bring down the two remaining zeros from 300.

$$
\begin{array}{r}
300 \\
\times 2 \\
\hline
6 \\
600 \qquad \text{Answer}
\end{array}
$$

(b) Multiply $4 \times 2 = 8$, then bring down the three remaining zeros from 40 and 200.

$$
\begin{array}{r}
200 \\
\times 40 \\
\hline
8 \\
8000 \qquad \text{Answer}
\end{array}
$$

(c) Multiply $2 \times 5 = 10$, then bring down the four remaining zeros from 200 and 500.

$$
\begin{array}{r}
500 \\
\times 200 \\
\hline
10 \\
100,000 \qquad \text{Answer}
\end{array}
$$

The procedure illustrated in this example can be described as follows: first multiply, ignoring the zeros at the tail ends of the factors; then adjoin those zeros to the resulting product.

Understanding the Procedure. To understand why the shortcut works, consider the multiplication 40×200. Since $40 = 4 \times 10$ and $200 = 2 \times 100$, then

$$40 \times 200 = 4 \times 10 \times 2 \times 100$$
$$= 4 \times 2 \times 10 \times 100 \qquad \text{(Rearrange the factors)}$$
$$= \quad 8 \quad \times \quad 1000$$
$$= \quad 8000$$

Multiplying Multiple-Digit Factors. To multiply a pair of factors, each with multiple digits, the factors are arranged vertically so that digits with the same place value are aligned, usually with the factor with fewer digits on the bottom. The procedure will be explained with examples.

EXAMPLE 1.18 Calculate the product 82×23.

1. Arrange the factors vertically so that digits
    of the same place value are aligned.

$$
\begin{array}{r}
82 \\
\times 23 \\
\end{array}
$$

2. Multiply the top factor by the ones digit of
    the bottom factor.

$$\begin{array}{r} 82 \\ \times 23 \\ \hline 246 \end{array} \leftarrow 3 \times 82$$

3. Multiply the top factor by the tens digit of the
    bottom factor. The result is written on the line
    below the first line but shifted one place to
    the left.

$$\begin{array}{r} 82 \\ \times 23 \\ \hline 246 \\ 164 \end{array} \leftarrow 2 \times 82$$

4. Add the resulting products.

$$\begin{array}{r} 82 \\ \times 23 \\ \hline 246 \\ 164 \\ \hline 1886 \end{array} \quad \text{Answer}$$

Understanding the Procedure.   The multiplication procedure outlined above can be understood by writing the factor 23 in expanded form, then applying the distributive property.

$$\begin{aligned} 82 \times 23 &= 82 \times (20 + 3) \\ &= 82 \times 20 + 82 \times 3 \quad \text{(These are the multiplications of Step 2 and Step 3)} \\ &= 1640 + 246 \quad \text{(This is the addition that was performed in Step 4)} \\ &= 1886 \end{aligned}$$

EXAMPLE 1.19   Calculate the product 516×7208.

1. Arrange the factors so that digits of the same
    place value are aligned, with the 7208 on top.

$$\begin{array}{r} 7208 \\ \times 516 \end{array}$$

2. Multiply 7208 by the ones digit.

$$\begin{array}{r} 7208 \\ \times 516 \\ \hline 43\ 248 \end{array} \leftarrow 6 \times 7208$$

3. Multiply 7208 by the tens digit.

$$\begin{array}{r} 7208 \\ \times 516 \\ \hline 43\ 248 \\ 72\ 08 \end{array} \leftarrow 1 \times 7208$$

4. Multiply 7208 by the hundreds digit.

$$\begin{array}{r} 7208 \\ \times 516 \\ \hline 43\ 248 \\ 72\ 08 \\ 3\ 604\ 0 \end{array} \leftarrow 5 \times 7208$$

5. Add the resulting products.

$$\begin{array}{r} 7208 \\ \times 516 \\ \hline 43\ 248 \\ 72\ 08 \\ 3\ 604\ 0 \\ \hline 3,719,328 \end{array} \quad \text{Answer}$$

EXAMPLE 1.20   Calculate the product 370×460.

1.   Multiply 37×46 disregarding the two zeros.

$$\begin{array}{r} 460 \\ \times 370 \\ \hline 322 \\ 138 \\ \hline 1702 \end{array}$$

2.   Then bring down the two zeros.   170,200   Answer

1.10   DIVISION OF WHOLE NUMBERS

To *divide* 15 by 3 means to find the number which when multiplied by 3 gives 15. The answer is 5 since $3 \times 5 = 15$. Thus we write $15 \div 3 = 5$. When one number is divided by another, the result is called a *quotient*. The number divided by is called the *divisor* and the number being divided is called the *dividend*. Thus, in $15 \div 3 = 5$, 15 is the dividend, 3 is the divisor, and 5 is the quotient.

Division as Repeated Subtraction.   Division does not always have a whole number quotient. For example, there is no whole number equal to $9 \div 4$, since there is no whole number which when multiplied by 4 gives 9. However, such a division can be understood as repeated subtraction. Thus, the division $9 \div 4$ tells how many times 4 can be subtracted from 9. The answer is 2 with a remainder of 1.

$$\begin{array}{r} 9 \\ -4 \\ \hline 5 \\ -4 \\ \hline 1 \end{array}$$ 2 Subtractions

$1 \leftarrow$ Remainder

The Division Procedure (Single-Digit Quotient).   To perform a division, the division is first set up in the form

$$\text{Divisor})\overline{\text{Dividend}}$$

Thus, the division $9 \div 4$ is set up $4\overline{)9}$. The division for a single-digit answer is as follows.

EXAMPLE 1.21   Perform the division $9 \div 4$.

(a) *Divide*   (b) *Multiply*   (c) *Subtract*
4 goes into 9 two times $2 \times 4 = 8$ $9 - 8 = 1$
$\begin{array}{r} 2 \\ 4\overline{)9} \end{array}$ $\begin{array}{r} 2 \\ 4\overline{)9} \\ 8 \end{array}$ $\begin{array}{r} 2 \\ 4\overline{)9} \\ 8 \\ \hline 1 \end{array}$ Quotient Remainder

The steps outlined above give the *quotient* (the number of times the divisor goes into the dividend) and the *remainder* (the difference that remains).

The Division Procedure (Multiple-Digit Quotient).   The steps labeled (a), (b), and (c) are the first three steps in any division. In this procedure, after the division has been set up, the quotient is found one digit at a time starting from the largest place value. It is written above the dividend so that its place values are aligned with the place values of the dividend: ones digit over ones digit, tens digit over tens digit, and so on. When there are two or more digits in the answer, there is a fourth step (d), as in Example 1.22. These steps (a) through (d) are repeated in any division until the division is ended.

EXAMPLE 1.22   Perform the division $94 \div 4$.

1.   Set up the division:

$$4\overline{)94}$$

2.   How many *tens* in the quotient?

(*a*)	*Divide*	(*b*)	*Multiply*	(*c*)	*Subtract*	(*d*)	*Bring down*

      (*a*) *Divide*   4 goes into 9 two times

                   2
$$4\overline{)94}$$

  (*b*) *Multiply* $2 \times 4 = 8$

               2
$$4\overline{)94}$$
                  8

  (*c*) *Subtract* $9 - 8 = 1$

               2
$$4\overline{)94}$$
                 8
                 1

  (*d*) *Bring down*   Bring down the next digit, 4

               2
$$4\overline{)94}$$
                8
              14

3.   How many *ones* in the quotient? The steps are now repeated using 14, the result of bringing down the 4, as the dividend.

  (*a*) *Divide*   4 goes into 14 three times

               23
$$4\overline{)94}$$
              8
             14

  (*b*) *Multiply* $4 \times 3 = 12$

           23
$$4\overline{)94}$$
          8
         14
         12

  (*c*) *Subtract* $14 - 12 = 2$

          23   Quotient
$$4\overline{)94}$$
        8
      14
      12
       2   Remainder

  (*d*) *Bring down*   There are no more digits to bring down. The division is complete.

EXAMPLE 1.23   Perform the division $273 \div 6$.

1.   Set up the division:

$$6\overline{)273}$$

In this division the divisor 6 will not go into the hundreds digit 2; therefore the quotient will start at the tens digit. The first division is 6 into 27.

2.   How many *tens* in the quotient?

  (*a*) *Divide*   6 goes into 27 four times

         4
$$6\overline{)273}$$

  (*b*) *Multiply* $6 \times 4 = 24$

         4
$$6\overline{)273}$$
      24

  (*c*) *Subtract* $27 - 24 = 3$

         4
$$6\overline{)273}$$
      24
       3

  (*d*) *Bring down*   Bring down the next digit, 3

         4
$$6\overline{)273}$$
      24
      33

3.   How many *ones* in the quotient?

  (*a*) *Divide*   6 goes into 33 five times

         45
$$6\overline{)273}$$
      24
      33

  b) *Multiply* $6 \times 5 = 30$

         45
$$6\overline{)273}$$
      24
      33
      30

  (*c*) *Subtract* $33 - 30 = 3$

         45   Quotient
$$6\overline{)273}$$
      24
      33
      30
       3   Remainder

EXAMPLE 1.24   Perform the division $3566 \div 52$.
Set up the division:

$$52\overline{)3566}$$

Before we start the division, two things must be observed: first, the divisor is now a two-digit number but the procedure is the same; second, the quotient must start at the tens place since the first division is 52 into 356. This division is not easy to do and requires guessing. Trial and error will show that the largest multiple of 52 that is less than 356 is $52 \times 6 = 312$ (because $52 \times 7 = 364$, which is too large). Thus the first calculations (divide, multiply, subtract, and bring down) are

$$
\begin{array}{r}
6 \\
52\overline{)3566} \\
\underline{312} \\
446
\end{array}
$$

The next calculations, starting with 52 into 446, give the answer:

$$
\begin{array}{rl}
68 & \text{Quotient} \\
52\overline{)3566} & \\
\underline{312} & \\
446 & \\
\underline{416} & \\
30 & \text{Remainder}
\end{array}
$$

At each step, remember that *each subtraction must result in a remainder that is less than the divisor*. Otherwise, the partial quotient at that step will be too small.

EXAMPLE 1.25   Perform the division $7368 \div 24$.

1. How many hundreds?

$$
\begin{array}{r}
3 \\
24\overline{)7368} \\
\underline{72} \\
16
\end{array}
$$

2. After bringing down the 6, we see that 24 goes into 16 zero times. Thus to answer the question "How many tens?" a 0 is put in the tens position of the quotient, and the next digit is brought down.

$$
\begin{array}{rl}
30 & \text{(Write 0 in the quotient and} \\
24\overline{)7368} & \text{bring down the 8)} \\
\underline{72} & \\
168 &
\end{array}
$$

3. How many ones?

$$
\begin{array}{rl}
307 & \text{Quotient} \\
24\overline{)7368} & \\
\underline{72} & \\
168 & \\
\underline{168} &
\end{array}
$$

The remainder is 0. Whenever the remainder is 0, it need not be written. When the remainder is 0, the division is said to be *exact*. Thus it is said that 24 divides into 7368 *exactly*, or that 7368 is *exactly divisable* by 24.

1.11   DIVISORS AND PRIME NUMBERS

A *divisor* of a number is any number that divides it exactly. Thus 3 is a divisor of 6, since 3 divides 6 exactly ($6 \div 3 = 2$). The numbers 1, 2, 3, and 6, and only these numbers, are the divisors of 6 since each divides 6 exactly and no other numbers do so. Any number has both 1 and itself as divisors; for example, both 1 and 6 are divisors of 6. Any number that has exactly two divisors—1 and itself, but no more—is called a *prime number*. Thus 6 is *not* a prime number. The number 5, however, *is* a prime number, since its only divisors are 1 and 5. The first 12 prime numbers are: 2, 3, 5, 7, 11, 13, 17, 19, 23, 29, 31, and 37. The list of prime numbers goes on indefinitely.

1.12 THE GREATEST COMMON DIVISOR (GCD)

A *common divisor* of two or more numbers is any number that is a divisor of each of the numbers. Thus a common divisor of 4 and 6 is 2, since it is a divisor of both ($4 \div 2 = 2$, and $6 \div 2 = 3$). A common divisor of 6, 9, and 12 is 3, since it is a divisor of each ($6 \div 3 = 2$, $9 \div 3 = 3$, and $12 \div 3 = 4$). Any set of numbers always has 1 as a common divisor.

A set of numbers may have common divisors. For example, 12 and 18 have the numbers 1, 2, 3, and 6 as common divisors. The number 6 is the greatest of these common divisors. Thus 6 is called the *greatest common divisor* (GCD) of 12 and 18. The GCD of any set of numbers is the greatest number which divides all the numbers exactly.

EXAMPLE 1.26 Find the GCD of the following sets of numbers: (*a*) 8 and 12; (*b*) 5 and 6; (*c*) 4 and 8; (*d*) 30, 40, and 20.

(*a*) The greatest number that divides both 8 and 12 exactly is 4 ($8 \div 4 = 2$ and $12 \div 4 = 3$). Thus, the GCD = 4.

(*b*) The greatest number that divides both 5 and 6 exactly is 1 ($5 \div 1 = 5$ and $6 \div 1 = 6$). Thus, the GCD = 1.

(*c*) The greatest number that divides both 4 and 8 exactly is 4 ($4 \div 4 = 1$ and $8 \div 4 = 2$). Thus, the GCD = 4.

(*d*) The greatest number that divides all three numbers 30, 40, and 20 is 10 ($30 \div 10 = 3$, $40 \div 10 = 4$, and $20 \div 10 = 2$). Thus, the GCD = 10.

A systematic method of finding the GCD of any two numbers is called the *Euclidean algorithm*. The method is as follows.

1. Divide the smaller number into the larger. If the remainder is zero, then stop.

2. If the remainder is not zero, repeat the first step with the remainder divided into the previously used divisor.

The steps are repeated until a remainder of zero is found. The last divisor used is then the GCD of the two originally given numbers.

EXAMPLE 1.27 Find the GCD of 63 and 84.

1. Divide 63 into 84.

$$
\begin{array}{r}
1 \\
63\overline{)84} \\
\underline{63} \\
21 \quad \text{Remainder}
\end{array}
$$

The remainder is not zero, so we divide again.
The remainder is divided into the previous divisor.

2. Divide 21 into 63.

$$
\begin{array}{r}
3 \\
21\overline{)63} \\
\underline{63} \\
0 \quad \text{Remainder}
\end{array}
$$

The remainder is 0. Therefore we stop. The GCD of 63 and 84 is 21 (the last divisor used).

EXAMPLE 1.28 Find the GCD of 105 and 91.

1. Divide 91 into 105.

$$
\begin{array}{r}
1 \\
9\overline{)105} \\
\underline{91} \\
14 \quad \text{Remainder}
\end{array}
$$

2. Divide 14 into 91.

$$
\begin{array}{r}
6 \\
14\overline{)91} \\
\underline{84} \\
7 \quad \text{Remainder}
\end{array}
$$

3. Divide 7 into 14.

$$\begin{array}{r} 2 \\ 7\overline{)14} \\ \underline{14} \\ 0 \quad \text{Remainder} \end{array}$$

The GCD of 91 and 105 is 7.

1.13   THE LEAST COMMON MULTIPLE (LCM)

A *common multiple* of two or more numbers is a number that is a multiple of each of the given numbers. For example, 18 is a common multiple of 6 and 9 since it is a multiple of both:

$$6 \times 3 = 18$$
$$9 \times 2 = 18$$

Here 18 is also the least number that is a multiple of both 6 and 9. It is thus called their *least common multiple* (LCM). The LCM of a set of numbers is the least number into which each of the numbers divides exactly.

EXAMPLE 1.29   Find the least common multiple (LCM) of the following sets of numbers: (*a*) 4 and 6; (*b*) 4 and 7; (*c*) 8 and 16; (*d*) 9, 6, and 12.

(*a*)   The least number into which both 4 and 6 divide exactly is 12 ($12 \div 4 = 3$ and $12 \div 6 = 2$). Thus, their LCM = 12.

(*b*)   The least number into which both 4 and 7 divide exactly is 28 ($28 \div 4 = 7$ and $28 \div 7 = 4$). Thus, their LCM = 28.

(*c*)   The least number into which both 8 and 16 divide exactly is 16 ($16 \div 8 = 2$ and $16 \div 16 = 1$). Thus, their LCM = 16.

(*d*)   The least number into which all three numbers 9, 6, and 12 divide exactly is 36 ($36 \div 9 = 4$, $36 \div 6 = 6$, and $36 \div 12 = 3$). Thus, their LCM = 36.

The next example illustrates a method of finding the LCM of a set of numbers if their GCD can be found. This is useful because it is usually much easier to find the GCD of a set of numbers than their LCM. The method is based on the fact that *the LCM of two numbers is equal to their product divided by their GCD*.

$$\text{LCM of } A \text{ and } B = (A \times B) \div \text{GCD}$$

EXAMPLE 1.30   Find the LCM of 63 and 84.

1. Find the GCD of 63 and 84. This was done in Example 1.27; their GCD = 21.

2. Now calculate LCM = $(63 \times 84) \div 21$. This can be done most easily by first dividing the GCD into either of the factors (63 or 84), and then multiplying the quotient by the other factor:

$$\text{LCM} = (63 \div 21) \times 84 = 3 \times 84 = 252$$

EXAMPLE 1.31   Find the LCM of 40 and 56.

1. Find the GCD of 40 and 56 by the Euclidean algorithm (see Sec. 1.12).

$$\begin{array}{ccc}
\begin{array}{r} 1 \\ 40\overline{)56} \\ \underline{40} \\ 16 \quad \text{Remainder} \end{array} &
\begin{array}{r} 2 \\ 16\overline{)40} \\ \underline{32} \\ 8 \quad \text{Remainder} \end{array} &
\begin{array}{r} 2 \\ 8\overline{)16} \\ \underline{16} \\ 0 \quad \text{Remainder} \quad \text{GCD} = 8 \end{array}
\end{array}$$

2. Now calculate LCM = $(40 \div 8) \times 56 = 5 \times 56 = 280$.

There are two special cases that are useful to know. One case is when the GCD of the two numbers is 1. In this case, the LCM is simply the product of the numbers.

EXAMPLE 1.32   Find the LCM of 8 and 9.
Since the GCD of 8 and 9 is 1, their LCM is simply their product:

$$LCM = 8 \times 9 = 72$$

The second case is when each of the numbers is a divisor of the largest of the numbers. In this case, the LCM is simply the largest of the numbers.

EXAMPLE 1.33   Find the LCM of 2, 6, and 12.
Since each of the numbers is a divisor of 12, the LCM = 12.

EXAMPLE 1.34   Find the LCM of 8, 12, and 20.
To find the LCM of any three numbers, find the LCM of two of them, and then find the LCM of the result of the first two and the third number.

1.   Find the GCD of 12 and 8: GCD = 4.
2.   Find the LCM of 12 and 8: LCM = $(12 \div 4) \times 8 = 3 \times 8 = 24$. This is used in the next step.
3.   Now find the GCD of 24 and 20: GCD = 4.
4.   Finally, find the LCM of 24 and 20: LCM = $(24 \div 4) \times 20 = 6 \times 20 = 120$.

Thus, the LCM of 8, 12, and 20 is 120.

← LCM

Solved Problems

1.1   Write the following numerals in words.

(a) 374	(c) 5608	(e) 23,400	(g) 2,450,000
(b) 902	(d) 1016	(f) 160,000	(h) 80,030,000

Solution

(a)   374 = three hundred seventy-four
(b)   902 = nine hundred two
(c)   5608 = five thousand, six hundred eight
(d)   1016 = one thousand, sixteen
(e)   23,400 = twenty-three thousand, four hundred
(f)   160,000 = one hundred sixty thousand
(g)   2,450,000 = two million, four hundred fifty thousand
(h)   80,030,000 = eighty million, thirty thousand

1.2   Write the following as base ten numerals.

(a) Nine hundred seventeen	(e) Fifty-two thousand, six
(b) Six hundred five	(f) Four hundred two thousand, one hundred
(c) Seven thousand, three hundred thirty	(g) Eight million, thirty thousand
(d) Two thousand, fifty	(h) Four hundred twenty million

Solution

(a) 917   (c) 7330   (e) 52,006   (g) 8,030,000

(b) 605   (d) 2050   (f) 402,100   (h) 420,000,000

1.3   Write the following numbers in expanded form in two ways.

(a) 72   (c) 594   (e) 7325   (g) 8003

(b) 27   (d) 408   (f) 6200   (h) 35,420

Solution

(a) $72 = 7$ tens $+ 2$ ones $= 70 + 2$

(b) $27 = 2$ tens $+ 7$ ones $= 20 + 7$

(c) $594 = 5$ hundreds $+ 9$ tens $+ 4$ ones $= 500 + 90 + 4$

(d) $408 = 4$ hundreds $+ 8$ ones $= 400 + 8$

(e) $7325 = 7$ thousands $+ 3$ hundreds $+ 2$ tens $+ 5$ ones
       $= 7000 + 300 + 20 + 5$

(f) $6200 = 6$ thousands $+ 2$ hundreds $= 6000 + 200$

(g) $8003 = 8$ thousands $+ 3$ ones $= 8000 + 3$

(h) $35,420 = 3$ ten thousands $+ 5$ thousands $+ 4$ hundreds $+ 2$ tens
       $= 30,000 + 5000 + 400 + 20$

1.4   Perform the following calculations.

(a) $3 + (1 + 6)$ (d) $5 \times (2 + 4)$ (g) $4 \times 1 + 3 \times 3$

(b) $(3 + 1) + 6$ (e) $3 + 2 \times 5$ (h) $4 + 2 \times 3 + 7$

(c) $5 \times 2 + 4$ (f) $(3 + 2) \times 5$ (i) $(7 + 3) \times (4 + 6)$

Solution

(a) $3 + (1 + 6)$ (d) $5 \times (2 + 4)$ (g) $4 \times 1 + 3 \times 3$

   $= 3 + 7$ $= 5 \times 6$ $= 4 + 9$

   $= 10$ $= 30$ $= 13$

(b) $(3 + 1) + 6$ (e) $3 + 2 \times 5$ (h) $4 + 2 \times 3 + 7$

   $= 4 + 6$ $= 3 + 10$ $= 4 + 6 + 7$

   $= 10$ $= 13$ $= 17$

(c) $5 \times 2 + 4$ (f) $= (3 + 2) \times 5$ (i) $= (7 + 3) \times (4 + 6)$

   $= 10 + 4$ $= 5 \times 5$ $= 10 \times 10$

   $= 14$ $= 25$ $= 100$

1.5   Calculate the following sums.

(a) $42 + 36$ (h) $3912 + 859$ (o) $47 + 564 + 9879$

(b) $83 + 54$ (i) $6987 + 934$ (p) $9984 + 32 + 513$

(c) $56 + 39$ (j) $23 + 30 + 32$ (q) $765 + 898 + 673$

(d) $713 + 924$ (k) $51 + 34 + 82$ (r) $9706 + 892 + 584$

(e) $383 + 167$ (l) $43 + 29 + 15$ (s) $8478 + 12,947 + 584$

(f) $568 + 74$ (m) $560 + 14 + 813$ (t) $493 + 8067 + 92,956$

(g) $6513 + 8072$ (n) $352 + 83 + 924$

Solution

(a)	$\begin{array}{r}42\\ +36\\ \hline 78\end{array}$	(e)	$\begin{array}{r}^{11}\\383\\ +167\\ \hline 550\end{array}$	(i)	$\begin{array}{r}^{111}\\6987\\ +934\\ \hline 7921\end{array}$	(m)	$\begin{array}{r}560\\14\\ +813\\ \hline 1387\end{array}$	(q)	$\begin{array}{r}^{21}\\765\\898\\ +673\\ \hline 2336\end{array}$

(b) $\begin{array}{r}83\\ +54\\ \hline 137\end{array}$ (f) $\begin{array}{r}^{11}\\568\\ +74\\ \hline 642\end{array}$ (j) $\begin{array}{r}23\\30\\ +32\\ \hline 85\end{array}$ (n) $\begin{array}{r}^{1}\\352\\83\\ +924\\ \hline 1359\end{array}$ (r) $\begin{array}{r}^{211}\\9706\\892\\ +584\\ \hline 11{,}182\end{array}$

(c) $\begin{array}{r}^{1}\\56\\ +39\\ \hline 95\end{array}$ (g) $\begin{array}{r}6513\\ +8072\\ \hline 14{,}585\end{array}$ (k) $\begin{array}{r}51\\34\\ +82\\ \hline 167\end{array}$ (o) $\begin{array}{r}^{112}\\47\\564\\ +9879\\ \hline 10{,}490\end{array}$ (s) $\begin{array}{r}^{1221}\\8478\\12{,}947\\ +584\\ \hline 22{,}009\end{array}$

(d) $\begin{array}{r}713\\ +924\\ \hline 1637\end{array}$ (h) $\begin{array}{r}^{1\ 1}\\3912\\ +859\\ \hline 4771\end{array}$ (l) $\begin{array}{r}^{1}\\43\\29\\ +15\\ \hline 87\end{array}$ (p) $\begin{array}{r}^{11}\\9984\\32\\ +513\\ \hline 10{,}529\end{array}$ (t) $\begin{array}{r}^{1121}\\493\\8067\\ +92{,}956\\ \hline 101{,}516\end{array}$

1.6 Calculate the following differences.

(a)	$79 - 54$	(h)	$8746 - 503$	(o)	$6000 - 1346$
(b)	$83 - 28$	(i)	$403 - 287$	(p)	$92{,}840 - 10{,}201$
(c)	$367 - 351$	(j)	$507 - 98$	(q)	$84{,}583 - 18{,}665$
(d)	$420 - 318$	(k)	$3076 - 1015$	(r)	$42{,}530 - 9999$
(e)	$489 - 82$	(l)	$3156 - 1248$	(s)	$35{,}046 - 8053$
(f)	$526 - 379$	(m)	$7413 - 356$	(t)	$10{,}053 - 4265$
(g)	$562 - 95$	(n)	$8205 - 7528$		

Solution

(a) $\begin{array}{r}79\\ -54\\ \hline 25\end{array}$ (e) $\begin{array}{r}489\\ -82\\ \hline 407\end{array}$ (i) $\begin{array}{r}^{3\ 9}\\4\cancel{0}^{1}3\\ -28\ 7\\ \hline 11\ 6\end{array}$ (m) $\begin{array}{r}^{3}{}^{1}0\\7\cancel{4}\ \cancel{1}^{1}3\\ -3\ 5\ 6\\ \hline 70\ 5\ 7\end{array}$ (q) $\begin{array}{r}^{7}{}^{1}3\ \ ^{7}\\\cancel{8}\ \cancel{4},{}^{1}5\cancel{8}^{1}3\\ -1\ 8,66\ 5\\ \hline 6\ 5,91\ 8\end{array}$

(b) $\begin{array}{r}^{7}\\\cancel{8}^{1}3\\ -2\ 8\\ \hline 5\ 5\end{array}$ (f) $\begin{array}{r}^{4}{}^{1}1\\\cancel{5}\ \cancel{2}^{1}6\\ -3\ 7\ 9\\ \hline 1\ 4\ 7\end{array}$ (j) $\begin{array}{r}^{4\ 9}\\\cancel{5}\cancel{0}^{1}7\\ -9\ 8\\ \hline 40\ 9\end{array}$ (n) $\begin{array}{r}^{7}{}^{1}19\\\cancel{8}\ \cancel{2}\cancel{0}^{1}5\\ -752\ 8\\ \hline 67\ 7\end{array}$ (r) $\begin{array}{r}^{3}{}^{1}1\ ^{1}4\ ^{1}2\\4\cancel{2},\cancel{5}\ \cancel{3}^{1}0\\ -9\ 9\ 9\ 9\\ \hline 3\ 2,5\ 3\ 1\end{array}$

(c) $\begin{array}{r}367\\ -351\\ \hline 16\end{array}$ (g) $\begin{array}{r}^{4}{}^{1}5\\\cancel{5}\ \cancel{6}^{1}2\\ -9\ 5\\ \hline 4\ 6\ 7\end{array}$ (k) $\begin{array}{r}3076\\ -1015\\ \hline 2061\end{array}$ (o) $\begin{array}{r}^{5\ 9\ 9}\\\cancel{6}\cancel{0}\cancel{0}^{1}0\\ -134\ 6\\ \hline 465\ 4\end{array}$ (s) $\begin{array}{r}^{2}{}^{1}4\ 9\\\cancel{3}\ \cancel{5},\cancel{0}^{1}46\\ -8\ 0\ 53\\ \hline 2\ 6,9\ 93\end{array}$

(d) $\begin{array}{r}^{1}\\4\cancel{2}^{1}0\\ -31\ 8\\ \hline 10\ 2\end{array}$ (h) $\begin{array}{r}8746\\ -503\\ \hline 8243\end{array}$ (l) $\begin{array}{r}^{2\ \ 4}\\\cancel{3}^{1}1\cancel{5}^{1}6\\ -1\ 24\ 8\\ \hline 1\ 90\ 8\end{array}$ (p) $\begin{array}{r}^{3}\\92{,}8\cancel{4}^{1}0\\ -10{,}20\ 1\\ \hline 82{,}63\ 9\end{array}$ (t) $\begin{array}{r}^{0\ 9\ 9}{}^{1}4\\\cancel{1}\cancel{0}\cancel{0}\ \cancel{5}^{1}3\\ -42\ 6\ 5\\ \hline 57\ 8\ 8\end{array}$

1.7 Calculate the following products.

(a)	23×3	(d)	47×8	(g)	462×5	(j)	386×7
(b)	60×4	(e)	314×2	(h)	194×7	(k)	8097×6
(c)	35×6	(f)	600×3	(i)	530×9	(l)	7693×8

Solution

(a) $\begin{array}{r} 23 \\ \times 3 \\ \hline 69 \end{array}$ (d) $\begin{array}{r} 47 \\ \times 8 \\ \hline 376 \end{array}$ (g) $\begin{array}{r} 462 \\ \times 5 \\ \hline 2310 \end{array}$ (j) $\begin{array}{r} 386 \\ \times 7 \\ \hline 2702 \end{array}$

(b) $\begin{array}{r} 60 \\ \times 4 \\ \hline 240 \end{array}$ (e) $\begin{array}{r} 314 \\ \times 2 \\ \hline 628 \end{array}$ (h) $\begin{array}{r} 194 \\ \times 7 \\ \hline 1358 \end{array}$ (k) $\begin{array}{r} 8097 \\ \times 6 \\ \hline 48{,}582 \end{array}$

(c) $\begin{array}{r} 36 \\ \times 6 \\ \hline 210 \end{array}$ (f) $\begin{array}{r} 600 \\ \times 3 \\ \hline 1800 \end{array}$ (i) $\begin{array}{r} 530 \\ \times 9 \\ \hline 4770 \end{array}$ (l) $\begin{array}{r} 7693 \\ \times 8 \\ \hline 61{,}544 \end{array}$

1.8 Calculate the following products.

(a) 52×31 (e) 902×432 (i) 540×80 (m) 3800×28

(b) 60×30 (f) 86×24 (j) 800×510 (n) 3040×1700

(c) 302×12 (g) 59×37 (k) 773×218 (o) 4800×7900

(d) 700×30 (h) 618×63 (l) 9607×417

Solution

(a) $\begin{array}{r} 52 \\ \times 31 \\ \hline 52 \\ 156 \\ \hline 1612 \end{array}$ (e) $\begin{array}{r} 902 \\ \times 432 \\ \hline 1\,804 \\ 27\,06 \\ 360\,8 \\ \hline 389{,}664 \end{array}$ (i) $\begin{array}{r} 540 \\ \times 80 \\ \hline 43{,}200 \end{array}$ (m) $\begin{array}{r} 3800 \\ \times 28 \\ \hline 30\,4 \\ 76 \\ \hline 106{,}400 \end{array}$

(b) $\begin{array}{r} 60 \\ \times 30 \\ \hline 1800 \end{array}$ (f) $\begin{array}{r} 86 \\ \times 24 \\ \hline 344 \\ 172 \\ \hline 2064 \end{array}$ (j) $\begin{array}{r} 510 \\ \times 800 \\ \hline 408{,}000 \end{array}$ (n) $\begin{array}{r} 3040 \\ \times 1700 \\ \hline 2\,128 \\ 3\,04 \\ \hline 5{,}168{,}000 \end{array}$

(c) $\begin{array}{r} 302 \\ \times 12 \\ \hline 604 \\ 302 \\ \hline 3624 \end{array}$ (g) $\begin{array}{r} 59 \\ \times 37 \\ \hline 413 \\ 177 \\ \hline 2183 \end{array}$ (k) $\begin{array}{r} 773 \\ \times 218 \\ \hline 6\,184 \\ 7\,73 \\ 154\,6 \\ \hline 168{,}514 \end{array}$ (o) $\begin{array}{r} 4800 \\ \times 7900 \\ \hline 4\,32 \\ 33\,6 \\ \hline 37{,}920{,}000 \end{array}$

(d) $\begin{array}{r} 700 \\ \times 30 \\ \hline 21{,}000 \end{array}$ (h) $\begin{array}{r} 618 \\ \times 63 \\ \hline 1\,854 \\ 37\,08 \\ \hline 38{,}934 \end{array}$ (l) $\begin{array}{r} 9607 \\ \times 417 \\ \hline 67\,249 \\ 96\,07 \\ 3\,842\,8 \\ \hline 4{,}006{,}119 \end{array}$

1.9 Perform the following divisions.

(a) $7 \div 3$ (f) $616 \div 8$ (k) $2782 \div 13$ (p) $9013 \div 375$

(b) $17 \div 5$ (g) $3624 \div 9$ (l) $7371 \div 24$ (q) $56{,}249 \div 172$

(c) $52 \div 3$ (h) $7200 \div 8$ (m) $2220 \div 37$ (r) $30{,}265 \div 802$

(d) $656 \div 4$ (i) $395 \div 16$ (n) $51{,}130 \div 17$ (s) $55{,}044 \div 417$

(e) $923 \div 3$ (j) $257 \div 63$ (o) $44{,}800 \div 32$ (t) $71{,}136 \div 342$

Solution

(a)
```
      2
   3)7
      6
      1
```

(e)
```
      307
   3)923
      9
      23
      21
       2
```

(i)
```
       24
   16)395
       32
       75
       64
       11
```

(m)
```
        60
   37)2220
       222
         0
```

(q)
```
         327
   172)56249
        516
        464
        344
       1209
       1204
          5
```

(b)
```
      3
   5)17
     15
      2
```

(f)
```
      77
   8)616
     56
     56
     56
```

(j)
```
       4
   63)257
      252
        5
```

(n)
```
       3007
   17)51130
      51
       130
       119
        11
```

(r)
```
         37
   802)30265
       2406
       6205
       5614
        591
```

(c)
```
      17
   3)52
     3
     22
     21
      1
```

(g)
```
       402
   9)3624
     36
       24
       18
        6
```

(k)
```
        214
   13)2782
      26
       18
       13
        52
        52
```

(o)
```
       1400
   32)44800
      32
       128
       128
```

(s)
```
         132
   417)55044
       417
       1334
       1251
        834
        834
```

(d)
```
      164
   4)656
     4
     25
     24
      16
      16
```

(h)
```
       900
   8)7200
     72
       00
```

(l)
```
        307
   24)7371
      72
       171
       168
         3
```

(p)
```
        24
   375)9013
       750
      1513
      1500
        13
```

(t)
```
         208
   342)71136
       684
       2736
       2736
```

1.10 Find the GCD for the following sets of numbers.

(a) 3 and 5   (f) 25 and 20   (k) 29 and 28
(b) 8 and 6   (g) 9 and 18   (l) 6, 8, and 10
(c) 12 and 15   (h) 56 and 72   (m) 12, 18, and 30
(d) 12 and 16   (i) 120 and 250   (n) 5, 6, and 7
(e) 18 and 20   (j) 91 and 112   (o) 6, 12, and 24

Solution

(a) GCD = 1

(d)
```
        1        3
   12)16     4)12
      12       12
       4        0     GCD = 4
```

(b)
```
       1       3
    6)8     2)6
      6       6
      2       0     GCD = 2
```

(e)
```
        1        9
   18)20     2)18
      18       18
       2        0     GCD = 2
```

(c)
```
        1        4
   12)15     3)12
      12       12
       3        0     GCD = 3
```

(f)
```
        1        4
   20)25     5)20
      20       20
       5        0     GCD = 5
```

(g)   2
        9)18
          18
           0   GCD = 9

(j)   1   4   3
        91)112   21)91   7)21
           91   84   21
           21   7   0   GCD = 7

(h)   1   3   2
        56)72   16)56   8)16
           56   48   16
           16   8   0   GCD = 8

(k)   GCD = 1

(i)   2   12
       120)250 10)120
          240   10
           10   20
                   20
                    0   GCD = 10

(l)   1   3
         6)8   2)6
           6   6
           2   0   GCD of 6 and 8 is 2.
        Since 2 also divides into 10 exactly, the GCD of 6, 8,
        and 10 is 2.

(m)   1   2
        12)18   6)12
           12   12
            6   0   GCD of 12 and 18 is 6. Since 6 also divides into 30
                             exactly, the GCD of 12, 18, and 30 is 6.

(n)   GCD = 1

(o)   Since 6 divides into both 12 and 24 exactly, the GCD of 6, 12, and 24 is 6.

1.11   Find the LCM of the following sets of numbers.

(a)   3 and 5   (f)   25 and 20   (k)   29 and 28
(b)   8 and 6   (g)   9 and 18   (l)   6, 8, and 10
(c)   12 and 15   (h)   56 and 72   (m)   12, 18, and 30
(d)   12 and 16   (i)   120 and 250   (n)   5, 6, and 7
(e)   18 and 20   (j)   91 and 112   (o)   6, 12, and 24

Solution

See the solutions for Prob. 1.10 for the GCD of each set of numbers.

(a)   GCD of 3 and 5 is 1. Therefore, LCM $= 3 \times 5 = 15$.

(b)   GCD $= 2$. Therefore, LCM $= (8 \div 2) \times 6 = 4 \times 6 = 24$.

(c)   GCD $= 3$. Therefore, LCM $= (12 \div 3) \times 15 = 4 \times 15 = 60$.

(d)   GCD $= 4$. Therefore, LCM $= (12 \div 4) \times 16 = 3 \times 16 = 48$.

(e)   GCD $= 2$. Therefore, LCM $= (18 \div 2) \times 20 = 9 \times 20 = 180$.

(f)   GCD $= 5$. Therefore, LCM $= (25 \div 5) \times 20 = 5 \times 20 = 100$.

(g)   9 divides into 18 exactly. Therefore, LCM $= 18$.

(h)   GCD $= 8$. Therefore, LCM $= (56 \div 8) \times 72 = 7 \times 72 = 504$.

(i)   GCD $= 10$. Therefore, LCM $= (120 \div 10) \times 250 = 12 \times 250 = 3000$.

(j)   GCD $= 7$. Therefore, LCM $= (91 \div 7) \times 112 = 13 \times 112 = 1456$.

(k)   GCD $= 1$. Therefore, LCM $= 29 \times 28 = 812$.

(l)   For 6, 8, and 10, find the LCM of 6 and 8 first: GCD $= 2$. Therefore, LCM $= (6 \div 2) \times 8 = 3 \times 8 = 24$. Then find the LCM of 24 and 10: GCD $= 2$. Therefore, LCM $= (24 \div 2) \times 10 = 12 \times 10 = 120$.

(m)   For 12, 18, and 30, find the LCM of 12 and 18 first: GCD $= 6$. Therefore, LCM $= (12 \div 6) \times 18 = 2 \times 18 = 36$. Then find the LCM of 36 and 30: GCD $= 6$. Therefore, LCM $= (36 \div 6) \times 30 = 6 \times 30 = 180$.

(*n*) For 5, 6, and 7, find the LCM of 5 and 6 first: GCD = 1. Therefore, LCM = 5 × 6 = 30. Then find the LCM of 30 and 7: GCD = 1. Therefore, LCM = 30 × 7 = 210.

(*o*) Both 6 and 12 divide into 24 exactly. Therefore, LCM = 24.

Supplementary Problems

1.12 Write the following numerals in words.

(*a*) 503   (*c*) 4117   (*e*) 20,208   (*g*) 3,000,021

(*b*) 619   (*d*) 6053   (*f*) 701,033   (*h*) 89,601,000

1.13 Write the following as base ten numerals.

(*a*) Six hundred forty

(*b*) Three hundred three

(*c*) Four thousand, eighty-two

(*d*) Twenty-two thousand, six hundred one

(*e*) One hundred twelve thousand, sixty

(*f*) Three million, twenty thousand

(*g*) Eight hundred sixty-two million, two hundred thousand

(*h*) One billion, three hundred ninety million

1.14 Write the following numbers in expanded form in two ways.

(*a*) 35   (*c*) 603   (*e*) 3302   (*g*) 3005

(*b*) 77   (*d*) 630   (*f*) 7100   (*h*) 20,304

1.15 Perform the following calculations.

(*a*) $8 + (2 + 4)$ (*f*) $(4 + 5) \times 3$ (*k*) $(4 + 5) \times (3 + 3)$

(*b*) $(5 + 4) + 7$ (*g*) $9 + 3 \times 3$ (*l*) $3 + 1 \times (4 + 6)$

(*c*) $4 \times 2 + 5$ (*h*) $4 \times (2 + 5)$ (*m*) $3 \times (1 + 2) + 6$

(*d*) $(5 + 2) \times 4$ (*i*) $3 \times 2 + 3 \times 3$ (*n*) $4 + 2 \times (3 + 2)$

(*e*) $5 + 2 \times 4$ (*j*) $3 + 2 \times 2 + 5$ (*o*) $(2 + 3) \times 4 + 6$

1.16 Calculate the following sums.

(*a*) $32 + 14$ (*h*) $4713 + 1619$ (*o*) $438 + 93 + 5279$

(*b*) $83 + 94$ (*i*) $8999 + 999$ (*p*) $9894 + 78 + 988$

(*c*) $47 + 38$ (*j*) $42 + 15 + 31$ (*q*) $587 + 978 + 9699$

(*d*) $652 + 847$ (*k*) $52 + 16 + 39$ (*r*) $8452 + 908 + 7657$

(*e*) $783 + 267$ (*l*) $96 + 78 + 29$ (*s*) $7506 + 18,097 + 870$

(*f*) $927 + 87$ (*m*) $323 + 15 + 951$ (*t*) $98,578 + 9750 + 6263$

(*g*) $8206 + 1372$ (*n*) $486 + 775 + 63$

1.17 Calculate the following differences.

(a)	$68 - 25$	(h)	$2912 - 610$
(b)	$56 - 48$	(i)	$504 - 276$
(c)	$482 - 251$	(j)	$602 - 79$
(d)	$523 - 209$	(k)	$5028 - 3963$
(e)	$376 - 66$	(l)	$2123 - 1987$
(f)	$815 - 608$	(m)	$4212 - 976$
(g)	$428 - 89$	(n)	$7002 - 4657$

(o)	$8000 - 4274$
(p)	$68,590 - 40,402$
(q)	$57,235 - 7946$
(r)	$73,490 - 69,999$
(s)	$40,052 - 12,065$
(t)	$10,006 - 9259$

1.18 Calculate the following products.

(a)	34×2	(h)	37×16
(b)	72×3	(i)	40×80
(c)	302×3	(j)	36×56
(d)	900×3	(k)	39×480
(e)	37×4	(l)	87×492
(f)	467×8	(m)	730×560
(g)	5206×7	(n)	18×4900

(o)	475×816
(p)	57×5230
(q)	204×4198
(r)	230×7430
(s)	1200×6705
(t)	6100×3500

1.19 Perform the following divisions.

(a)	$8 \div 5$	(h)	$4800 \div 6$
(b)	$19 \div 4$	(i)	$296 \div 12$
(c)	$74 \div 3$	(j)	$197 \div 73$
(d)	$623 \div 5$	(k)	$5619 \div 24$
(e)	$816 \div 4$	(l)	$7870 \div 38$
(f)	$507 \div 7$	(m)	$4026 \div 61$
(g)	$4602 \div 8$	(n)	$71,034 \div 18$

(o)	$52,700 \div 47$
(p)	$8110 \div 340$
(q)	$60,250 \div 189$
(r)	$18,627 \div 910$
(s)	$40,219 \div 396$
(t)	$87,052 \div 912$

1.20 Find the GCD of the following sets of numbers.

(a)	1 and 6	(h)	35 and 9
(b)	9 and 12	(i)	7 and 35
(c)	7 and 9	(j)	25 and 100
(d)	10 and 15	(k)	42 and 56
(e)	16 and 20	(l)	300 and 200
(f)	8 and 16	(m)	68 and 51
(g)	30 and 40	(n)	72 and 54

(o)	9, 16, and 15
(p)	16, 20, and 12
(q)	5, 10, and 15
(r)	8, 15, and 18
(s)	27, 18, and 36
(t)	39, 52, and 65

1.21 Find the LCM of the following sets of numbers.

(a)	1 and 6	(e)	16 and 20	(i)	7 and 35
(b)	9 and 12	(f)	8 and 16	(j)	25 and 100
(c)	7 and 9	(g)	30 and 40	(k)	42 and 56
(d)	10 and 15	(h)	35 and 9	(l)	300 and 200

(m)	68 and 51	(p)	16, 20, and 12	(s)	27, 18, and 36
(n)	72 and 54	(q)	5, 10, and 15	(t)	39, 52, and 65
(o)	9, 16, and 15	(r)	8, 15, and 18		

Answers to Supplementary Problems

1.12
(a) Five hundred three
(b) Six hundred nineteen
(c) Four thousand, one hundred seventeen
(d) Six thousand, fifty-three
(e) Twenty thousand, two hundred eight
(f) Seven hundred one thousand, thirty-three
(g) Three million, twenty-one
(h) Eighty-nine million, six hundred one thousand

1.13
(a)	640	(c)	4082	(e)	112,060	(g)	862,200,000
(b)	303	(d)	22,601	(f)	3,020,000	(h)	1,390,000,000

1.14
(a) $35 = 3$ tens $+ 5$ ones $= 30 + 5$
(b) $77 = 7$ tens $+ 7$ ones $= 70 + 7$
(c) $603 = 6$ hundreds $+ 3$ ones $= 600 + 3$
(d) $630 = 6$ hundreds $+ 3$ tens $= 600 + 30$
(e) $3302 = 3$ thousands $+ 3$ hundreds $+ 2$ ones $= 3000 + 300 + 2$
(f) $7100 = 7$ thousands $+ 1$ hundred $= 7000 + 100$
(g) $3005 = 3$ thousands $+ 5$ ones $= 3000 + 5$
(h) $20,304 = 2$ ten thousands $+ 3$ hundreds $+ 4$ ones $= 20,000 + 300 + 4$

1.15
(a)	14	(d)	28	(g)	18	(j)	12	(m)	15
(b)	16	(e)	13	(h)	28	(k)	54	(n)	14
(c)	13	(f)	27	(i)	15	(l)	13	(o)	26

1.16
(a)	46	(e)	1050	(i)	9998	(m)	1289	(q)	11,264
(b)	177	(f)	1014	(j)	88	(n)	1324	(r)	17,017
(c)	85	(g)	9578	(k)	107	(o)	5810	(s)	26,473
(d)	1499	(h)	6332	(l)	203	(p)	10,960	(t)	114,591

1.17
(a)	43	(e)	310	(i)	228	(m)	3236	(q)	49,289
(b)	8	(f)	207	(j)	523	(n)	2345	(r)	3491
(c)	231	(g)	339	(k)	1065	(o)	3726	(s)	27,987
(d)	314	(h)	2302	(l)	136	(p)	28,188	(t)	747

1.18
(a)	68	(e)	148	(i)	3200	(m)	408,800	(q)	856,392
(b)	216	(f)	3736	(j)	2016	(n)	88,200	(r)	1,798,900
(c)	906	(g)	36,442	(k)	18,720	(o)	387,600	(s)	8,046,000
(d)	2700	(h)	592	(l)	42,804	(p)	298,110	(t)	21,350,000

1.19 (*a*) Quotient: 1   (*h*) Quotient: 800   (*o*) Quotient: 1121
          Remainder: 3   Remainder: 13

       (*b*) Quotient: 4   (*i*) Quotient: 24   (*p*) Quotient: 23
          Remainder: 3   Remainder: 8   Remainder: 290

       (*c*) Quotient: 24   (*j*) Quotient: 2   (*q*) Quotient: 318
          Remainder: 2   Remainder: 51   Remainder: 148

       (*d*) Quotient: 124   (*k*) Quotient: 234   (*r*) Quotient: 20
          Remainder: 3   Remainder: 3   Remainder: 427

       (*e*) Quotient: 204   (*l*) Quotient: 207   (*s*) Quotient: 101
                                    Remainder: 4   Remainder: 223

       (*f*) Quotient: 72   (*m*) Quotient: 66   (*t*) Quotient: 95
          Remainder: 3   Remainder: 412

       (*g*) Quotient: 575   (*n*) Quotient: 3946
          Remainder: 2   Remainder: 6

1.20 (*a*) GCD = 1   (*f*) GCD = 8   (*k*) GCD = 14   (*p*) GCD = 4
       (*b*) GCD = 3   (*g*) GCD = 10   (*l*) GCD = 100   (*q*) GCD = 5
       (*c*) GCD = 1   (*h*) GCD = 1   (*m*) GCD = 17   (*r*) GCD = 1
       (*d*) GCD = 5   (*i*) GCD = 7   (*n*) GCD = 18   (*s*) GCD = 9
       (*e*) GCD = 4   (*j*) GCD = 25   (*o*) GCD = 1   (*t*) GCD = 13

1.21 (*a*) LCM = 6   (*f*) LCM = 16   (*k*) LCM = 168   (*p*) LCM = 240
       (*b*) LCM = 36   (*g*) LCM = 120   (*l*) LCM = 600   (*q*) LCM = 30
       (*c*) LCM = 63   (*h*) LCM = 315   (*m*) LCM = 204   (*r*) LCM = 360
       (*d*) LCM = 30   (*i*) LCM = 35   (*n*) LCM = 216   (*s*) LCM = 108
       (*e*) LCM = 80   (*j*) LCM = 100   (*o*) LCM = 720   (*t*) LCM = 780

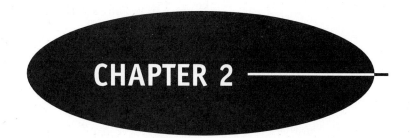

CHAPTER 2

Working with Fractions

2.1 THE MEANING OF FRACTIONS

The symbol $\frac{A}{B}$ (also written A/B), where A and B are whole numbers, is called a *fraction* and represents the division A divided by B ($A \div B$). Since division by zero is not allowed, B cannot be zero. The line between the numbers is called a *fraction bar*. The number above the bar is called the *numerator* and the number below the bar the *denominator*.

If the numerator is less than the denominator, the fraction is said to be *proper*. Thus, $\frac{3}{8}$ is a proper fraction. If the numerator is greater than or equal to the denominator, the fraction is said to be *improper*. The fractions $\frac{9}{5}$ and $\frac{4}{4}$ are thus improper fractions.

One use of fractions is to describe the relationship between a whole and its parts. When a whole is divided into smaller equal units, and a certain number of these are compared to the whole, this part is said to make up a *fraction of the whole*. The denominator of the fraction is the total number of units making up the whole, and the numerator is the number of units in the part. That is,

$$\text{Fraction of the whole} = \frac{\text{number of units in the part}}{\text{number of units in the whole}}$$

EXAMPLE 2.1 What fraction of the whole circle in Fig. 2-1 is the shaded part?

The circle is divided into four equal units. Thus, the denominator is 4. Three of these units are shaded, so the numerator is 3. Thus, the fraction is $\frac{3}{4}$ (three-fourths).

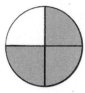

Fig. 2-1

EXAMPLE 2.2   A 12-ounce bottle has 7 ounces of liquid in it (see Fig. 2-2). What fraction of the bottle is filled?

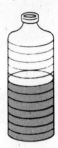

Fig. 2-2

The bottle (the whole) is divided into 12 ounces (the denominator), of which 7 ounces (the numerator) is filled. Thus, $\frac{7}{12}$ (seven-twelfths) of the bottle is filled.

Examples 2.1 and 2.2 resulted in proper fractions. Improper fractions result when the total number of units counted is greater than or equal to the number of units in a whole.

EXAMPLE 2.3   If each of the equal circles in Fig. 2-3 is a whole, what fraction of a whole is the shaded area?
Since each whole is divided into 3 equal units, the denominator is 3. There are 5 units shaded, so the numerator is

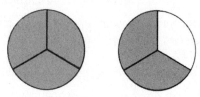

Fig. 2-3

5. Thus, the shaded part is $\frac{5}{3}$ (five-thirds) of a whole.

Any whole number can be represented as a fraction with a denominator of 1. The whole number 5, for example, can be represented by the fraction $\frac{5}{1}$.

2.2   EQUIVALENT FRACTIONS

Fractions that represent the same part of a whole are said to be *equivalent*.

EXAMPLE 2.4

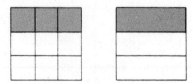

Fig. 2-4

The square on the left in Fig. 2-4 is divided into nine equal units. The shaded part is thus represented by the fraction $\frac{3}{9}$. The same square can also be divided into three equal units, as shown on the right, in which case the same shaded part is represented by the fraction $\frac{1}{3}$. Since the fractions $\frac{3}{9}$ and $\frac{1}{3}$ represent the same part of the whole, they are equivalent. That is, $\frac{3}{9} = \frac{1}{3}$.

2.3 REDUCING FRACTIONS

To *reduce* a fraction means to change it to an equivalent fraction by dividing both numerator and denominator by a common divisor greater than 1. The result is an equivalent fraction with a smaller numerator and denominator. A fraction is said to be in *lowest terms* if it cannot be reduced. The fraction $\frac{3}{4}$ is in lowest terms since 3 and 4 have no common divisors. However, the fraction $\frac{15}{20}$ is not in lowest terms since 15 and 20 have the common divisor 5. The fraction $\frac{15}{20}$ can be reduced to lowest terms by dividing both numerator and denominator by the common divisor 5:

$$\frac{15}{20} = \frac{15 \div 5}{20 \div 5} = \frac{3}{4}$$

This illustrates the following principle: *To reduce a fraction to lowest terms, divide both numerator and denominator by their greatest common divisor (GCD).*

EXAMPLE 2.5 Reduce the fraction $\frac{24}{36}$ to lowest terms.

The GCD of 24 and 36 is 12. Therefore, we divide both numerator and denominator by 12:

$$\frac{24}{36} = \frac{24 \div 12}{36 \div 12} = \frac{2}{3}$$

For brevity, this is often written as follows:

$$\frac{\overset{2}{\cancel{24}}}{\underset{3}{\cancel{36}}} = \frac{2}{3} \qquad \text{(Dividing both numerator and denominator by 12)}$$

EXAMPLE 2.6 Reduce the fraction $\frac{630}{140}$ to lowest terms.

1. Use the Euclidean algorithm (Sec. 1.12) to find the GCD of 140 and 630.

$$\begin{array}{r} 4 \\ 140\overline{)630} \\ 560 \\ \hline 70 \end{array} \qquad \begin{array}{r} 2 \\ 70\overline{)140} \\ 140 \\ \hline 0 \end{array} \qquad \text{GCD} = 70$$

2. Divide both numerator and denominator by 70.

$$\frac{630}{140} = \frac{630 \div 70}{140 \div 70} = \frac{9}{2}$$

EXAMPLE 2.7 Reduce the fraction $\frac{148}{185}$ to lowest terms.

1. Use the Euclidean algorithm to find the GCD of 148 and 185.

$$\begin{array}{r} 1 \\ 148\overline{)185} \\ 148 \\ \hline 37 \end{array} \qquad \begin{array}{r} 4 \\ 37\overline{)148} \\ 148 \\ \hline 0 \end{array} \qquad \text{GCD} = 37$$

2. Divide both numerator and denominator by 37.

$$\frac{\overset{4}{\cancel{148}}}{\underset{5}{\cancel{185}}} = \frac{4}{5}$$

2.4 BUILDING UP FRACTIONS

To *build up* a fraction means to change it to an equivalent fraction by multiplying both numerator and denominator by a factor greater than 1. The result is a fraction with a larger numerator and denominator. The process of building up a fraction is the reverse of reducing a fraction. A fraction is usually built up in order to write it as an equivalent fraction with a given denominator which is a multiple of the original denominator.

EXAMPLE 2.8 Build up the fraction $\frac{3}{8}$ to have a denominator of 24.

1. We are looking for a fraction with a denominator of 24 that is equivalent to $\frac{3}{8}$.

$$\frac{3}{8} = \frac{?}{24}$$

2. A fraction is built up by multiplying both parts by the same number. To build up the denominator 8 to 24 we must ask, "8 multiplied by what number gives 24?" We divide 8 into 24 to get the answer.

$$\overset{3}{8\overline{)24}} \leftarrow \text{This is the multiplier}$$

3. Since the denominator is multiplied by 3, the numerator must also be multiplied by 3.

$$\frac{3}{8} = \frac{3 \times 3}{8 \times 3} = \frac{9}{24} \qquad \text{Answer}$$

EXAMPLE 2.9 Build up the fraction $\frac{5}{12}$ to have a denominator of 300.

1. We are looking for a fraction with a denominator of 300 that is equivalent to $\frac{5}{12}$.

$$\frac{5}{12} = \frac{?}{300}$$

2. What number multiplied by 12 gives 300? Divide 12 into 300 to get the answer.

$$\overset{25}{12\overline{)300}} \leftarrow \text{This is the multiplier}$$

3. Both numerator and denominator must be multiplied by 25.

$$\frac{5}{12} = \frac{5 \times 25}{12 \times 25} = \frac{125}{300} \qquad \text{Answer}$$

EXAMPLE 2.10 Express the whole number 6 as an equivalent fraction with a denominator of 5.

1. We are looking for a fraction with a denominator of 5.

$$6 = \frac{?}{5}$$

2. This can be solved as a problem in building up fractions, since $6 = \frac{6}{1}$.

$$\frac{6}{1} = \frac{?}{5}$$

3. Since $1 \times 5 = 5$, both the numerator and denominator must be multiplied by 5.

$$\frac{6}{1} = \frac{6 \times 5}{1 \times 5} = \frac{30}{5} \qquad \text{Answer}$$

2.5 MULTIPLICATION OF FRACTIONS

The product of two or more fractions is equal to the product of their numerators over the product of their denominators. That is, if $\dfrac{A}{B}$ and $\dfrac{C}{D}$ are fractions, then

$$\frac{A}{B} \times \frac{C}{D} = \frac{A \times C}{B \times D}$$

EXAMPLE 2.11 Calculate the product $\dfrac{5}{3} \times \dfrac{2}{7}$.

According to the rule for multiplying fractions, we multiply the numerators and multiply the denominators.

$$\frac{5}{3} \times \frac{2}{7} = \frac{5 \times 2}{3 \times 7} = \frac{10}{21}$$

When multiplying fractions, it is usually desirable to reduce the answer to lowest terms. This can be done conveniently by dividing out common divisors between numerator and denominator *before* performing the multiplication.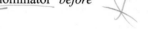

EXAMPLE 2.12 Calculate the product $\dfrac{3}{8} \times \dfrac{4}{3}$.

1. The multiplication to be done is:

$$\frac{3}{8} \times \frac{4}{3} = \frac{3 \times 4}{8 \times 3}$$

2. But before multiplying, divide out the common divisor 3.

$$\frac{\cancel{3}^{1} \times 4}{8 \times \cancel{3}_{1}} = \frac{1 \times 4}{8 \times 1}$$

3. 4 is also a common divisor that can be divided out.

$$= \frac{1 \times \cancel{4}^{1}}{\cancel{8}_{2} \times 1}$$

4. Now multiply.

$$= \frac{1 \times 1}{2 \times 1} = \frac{1}{2}$$

When dividing out common divisors in a product of fractions, it is important to remember that a divisor common to any numerator and any denominator can be divided out—the numerator and denominator need not be in the same fraction. However, a divisor that is common to two numerators or to two denominators *cannot* be divided out.

EXAMPLE 2.13 Calculate the product $\dfrac{25}{36} \times \dfrac{16}{20}$.

1. Reduce by dividing out common divisors between numerator and denominator.

$$\frac{25}{36} \times \frac{\cancel{16}^{4}}{\cancel{20}_{5}} = \frac{25}{36} \times \frac{4}{5} \qquad \text{(Divide by 4)}$$

$$= \frac{\cancel{25}^{5}}{36} \times \frac{4}{\cancel{5}_{1}} \qquad \text{(Divide by 5)}$$

$$= \frac{5}{\cancel{36}_{9}} \times \frac{\cancel{4}^{1}}{1} \qquad \text{(Divide by 4)}$$

2. Perform the multiplication.

$$= \frac{5}{9} \times \frac{1}{1} = \frac{5 \times 1}{9 \times 1} = \frac{5}{9}$$

EXAMPLE 2.14 Perform the multiplication $\dfrac{5}{8} \times \dfrac{7}{25} \times \dfrac{12}{21}$.

1. Reduce first.

$$\dfrac{\overset{1}{\cancel{5}}}{8} \times \dfrac{7}{\underset{5}{\cancel{25}}} \times \dfrac{12}{21} = \dfrac{1}{8} \times \dfrac{7}{5} \times \dfrac{12}{21} \qquad \text{(Divide by 5)}$$

$$= \dfrac{1}{8} \times \dfrac{\overset{1}{\cancel{7}}}{5} \times \dfrac{12}{\underset{3}{\cancel{21}}} \qquad \text{(Divide by 7)}$$

$$= \dfrac{1}{\underset{2}{\cancel{8}}} \times \dfrac{1}{5} \times \dfrac{\overset{3}{\cancel{12}}}{3} \qquad \text{(Divide by 4)}$$

$$= \dfrac{1}{2} \times \dfrac{1}{5} \times \dfrac{\overset{1}{\cancel{3}}}{\underset{1}{\cancel{3}}} \qquad \text{(Divide by 3)}$$

2. Then multiply.

$$= \dfrac{1 \times 1 \times 1}{2 \times 5 \times 1} = \dfrac{1}{10}$$

EXAMPLE 2.15 Perform the multiplication $6 \times \dfrac{2}{3}$.

1. Change the problem into multiplying fractions by expressing 6 as $\dfrac{6}{1}$.

$$6 \times \dfrac{2}{3}$$

$$= \dfrac{6}{1} \times \dfrac{2}{3}$$

2. Reduce first, then multiply.

$$= \dfrac{\overset{2}{\cancel{6}}}{1} \times \dfrac{2}{\underset{1}{\cancel{3}}} = \dfrac{2 \times 2}{1 \times 1} = \dfrac{4}{1} = 4$$

2.6 DIVISION OF FRACTIONS

To *invert* a fraction means to interchange the numerator and denominator. For example, to invert $\dfrac{2}{3}$, change it to the fraction $\dfrac{3}{2}$. The result of inverting a fraction is called its *reciprocal*. Thus, the reciprocal of $\dfrac{2}{3}$ is $\dfrac{3}{2}$. The reciprocal of the fraction $\dfrac{1}{6}$ is $\dfrac{6}{1} = 6$. Since we can write the whole number 4 as $\dfrac{4}{1}$, the reciprocal of 4 is $\dfrac{1}{4}$.

To divide one fraction by another, the dividend is multiplied by the reciprocal of the divisor. In other words, *to divide one fraction by another, invert the divisor and change the operation to multiplication.*

$$\dfrac{A}{B} \div \dfrac{C}{D} = \dfrac{A}{B} \times \dfrac{D}{C} = \dfrac{A \times D}{B \times C}$$

EXAMPLE 2.16 Perform the division $\dfrac{3}{4} \div \dfrac{5}{2}$.

1. Invert the divisor and change the operation to multiplication.

$$\dfrac{3}{4} \div \dfrac{5}{2} = \dfrac{3}{4} \times \dfrac{2}{5}$$

2. Reduce.

$$= \dfrac{3}{\underset{2}{\cancel{4}}} \times \dfrac{\overset{1}{\cancel{2}}}{5}$$

3. Perform the multiplication.

$$= \frac{3}{2} \times \frac{1}{5} = \frac{3}{10}$$

EXAMPLE 2.17 Perform the division $\frac{72}{50} \div \frac{200}{35}$.

1. Invert the divisor and change the operation to multiplication.

$$\frac{72}{50} \div \frac{200}{35} = \frac{72}{50} \times \frac{35}{200}$$

2. Reduce and perform the multiplication.

$$= \frac{\overset{9}{\cancel{72}}}{50} \times \frac{35}{\underset{25}{\cancel{200}}}$$

$$= \frac{9}{50} \times \frac{\overset{7}{\cancel{35}}}{\underset{5}{\cancel{25}}}$$

$$= \frac{9}{50} \times \frac{7}{5} = \frac{63}{250}$$

EXAMPLE 2.18 Perform the division $18 \div \frac{3}{4}$.

1. Invert the divisor and change the operation to multiplication.

$$18 \div \frac{3}{4} = 18 \times \frac{4}{3}$$

2. Write 18 as $\frac{18}{1}$.

$$= \frac{18}{1} \times \frac{4}{3}$$

3. Reduce.

$$= \frac{\overset{6}{\cancel{18}}}{1} \times \frac{4}{\underset{1}{\cancel{3}}}$$

4. Multiply.

$$= \frac{6}{1} \times \frac{4}{1} = \frac{24}{1} = 24$$

EXAMPLE 2.19 Perform the division $\frac{5}{8} \div 10$.

1. Write 10 as $\frac{10}{1}$.

$$\frac{5}{8} \div 10 = \frac{5}{8} \div \frac{10}{1}$$

2. Invert the divisor and change the operation to multiplication.

$$= \frac{5}{8} \times \frac{1}{10}$$

3. Reduce and multiply.

$$= \frac{\overset{1}{\cancel{5}}}{8} \times \frac{1}{\underset{2}{\cancel{10}}} = \frac{1 \times 1}{8 \times 2} = \frac{1}{16}$$

2.7 COMPLEX FRACTIONS

A *complex fraction* is a fraction in which the numerator or denominator is itself a fraction. For example,

$$\frac{\frac{2}{3}}{5} \qquad \frac{\frac{7}{2}}{\frac{1}{4}} \qquad \frac{13}{\frac{9}{10}}$$

are all complex fractions. To *simplify* a complex fraction means to write it as an equivalent fraction with whole number numerator and denominator. This can be done by performing the division indicated by the complex fraction.

EXAMPLE 2.20   Simplify the complex fraction $\dfrac{7/8}{3/4}$.

1. The fraction $\dfrac{7/8}{3/4}$ means:

$$\frac{7}{8} \div \frac{3}{4}$$

2. Invert and multiply.

$$= \frac{7}{8} \times \frac{4}{3} = \frac{7}{\overset{}{\underset{2}{8}}} \times \frac{\overset{1}{4}}{3} = \frac{7 \times 1}{2 \times 3} = \frac{7}{6}$$

EXAMPLE 2.21   Simplify the complex fraction $\dfrac{100}{\frac{2}{3}}$.

1. The fraction $\dfrac{100}{\frac{2}{3}}$ means:

$$100 \div \frac{2}{3}$$

2. Invert and multiply.

$$= 100 \times \frac{3}{2}$$

$$= \frac{100}{1} \times \frac{3}{2} = \frac{\overset{50}{100}}{1} \times \frac{3}{\underset{1}{2}} = \frac{50 \times 3}{1 \times 1}$$

$$= \frac{150}{1} = 150$$

EXAMPLE 2.22   Simplify the complex fraction $\dfrac{\frac{1}{60}}{3}$.

1. The fraction $\dfrac{\frac{1}{60}}{3}$ means:

$$\frac{1}{60} \div 3 = \frac{1}{60} \div \frac{3}{1}$$

2. Invert and multiply.

$$= \frac{1}{60} \times \frac{1}{3} = \frac{1 \times 1}{60 \times 3} = \frac{1}{180}$$

Note that the main division in a complex fraction is indicated by the longest fraction bar. If the longest fraction bar is not clearly written, the meaning of the fraction bar will not be clear. For example,

$$\frac{1}{\frac{2}{3}}$$

could mean $1 \div \dfrac{2}{3}$ or $\dfrac{1}{2} \div 3$, which have different values, since $1 \div \dfrac{2}{3} = \dfrac{1}{1} \times \dfrac{3}{2} = \dfrac{3}{2}$, but $\dfrac{1}{2} \div 3 = \dfrac{1}{2} \times \dfrac{1}{3} = \dfrac{1}{6}$. To distinguish between the two meanings, a long fraction bar is used to indicate the main division:

$$1 \div \frac{2}{3} = \frac{1}{\frac{2}{3}} \qquad \text{and} \qquad \frac{1}{2} \div 3 = \frac{\frac{1}{2}}{3}$$

2.8   ADDITION AND SUBTRACTION OF FRACTIONS WITH A COMMON DENOMINATOR

Addition.   Two or more fractions with a common denominator are added by adding the numerators over the common denominator. That is, for two fractions $\dfrac{A}{C}$ and $\dfrac{B}{C}$, with common denominator C,

$$\frac{A}{C} + \frac{B}{C} = \frac{A+B}{C}$$

EXAMPLE 2.23   Perform the following additions.

$$(a) \quad \frac{5}{8} + \frac{1}{8} \qquad (b) \quad \frac{1}{50} + \frac{7}{50} + \frac{23}{50} \qquad (c) \quad \frac{11}{24} + \frac{25}{24}$$

According to the rule for adding fractions with a common denominator, the numerators are added over the common denominator.

$(a) \quad \dfrac{5}{8} + \dfrac{1}{8} = \dfrac{5+1}{8} = \dfrac{6}{8} = \dfrac{3}{4}$ (Reducing the answer)

$(b) \quad \dfrac{1}{50} + \dfrac{7}{50} + \dfrac{23}{50} = \dfrac{1+7+23}{50} = \dfrac{31}{50}$

$(c) \quad \dfrac{11}{24} + \dfrac{25}{24} = \dfrac{11+25}{24} = \dfrac{36}{24} = \dfrac{3}{2}$ (Reducing the answer)

Subtraction.   Two fractions with a common denominator are subtracted by subtracting the numerators over the common denominator.

$$\frac{A}{C} - \frac{B}{C} = \frac{A-B}{C}$$

EXAMPLE 2.24   Perform the subtraction $\dfrac{13}{24} - \dfrac{9}{24}$.

According to the rule for subtracting fractions with a common denominator, the numerators are subtracted over the common denominator.

$$\frac{13}{24} - \frac{9}{24} = \frac{13-9}{24} = \frac{4}{24} = \frac{1}{6} \qquad \text{(Reducing the answer)}$$

When additions and subtractions are combined, the numerators are added or subtracted as indicated.

EXAMPLE 2.25   Perform the following operations.

$$(a) \quad \frac{23}{24} - \frac{4}{24} - \frac{9}{24} \qquad (b) \quad \frac{17}{40} + \frac{33}{40} - \frac{25}{40}$$

$(a) \quad \dfrac{23}{24} - \dfrac{4}{24} - \dfrac{9}{24} = \dfrac{23-4-9}{24} = \dfrac{10}{24} = \dfrac{5}{12}$

$(b) \quad \dfrac{17}{40} + \dfrac{33}{40} - \dfrac{25}{40} = \dfrac{17+33-25}{40} = \dfrac{25}{40} = \dfrac{5}{8}$

2.9   THE LEAST COMMON DENOMINATOR (LCD)

Two fractions with different denominators cannot be added as they stand. For example, the sum $\dfrac{2}{3} + \dfrac{1}{4}$ cannot be calculated as it stands, since the rule stated previously for adding fractions applies only when the fractions have a common denominator. Thus, before fractions with different denominators can be added they must first be written as equivalent fractions with a common denominator. It is usually best to find the least (smallest) common denominator. The *least common denominator* (LCD) of two or more fractions is the least common multiple (LCM) of their denominators (see Sec. 1.13).

EXAMPLE 2.26   Find the least common denominator (LCD) for the following sets of fractions.

(a) $\dfrac{1}{3}$ and $\dfrac{2}{5}$ (c) $\dfrac{1}{6}$ and $\dfrac{5}{4}$ (e) $\dfrac{3}{4}, \dfrac{1}{5},$ and $\dfrac{1}{6}$

(b) $\dfrac{1}{4}$ and $\dfrac{1}{8}$ (d) $\dfrac{3}{16}$ and $\dfrac{7}{24}$

The LCD for each set of fractions is the least common multiple of their denominators.

(a) The LCM of 3 and 5 is $3 \times 5 = 15$. Thus, 15 is the LCD of $\dfrac{1}{3}$ and $\dfrac{2}{5}$.

(b) The LCM of 4 and 8 is 8. Thus, 8 is the LCD of $\dfrac{1}{4}$ and $\dfrac{1}{8}$.

(c) The LCM of 6 and 4 is 12. Thus, 12 is the LCD of $\dfrac{1}{4}$ and $\dfrac{1}{12}$.

(d) To find the LCM of 16 and 24, use the method shown in Example 1.31.

   1.   The GCD of 16 and 24 is 8
   2.   Calculate LCM $= (16 \div 8) \times 24 = 2 \times 24 = 48$

   Thus, 48 is the LCD of $\dfrac{3}{16}$ and $\dfrac{7}{24}$.

(e) To find the LCM of 4, 5, and 6, use the method shown in Example 1.33.

   1.   The LCM of 4 and 5 is $4 \times 5 = 20$
   2.   The LCM of 20 and 6 is $(20 \div 2) \times 6 = 10 \times 6 = 60$

   Thus, the LCD of $\dfrac{3}{4}, \dfrac{1}{5},$ and $\dfrac{1}{6}$ is 60.

2.10   ADDITION AND SUBTRACTION OF FRACTIONS WITH DIFFERENT DENOMINATORS

To add or subtract fractions with different denominators, use the following procedure:

1.   Find their least common denominator.
2.   Build up each fraction to have this denominator.
3.   Add or subtract the resulting fractions, reducing the answer if possible.

EXAMPLE 2.27   Perform the addition $\dfrac{3}{5} + \dfrac{2}{3}$.

Follow the procedure outlined above.

1.   Since the GCD of 3 and 5 is 1, the LCD of the fractions is the product of the denominators. $\text{LCD} = 3 \times 5 = 15$

2. Build up each fraction to have 15 as denominator (see Sec. 2.4).

$$\frac{3}{5} = \frac{3 \times 3}{5 \times 3} = \frac{9}{15}$$

$$\frac{2}{3} = \frac{2 \times 5}{3 \times 5} = \frac{10}{15}$$

3. Add the resulting fractions.

$$\frac{9 + 10}{15} = \frac{19}{15} \qquad \text{Answer}$$

EXAMPLE 2.28 Calculate the sum $\frac{5}{12} + \frac{1}{16}$.

1. Find the LCD. The GCD of 12 and 16 is 4; therefore,

$$\text{LCD} = (12 \div 4) \times 16 = 3 \times 16 = 48$$

2. Build up each fraction to have 48 as denominator.

$$\frac{5}{12} = \frac{5 \times 4}{12 \times 4} = \frac{20}{48}$$

$$\frac{1}{16} = \frac{1 \times 3}{16 \times 3} = \frac{3}{48}$$

3. Add the resulting fractions.

$$\frac{20 + 3}{48} = \frac{23}{48} \qquad \text{Answer}$$

EXAMPLE 2.29 Perform the subtraction $\frac{17}{36} - \frac{11}{90}$.

1. Find the LCD.

GCD of 36 and 90 is 18; therefore,
$$\text{LCD} = (36 \div 18) \times 90 = 2 \times 90 = 180.$$

2. Build up each fraction to have 180 as denominator.

$$\frac{17}{36} = \frac{17 \times 5}{36 \times 5} = \frac{85}{180}$$

$$\frac{11}{90} = \frac{11 \times 2}{90 \times 2} = \frac{22}{180}$$

3. Subtract the resulting fractions.

$$\frac{85 - 22}{180} = \frac{63}{180} = \frac{7}{20} \qquad \text{Answer}$$

EXAMPLE 2.30 Perform the indicated operations: $\frac{2}{9} + \frac{5}{6} - \frac{3}{8}$.

1. Find the LCD.

LCM of 9 and 6 is 18; LCM of 18 and 8 is 72.
Therefore, LCD = 72.

2. Build up each fraction to have 72 as denominator.

$$\frac{2}{9} = \frac{2 \times 8}{9 \times 8} = \frac{16}{72}$$

$$\frac{5}{6} = \frac{5 \times 12}{6 \times 12} = \frac{60}{72}$$

$$\frac{3}{8} = \frac{3 \times 9}{8 \times 9} = \frac{27}{72}$$

3. Add or subtract the numerators as indicated.

$$\frac{16 + 60 - 27}{72} = \frac{49}{72} \qquad \text{Answer}$$

EXAMPLE 2.31 Express the sum $5 + \dfrac{3}{8}$ as an improper fraction.

This is a problem in adding a whole number to a fraction. This can be done as a problem in adding fractions if we express the whole number 5 as the improper fraction $\dfrac{5}{1}$.

1. Express 5 as the equivalent fraction $\dfrac{5}{1}$. $5 + \dfrac{3}{8} = \dfrac{5}{1} + \dfrac{3}{8}$

2. Proceeding as before, find the LCD. $\text{LCD} = 8$

3. Build up each fraction to have the LCD 8.
$$\dfrac{3}{8} = \dfrac{3}{8}$$
$$\dfrac{5}{1} = \dfrac{5 \times 8}{1 \times 8} = \dfrac{40}{8}$$

4. Add the resulting fractions. $\dfrac{3 + 40}{8} = \dfrac{43}{8}$ Answer

2.11 MIXED NUMBERS

A *mixed number* is an abbreviated way of writing the sum of a whole number and a proper fraction. For example, $5\dfrac{2}{3}$ is a mixed number. It is an abbreviation for the sum $5 + \dfrac{2}{3}$.

Changing a Mixed Number into an Equivalent Improper Fraction. Since a mixed number is the sum of a whole number and a fraction, it can be written as an equivalent improper fraction by performing the addition (see Example 2.31).

EXAMPLE 2.32 Express the mixed number $3\dfrac{2}{5}$ as an improper fraction.

Perform the addition:

$$3\dfrac{2}{5} = 3 + \dfrac{2}{5} = \dfrac{3}{1} + \dfrac{2}{5} = \dfrac{15}{2} + \dfrac{2}{5} = \dfrac{17}{5}$$

The above steps can be abbreviated into the shortcut illustrated below:

1. Multiply the whole number part by the denominator. $3 \times 5 = 15$

2. Add the numerator. $15 + 2 = 17$

3. Write the answer over the denominator. $\dfrac{17}{5}$ Answer

EXAMPLE 2.33 Use the shortcut method to write the mixed number $7\dfrac{3}{16}$ as an improper fraction.

1. Multiply the whole number part by the denominator. $7 \times 16 = 112$

2. Add the numerator. $112 + 3 = 115$

3. Write the answer over the denominator. $\dfrac{115}{16}$ Answer

Changing an Improper Fraction into an Equivalent Whole or Mixed Number. Since the denominator of an improper fraction is less than or equal to the numerator, performing the division indicated by the fraction will result in a whole number quotient plus a remainder. If the remainder is zero, the improper fraction is equivalent to a whole number. If the remainder is not zero, the improper fraction is equivalent to a mixed number. The next example illustrates both cases.

EXAMPLE 2.34 Change each of the given improper fractions into equivalent mixed or whole numbers: (a) $\frac{53}{12}$; (b) $\frac{112}{16}$; (c) $\frac{83}{83}$.

(a) 1. The fraction $\frac{53}{12}$ means the division $53 \div 12$.

Perform this division.

$$\begin{array}{r} 4 \\ 12\overline{)53} \\ 48 \\ \hline 5 \end{array}$$ Quotient

Remainder

2. The quotient is the whole number part of the answer, and the remainder is the numerator of the fractional part.

$$\frac{53}{12} = 4\frac{5}{12}$$

(b) 1. The fraction $\frac{112}{16}$ means the division $112 \div 16$.

Perform this division.

$$\begin{array}{r} 7 \\ 16\overline{)112} \\ 112 \end{array}$$

2. The remainder is zero, so:

$$\frac{112}{16} = 7$$

(c) Any number divided by itself is equal to 1:

$$\frac{83}{83} = 1$$

An equivalence between an improper fraction and a mixed number, such as $1\frac{2}{3} = \frac{5}{3}$, has the meaning shown in Fig. 2-5.

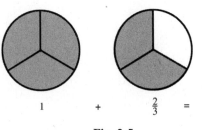

$$1 \quad + \quad \frac{2}{3} \quad = \quad \frac{5}{3}$$

Fig. 2-5

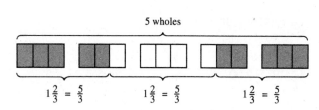

5 wholes

$$1\frac{2}{3} = \frac{5}{3} \qquad 1\frac{2}{3} = \frac{5}{3} \qquad 1\frac{2}{3} = \frac{5}{3}$$

Fig. 2-6

This equivalence can also be given the meaning shown in Fig. 2-6. This shows that when a group of 5 wholes is divided into 3 equal parts, each part is $1\frac{2}{3}$ of a whole.

EXAMPLE 2.35 The contents of a 15-ounce bottle are to be divided into 4 equal parts. How many ounces will there be in each part?

1. The total amount, 15 ounces, is to be divided into 4 equal parts. Thus, we divide 15 by 4.

   Each part is $\dfrac{15}{4}$ ounces

2. To see how many ounces this is, write it as the equivalent mixed number by performing the division.

$$\begin{array}{r} 3 \quad \text{Quotient} \\ 4\overline{)15} \\ \underline{12} \\ 3 \quad \text{Remainder} \end{array}$$

3. Thus, $\dfrac{15}{4}$ ounces is equal to:

   $3\dfrac{3}{4}$ ounces in each part

2.12 CALCULATIONS WITH MIXED NUMBERS

Multiplication and Division of Mixed Numbers. When multiplying or dividing mixed numbers, it is usually easiest first to change the mixed numbers into improper fractions, then multiply or divide as usual.

EXAMPLE 2.36 Perform the multiplication $2\dfrac{1}{3} \times 1\dfrac{1}{2}$, and write the answer both as an improper fraction and as a mixed number.

1. To perform the multiplication, change both mixed numbers into improper fractions.

$$2\frac{1}{3} \times 1\frac{1}{2} = \frac{7}{3} \times \frac{3}{2}$$

2. Perform the multiplication.

$$= \frac{7}{\overset{}{\underset{1}{\cancel{3}}}} \times \frac{\overset{1}{\cancel{3}}}{2} = \frac{7}{2} = 3\frac{1}{2}$$

EXAMPLE 2.37 Perform the division $\dfrac{5}{8} \div 2\dfrac{3}{4}$.

1. First change the mixed number to an improper fraction.

$$\frac{5}{8} \div 2\frac{3}{4} = \frac{5}{8} \div \frac{11}{4}$$

2. Perform the division.

$$= \frac{5}{\overset{}{\underset{2}{\cancel{8}}}} \times \frac{\overset{1}{\cancel{4}}}{11} = \frac{5}{22}$$

EXAMPLE 2.38 Write the complex fraction $2\dfrac{1}{2} \Big/ 3\dfrac{1}{3}$ as a simple fraction.

1. First change the mixed numbers to improper fractions.

$$\frac{2\frac{1}{2}}{3\frac{1}{3}} = \frac{\frac{5}{2}}{\frac{10}{3}}$$

2. Perform the indicated division.

$$= \frac{5}{2} \div \frac{10}{3} = \frac{\overset{1}{\cancel{5}}}{2} \times \frac{3}{\overset{}{\underset{2}{\cancel{10}}}} = \frac{3}{4}$$

EXAMPLE 2.39　Write the complex fraction $3\dfrac{1}{10}\Big/\dfrac{1}{200}$ as a simple fraction.

1. First change the mixed number to an improper fraction.

$$\dfrac{3\dfrac{1}{10}}{\dfrac{1}{200}}=\dfrac{\dfrac{31}{10}}{\dfrac{1}{200}}$$

2. Perform the indicated division.

$$=\dfrac{31}{10}\div\dfrac{1}{200}$$

$$=\dfrac{31}{\overset{}{\underset{1}{\cancel{10}}}}\times\dfrac{\overset{20}{\cancel{200}}}{1}=\dfrac{620}{1}=620$$

Addition of Mixed Numbers.　When adding mixed numbers, it is generally easier to leave the mixed numbers as they are if the answer is to be written as a mixed number also. The whole number parts and the fractional parts are added separately.

EXAMPLE 2.40　Perform the addition $4\dfrac{5}{8}+2\dfrac{1}{3}$.

1. A mixed number is the sum of the whole number part and the fractional part.

$$4\dfrac{5}{8}+2\dfrac{1}{3}=4+\dfrac{5}{8}+2+\dfrac{1}{3}$$

2. Add the whole numbers and the fractions separately.

$$=(4+2)+\left(\dfrac{5}{8}+\dfrac{1}{3}\right)$$

$$=\quad6\quad+\dfrac{15}{24}+\dfrac{8}{24}\quad(\text{LCD}=24)$$

$$=\quad6\quad+\dfrac{23}{24}$$

$$=6\dfrac{23}{24}$$

EXAMPLE 2.41　Perform the addition $5\dfrac{3}{4}+6\dfrac{5}{9}$.

1. Add the whole number and fractional parts separately.

$$5\dfrac{3}{4}+6\dfrac{5}{9}=11+\dfrac{3}{4}+\dfrac{5}{9}$$

$$=11+\dfrac{27}{36}+\dfrac{20}{36}\quad(\text{LCD}=36)$$

$$=11+\dfrac{47}{36}$$

2. Change the improper fraction $\dfrac{47}{36}$ to the mixed number $1\dfrac{11}{36}$, then add.

$$=11+1\dfrac{11}{36}=12\dfrac{11}{36}$$

Addition of mixed numbers may also be performed using a vertical format. This is illustrated in the next example.

EXAMPLE 2.42   Perform the addition $3\frac{1}{2} + 5\frac{2}{3}$.

1. Arrange the sum vertically.

$$
\begin{array}{r}
3\dfrac{1}{2} \\[1em]
+5\dfrac{2}{3} \\[0.5em]
\hline
\end{array}
$$

2. Write the fractional parts with a common denominator.

$$
\begin{array}{r}
3\dfrac{1}{2} = 3\dfrac{3}{6} \\[1em]
+5\dfrac{2}{3} = 5\dfrac{4}{6} \\[0.5em]
\hline
\end{array} \quad \text{(LCD} = 6)
$$

3. Add the whole number and fractional parts separately.

$$8\frac{7}{6}$$

4. Change the improper fraction $\frac{7}{6}$ to the mixed number $1\frac{1}{6}$, then add.

$$= 8 + 1\frac{1}{6} = 9\frac{1}{6}$$

Borrowing with Mixed Numbers.   Before subtraction of mixed numbers is discussed, the idea of borrowing when mixed numbers are involved must be understood. A mixed number such as $7\frac{5}{40}$ can be written as a mixed number with a larger fractional part as follows:

$$\text{Write } 7 = 6 + 1: \qquad 7\frac{5}{40} = 6 + 1\frac{5}{40}$$

$$\text{Write } 1\frac{5}{40} = \frac{45}{40}: \qquad\quad = 6 + \frac{45}{40}$$

This is written as $7\frac{5}{40} = 6\frac{45}{40}$. Note that $6\frac{45}{40}$ comes from $7\frac{5}{40}$ by subtracting 1 from the whole number part $(7 - 1 = 6)$ and adding the denominator to the numerator $(5 + 40 = 45)$. This is described as *borrowing 1* from the whole number to increase the fraction. This procedure will sometimes be necessary when subtracting mixed numbers.

Subtraction of Mixed Numbers

EXAMPLE 2.43   Perform the subtraction $7\frac{1}{8} - 3\frac{2}{5}$.

1. Arrange the subtraction vertically, and write the fractional parts with a common denominator.

$$
\begin{array}{r}
7\dfrac{1}{8} = 7\dfrac{5}{40} \\[1em]
-3\dfrac{2}{5} = -3\dfrac{16}{40} \\[0.5em]
\hline
\end{array} \quad \text{(LCD} = 40)
$$

2. The bottom fraction cannot be subtracted from the top one, so we must borrow 1 from the whole number.

$$7\frac{5}{40} = 6\frac{45}{40} \quad \text{Borrowed}$$
$$-3\frac{16}{40} = -3\frac{16}{40} \quad \text{Unchanged}$$
$$\overline{\phantom{-3\frac{16}{40}} \quad 3\frac{29}{40}}$$

3. Now the subtraction is performed.

EXAMPLE 2.44 Perform the calculation $4\frac{1}{5} + 3\frac{1}{4} - 5\frac{2}{3}$.

1. Arrange the calculation vertically, and write the fractional parts with a common denominator.

$$4\frac{1}{5} = 4\frac{12}{60}$$
$$+3\frac{1}{4} = +3\frac{15}{60} \quad (\text{LCD} = 60)$$
$$-5\frac{2}{3} = -5\frac{40}{60}$$

2. Perform the addition to get $7\frac{27}{60}$. We see that the subtraction cannot be done as is, so we borrow and then subtract.

$$7\frac{27}{60} = 6\frac{87}{60} \quad \text{Borrowed}$$
$$-5\frac{40}{60} = -5\frac{40}{60} \quad \text{Unchanged}$$
$$\overline{\phantom{-5\frac{40}{60}} \quad 1\frac{47}{60}}$$

2.13 COMPARING FRACTIONS

The mathematical symbols used to compare numbers are:

$$= \text{which means "is equal to"}$$
$$< \text{which means "is less than"}$$
$$> \text{which means "is greater than"}$$

For example,

$$3 + 2 = 5 \text{ is read "}3 + 2 \text{ is equal to 5"}$$
$$4 < 9 \text{ is read "4 is less than 9"}$$
$$7 > 2 \text{ is read "7 is greater than 2"}$$

Comparing Fractions with the Same Denominator. If two fractions have the same denominator, the lesser fraction is the one with the lesser numerator and the greater fraction is the one with the greater numerator.

EXAMPLE 2.45 Compare the fractions $\frac{7}{16}$ and $\frac{3}{16}$.

The two fractions have the same denominator. Since 3 is less than 7, then $\frac{3}{16}$ is less than $\frac{7}{16}$. In symbols, this is written $\frac{3}{16} < \frac{7}{16}$, since $3 < 7$. Equivalently, $\frac{7}{16} > \frac{3}{16}$, since $7 > 3$.

EXAMPLE 2.46 Compare the fractions $\dfrac{325}{1000}$ and $\dfrac{235}{1000}$.

The two fractions have the same denominator. Since 235 is less than 325 (235 < 325), then $\dfrac{235}{1000} < \dfrac{325}{1000}$, or equivalently, $\dfrac{325}{1000} > \dfrac{235}{1000}$.

Comparing Fractions with Different Denominators. When two fractions have different denominators, they can be compared by writing them as equivalent fractions with a common denominator.

EXAMPLE 2.47 Compare the fractions $\dfrac{5}{7}$ and $\dfrac{3}{4}$.

Write the fractions with a common denominator.

$$\frac{5}{7} = \frac{5 \times 4}{7 \times 4} = \frac{20}{28}$$
$$\frac{3}{4} = \frac{3 \times 7}{4 \times 7} = \frac{21}{28} \qquad (\text{LCD} = 28)$$

Compare the numerators, 20 < 21, so:

$$\frac{20}{28} < \frac{21}{28}$$

Therefore:

$$\frac{5}{7} < \frac{3}{4} \text{ or } \frac{3}{4} > \frac{5}{7}$$

EXAMPLE 2.48 Compare the fractions $\dfrac{3}{1000}$ and $\dfrac{1}{250}$.

Write the fractions with a common denominator.

$$\frac{3}{1000} = \frac{3}{1000}$$
$$\frac{1}{250} = \frac{1 \times 4}{250 \times 4} = \frac{4}{1000}$$

Compare numerators, 3 < 4, so:

$$\frac{3}{1000} < \frac{4}{1000}$$

Therefore:

$$\frac{3}{1000} < \frac{1}{250}$$

Two fractions can be compared by a shortcut method based on cross multiplying. If $\dfrac{A}{B}$ and $\dfrac{C}{D}$ are two fractions, then

$$\frac{A}{B} < \frac{C}{D} \text{ if, and only if, } A \times D < B \times C$$

The multiplications $A \times D$ and $B \times C$ are called *cross multiplications* because they are performed as indicated below:

$$\frac{A}{B} \bowtie \frac{C}{D}$$

Examples 2.47 and 2.48 can also be done by cross multiplying.

EXAMPLE 2.49   Compare the fractions $\frac{5}{7}$ and $\frac{3}{4}$.

1. Cross multiply.

   $$\frac{5}{7} \bowtie \frac{3}{4}$$

   $5 \times 4 = 20; 7 \times 3 = 21$

2. Compare.

   $20 < 21$

3. Therefore:

   $$\frac{5}{7} < \frac{3}{4}$$

EXAMPLE 2.50   Compare the fractions $\frac{1}{250}$ and $\frac{3}{1000}$.

1. Cross multiply.

   $$\frac{1}{250} \bowtie \frac{3}{1000}$$

   $1 \times 1000 = 1000; 250 \times 3 = 750$

2. Compare.

   $1000 > 750$

3. Therefore:

   $$\frac{1}{250} > \frac{3}{1000}$$

Solved Problems

2.1   Reduce the following fractions to lowest terms.

   (a) $\dfrac{8}{12}$ (f) $\dfrac{1000}{100}$ (k) $\dfrac{13}{52}$ (p) $\dfrac{84}{70}$

   (b) $\dfrac{10}{100}$ (g) $\dfrac{3}{27}$ (l) $\dfrac{64}{40}$ (q) $\dfrac{65}{39}$

   (c) $\dfrac{8}{2}$ (h) $\dfrac{9}{18}$ (m) $\dfrac{48}{100}$ (r) $\dfrac{160}{640}$

   (d) $\dfrac{36}{30}$ (i) $\dfrac{48}{16}$ (n) $\dfrac{50}{200}$ (s) $\dfrac{144}{288}$

   (e) $\dfrac{15}{15}$ (j) $\dfrac{12}{60}$ (o) $\dfrac{27}{72}$ (t) $\dfrac{480}{1200}$

Solution

   (a) Divide by the GCD 4.

   $$\frac{\overset{2}{\cancel{8}}}{\underset{3}{\cancel{12}}} = \frac{2}{3}$$

   (b) Divide by the GCD 10.

   $$\frac{\overset{1}{\cancel{10}}}{\underset{10}{\cancel{100}}} = \frac{1}{10}$$

   (c) Divide by the GCD 2.

   $$\frac{\overset{4}{\cancel{8}}}{\underset{1}{\cancel{2}}} = \frac{4}{1} = 4$$

(d) Divide by the GCD 6.

$$\frac{\overset{6}{\cancel{36}}}{\underset{5}{\cancel{30}}} = \frac{6}{5}$$

(e) Divide by the GCD 15.

$$\frac{\overset{1}{\cancel{15}}}{\underset{1}{\cancel{15}}} = \frac{1}{1} = 1$$

(f) Divide by the GCD 100.

$$\frac{\overset{10}{\cancel{1000}}}{\underset{1}{\cancel{100}}} = \frac{10}{1} = 10$$

(g) Divide by the GCD 3.

$$\frac{\overset{1}{\cancel{3}}}{\underset{9}{\cancel{27}}} = \frac{1}{9}$$

(h) Divide by the GCD 9.

$$\frac{\overset{1}{\cancel{9}}}{\underset{2}{\cancel{18}}} = \frac{1}{2}$$

(i) Divide by the GCD 16.

$$\frac{\overset{3}{\cancel{48}}}{\underset{1}{\cancel{16}}} = \frac{3}{1} = 3$$

(j) Divide by the GCD 12.

$$\frac{\overset{1}{\cancel{12}}}{\underset{5}{\cancel{60}}} = \frac{1}{5}$$

(k) Divide by the GCD 13.

$$\frac{\overset{1}{\cancel{13}}}{\underset{4}{\cancel{52}}} = \frac{1}{4}$$

(l) Divide by the GCD 8.

$$\frac{\overset{8}{\cancel{64}}}{\underset{5}{\cancel{40}}} = \frac{8}{5}$$

(m) Divide by the GCD 4.

$$\frac{\overset{12}{\cancel{48}}}{\underset{25}{\cancel{100}}} = \frac{12}{25}$$

(n) Divide by the GCD 50.

$$\frac{\overset{1}{\cancel{50}}}{\underset{4}{\cancel{200}}} = \frac{1}{4}$$

(o) Divide by the GCD 9.

$$\frac{\overset{3}{\cancel{27}}}{\underset{8}{\cancel{72}}} = \frac{3}{8}$$

(p) Divide by the GCD 14.

$$\frac{\overset{6}{\cancel{84}}}{\underset{5}{\cancel{70}}} = \frac{6}{5}$$

(q) Divide by the GCD 13.

$$\frac{\overset{5}{\cancel{65}}}{\underset{3}{\cancel{39}}} = \frac{5}{3}$$

(r) Divide by the GCD 160.

$$\frac{\overset{1}{\cancel{160}}}{\underset{4}{\cancel{640}}} = \frac{1}{4}$$

(s) Divide by the GCD 144.

$$\frac{\overset{1}{\cancel{144}}}{\underset{2}{\cancel{288}}} = \frac{1}{2}$$

(t) Divide by the GCD 240.

$$\frac{\overset{2}{\cancel{480}}}{\underset{5}{\cancel{1200}}} = \frac{2}{5}$$

2.2 Build up the given fractions to have the indicated denominators.

(a) $\dfrac{3}{8} = \dfrac{?}{40}$ (f) $\dfrac{3}{4} = \dfrac{?}{100}$ (k) $\dfrac{7}{10} = \dfrac{?}{500}$ (p) $\dfrac{1}{25} = \dfrac{?}{1000}$

(b) $\dfrac{4}{5} = \dfrac{?}{45}$ (g) $5 = \dfrac{?}{20}$ (l) $\dfrac{3}{100} = \dfrac{?}{1000}$ (q) $\dfrac{5}{16} = \dfrac{?}{64}$

(c) $8 = \dfrac{?}{1}$ (h) $\dfrac{3}{5} = \dfrac{?}{60}$ (m) $\dfrac{5}{12} = \dfrac{?}{60}$ (r) $\dfrac{1}{20} = \dfrac{?}{500}$

(d) $\dfrac{1}{25} = \dfrac{?}{100}$ (i) $\dfrac{1}{2} = \dfrac{?}{120}$ (n) $\dfrac{2}{15} = \dfrac{?}{300}$ (s) $\dfrac{1}{250} = \dfrac{?}{1000}$

(e) $7 = \dfrac{?}{10}$ (j) $\dfrac{1}{3} = \dfrac{?}{300}$ (o) $\dfrac{1}{30} = \dfrac{?}{150}$ (t) $\dfrac{7}{24} = \dfrac{?}{480}$

Solution

(a) $\dfrac{3}{8} = \dfrac{3 \times 5}{8 \times 5} = \dfrac{15}{40}$ (k) $\dfrac{7}{10} = \dfrac{7 \times 50}{10 \times 50} = \dfrac{350}{500}$

(b) $\dfrac{4}{5} = \dfrac{4 \times 9}{5 \times 9} = \dfrac{36}{45}$ (l) $\dfrac{3}{100} = \dfrac{3 \times 10}{100 \times 10} = \dfrac{30}{1000}$

(c) $8 = \dfrac{8}{1}$ (m) $\dfrac{5}{12} = \dfrac{5 \times 5}{12 \times 5} = \dfrac{25}{60}$

(d) $\dfrac{1}{25} = \dfrac{1 \times 4}{25 \times 4} = \dfrac{4}{100}$ (n) $\dfrac{2}{15} = \dfrac{2 \times 20}{15 \times 20} = \dfrac{40}{300}$

(e) $7 = \dfrac{7}{1} = \dfrac{7 \times 10}{1 \times 10} = \dfrac{70}{10}$ (o) $\dfrac{1}{30} = \dfrac{1 \times 5}{30 \times 5} = \dfrac{5}{150}$

(f) $\dfrac{3}{4} = \dfrac{3 \times 25}{4 \times 25} = \dfrac{75}{100}$ (p) $\dfrac{1}{25} = \dfrac{1 \times 40}{25 \times 40} = \dfrac{40}{1000}$

(g) $5 = \dfrac{5}{1} = \dfrac{5 \times 20}{1 \times 20} = \dfrac{100}{20}$ (q) $\dfrac{5}{16} = \dfrac{5 \times 4}{16 \times 4} = \dfrac{20}{64}$

(h) $\dfrac{3}{5} = \dfrac{3 \times 12}{5 \times 12} = \dfrac{36}{60}$ (r) $\dfrac{1}{20} = \dfrac{1 \times 25}{20 \times 25} = \dfrac{25}{500}$

(i) $\dfrac{1}{2} = \dfrac{1 \times 60}{2 \times 60} = \dfrac{60}{120}$ (s) $\dfrac{1}{250} = \dfrac{1 \times 4}{250 \times 4} = \dfrac{4}{1000}$

(j) $\dfrac{1}{3} = \dfrac{1 \times 100}{3 \times 100} = \dfrac{100}{300}$ (t) $\dfrac{7}{24} = \dfrac{7 \times 20}{24 \times 20} = \dfrac{140}{480}$

2.3 Calculate the following products. Give answers reduced to lowest terms.

(a) $\dfrac{1}{3} \times \dfrac{1}{5}$ (f) $\dfrac{25}{16} \times \dfrac{12}{10}$ (k) $\dfrac{1}{250} \times \dfrac{400}{3}$ (p) $9 \times \dfrac{5}{4} \times \dfrac{8}{50}$

(b) $\dfrac{5}{8} \times \dfrac{7}{3}$ (g) $5 \times \dfrac{3}{10}$ (l) $\dfrac{350}{4} \times \dfrac{1}{490}$ (q) $\dfrac{36}{15} \times \dfrac{56}{49} \times \dfrac{1}{100}$

(c) $\dfrac{1}{2} \times \dfrac{2}{3}$ (h) $\dfrac{8}{9} \times 3$ (m) $\dfrac{600}{2000} \times \dfrac{121}{44}$ (r) $200 \times \dfrac{1}{50} \times \dfrac{150}{20}$

(d) $\dfrac{6}{5} \times \dfrac{10}{9}$ (i) $\dfrac{16}{5} \times 5$ (n) $\dfrac{75}{130} \times 52$ (s) $300 \times \dfrac{1}{60} \times \dfrac{1}{250}$

(e) $\dfrac{8}{12} \times \dfrac{35}{15}$ (j) $\dfrac{8}{50} \times \dfrac{100}{64}$ (o) $\dfrac{5}{10} \times \dfrac{8}{18} \times \dfrac{7}{3}$ (t) $750 \times \dfrac{65}{4} \times \dfrac{1}{3000}$

Solution

(a) $\dfrac{1}{3} \times \dfrac{1}{5} = \dfrac{1 \times 1}{3 \times 5} = \dfrac{1}{15}$

(e) $\dfrac{8}{12} \times \dfrac{35}{15} = \dfrac{2}{3} \times \dfrac{35}{15} = \dfrac{2 \times 7}{3 \times 3} = \dfrac{14}{9}$

(b) $\dfrac{5}{8} \times \dfrac{7}{3} = \dfrac{5 \times 7}{8 \times 3} = \dfrac{35}{24}$

(f) $\dfrac{25}{16} \times \dfrac{12}{10} = \dfrac{5}{16} \times \dfrac{12}{2} = \dfrac{5 \times 3}{4 \times 2} = \dfrac{15}{8}$

(c) $\dfrac{1}{2} \times \dfrac{2}{3} = \dfrac{1 \times 1}{1 \times 3} = \dfrac{1}{3}$

(g) $5 \times \dfrac{3}{10} = \dfrac{5}{1} \times \dfrac{3}{10} = \dfrac{1 \times 3}{1 \times 2} = \dfrac{3}{2}$

(d) $\dfrac{6}{5} \times \dfrac{10}{9} = \dfrac{2}{3} \times \dfrac{10}{3} = \dfrac{2 \times 2}{1 \times 3} = \dfrac{4}{3}$

(h) $\dfrac{8}{9} \times 3 = \dfrac{8}{9} \times \dfrac{3}{1} = \dfrac{8 \times 1}{3 \times 1} = \dfrac{8}{3}$

(i) $\dfrac{16}{5} \times 5 = \dfrac{16}{5} \times \dfrac{5}{1} = \dfrac{16 \times 1}{1 \times 1} = \dfrac{16}{1} = 16$

(j) $\dfrac{8}{50} \times \dfrac{100}{64} = \dfrac{8}{1} \times \dfrac{2}{64} = \dfrac{1}{1} \times \dfrac{2}{8} = \dfrac{1 \times 1}{1 \times 4} = \dfrac{1}{4}$

(k) $\dfrac{1}{250} \times \dfrac{400}{3} = \dfrac{1 \times 8}{5 \times 3} = \dfrac{8}{15}$

(l) $\dfrac{350}{4} \times \dfrac{1}{490} = \dfrac{5 \times 1}{4 \times 7} = \dfrac{5}{28}$

(m) $\dfrac{600}{2000} \times \dfrac{121}{44} = \dfrac{3}{10} \times \dfrac{121}{44} = \dfrac{3 \times 11}{10 \times 4} = \dfrac{33}{40}$

(n) $\dfrac{75}{130} \times 52 = \dfrac{75}{130} \times \dfrac{52}{1} = \dfrac{15}{26} \times \dfrac{52}{1} = \dfrac{15 \times 2}{1 \times 1} = \dfrac{30}{1} = 30$

(o) $\dfrac{5}{10} \times \dfrac{8}{18} \times \dfrac{7}{3} = \dfrac{1}{2} \times \dfrac{8}{18} \times \dfrac{7}{3} = \dfrac{1}{1} \times \dfrac{4}{18} \times \dfrac{7}{3} = \dfrac{1 \times 2 \times 7}{1 \times 9 \times 3} = \dfrac{14}{27}$

(p) $9 \times \dfrac{5}{4} \times \dfrac{8}{50} = \dfrac{9}{1} \times \dfrac{5}{4} \times \dfrac{8}{50} = \dfrac{9}{1} \times \dfrac{1}{4} \times \dfrac{8}{10} = \dfrac{9}{1} \times \dfrac{1}{1} \times \dfrac{2}{10} = \dfrac{9 \times 1 \times 1}{1 \times 1 \times 5} = \dfrac{9}{5}$

(q) $\dfrac{36}{15} \times \dfrac{56}{49} \times \dfrac{1}{100} = \dfrac{12}{5} \times \dfrac{56}{49} \times \dfrac{1}{100} = \dfrac{12}{5} \times \dfrac{8}{7} \times \dfrac{1}{100} = \dfrac{12 \times 2 \times 1}{5 \times 7 \times 25} = \dfrac{24}{875}$

(r) $200 \times \dfrac{1}{50} \times \dfrac{150}{20} = \dfrac{200}{1} \times \dfrac{1}{50} \times \dfrac{150}{20} = \dfrac{10}{1} \times \dfrac{1}{50} \times \dfrac{150}{1} = \dfrac{10 \times 1 \times 3}{1 \times 1 \times 1} = \dfrac{30}{1} = 30$

(s) $300 \times \dfrac{1}{60} \times \dfrac{1}{250} = \dfrac{300}{1} \times \dfrac{1}{60} \times \dfrac{1}{250} = \dfrac{5}{1} \times \dfrac{1}{1} \times \dfrac{1}{250} = \dfrac{1 \times 1 \times 1}{1 \times 1 \times 50} = \dfrac{1}{50}$

(t) $750 \times \dfrac{65}{4} \times \dfrac{1}{3000} = \dfrac{750}{1} \times \dfrac{65}{4} \times \dfrac{1}{3000} = \dfrac{1 \times 65 \times 1}{1 \times 4 \times 4} = \dfrac{65}{16}$

2.4   Perform the following divisions. Give answers reduced to lowest terms.

(a) $\dfrac{1}{2} \div \dfrac{1}{3}$ (f) $1 \div \dfrac{1}{2}$ (k) $\dfrac{1}{200} \div \dfrac{1}{250}$ (p) $\dfrac{1}{500} \div 2$

(b) $\dfrac{4}{3} \div \dfrac{5}{3}$ (g) $9 \div \dfrac{3}{8}$ (l) $\dfrac{3}{8} \div \dfrac{24}{1000}$ (q) $\dfrac{2}{3} \div 200$

(c) $\dfrac{3}{4} \div \dfrac{1}{8}$ (h) $\dfrac{1}{30} \div 6$ (m) $\dfrac{27}{100} \div \dfrac{3}{500}$ (r) $\dfrac{5}{300} \div \dfrac{2}{150}$

(d) $\dfrac{1}{60} \div \dfrac{3}{10}$ (i) $\dfrac{1}{100} \div 10$ (n) $750 \div \dfrac{1}{2}$ (s) $\dfrac{1}{1000} \div \dfrac{1}{60}$

(e) $\dfrac{12}{16} \div \dfrac{1}{4}$ (j) $\dfrac{5}{300} \div \dfrac{1}{60}$ (o) $240 \div \dfrac{60}{5}$ (t) $\dfrac{3}{1000} \div \dfrac{1}{250}$

Solution

(a) $\dfrac{1}{2} \div \dfrac{1}{3} = \dfrac{1}{2} \times \dfrac{3}{1} = \dfrac{3}{2}$

(b) $\dfrac{4}{3} \div \dfrac{5}{3} = \dfrac{4}{3} \times \dfrac{3}{5} = \dfrac{4 \times 1}{1 \times 5} = \dfrac{4}{5}$

(c) $\dfrac{3}{4} \div \dfrac{1}{8} = \dfrac{3}{4} \times \dfrac{8}{1} = \dfrac{3 \times 2}{1 \times 1} = \dfrac{6}{1} = 6$

(d) $\dfrac{1}{60} \div \dfrac{3}{10} = \dfrac{1}{60} \times \dfrac{10}{3} = \dfrac{1 \times 1}{6 \times 3} = \dfrac{1}{18}$

(e) $\dfrac{12}{16} \div \dfrac{1}{4} = \dfrac{12}{16} \times \dfrac{4}{1} = \dfrac{12}{4} \times \dfrac{1}{1} = \dfrac{3 \times 1}{1 \times 1} = \dfrac{3}{1} = 3$

(f) $1 \div \dfrac{1}{2} = \dfrac{1}{1} \times \dfrac{2}{1} = \dfrac{1 \times 2}{1 \times 1} = \dfrac{2}{1} = 2$

(g) $9 \div \dfrac{3}{8} = \dfrac{9}{1} \times \dfrac{8}{3} = \dfrac{3 \times 8}{1 \times 1} = \dfrac{24}{1} = 24$

(h) $\dfrac{1}{30} \div 6 = \dfrac{1}{30} \times \dfrac{1}{6} = \dfrac{1 \times 1}{30 \times 6} = \dfrac{1}{180}$

(i) $\dfrac{1}{100} \div 10 = \dfrac{1}{100} \times \dfrac{1}{10} = \dfrac{1 \times 1}{100 \times 10} = \dfrac{1}{1000}$

(j) $\dfrac{5}{300} \div \dfrac{1}{60} = \dfrac{5}{300} \times \dfrac{60}{1} = \dfrac{5}{5} \times \dfrac{1}{1} = \dfrac{1 \times 1}{1 \times 1} = \dfrac{1}{1} = 1$

(k) $\dfrac{1}{200} \div \dfrac{1}{250} = \dfrac{1}{200} \times \dfrac{250}{1} = \dfrac{1 \times 5}{4 \times 1} = \dfrac{5}{4}$

(l) $\dfrac{3}{8} \div \dfrac{24}{1000} = \dfrac{3}{8} \times \dfrac{1000}{24} = \dfrac{1}{8} \times \dfrac{1000}{8} = \dfrac{1 \times 125}{8 \times 1} = \dfrac{125}{8}$

(m) $\dfrac{27}{100} \div \dfrac{3}{500} = \dfrac{27}{100} \times \dfrac{500}{3} = \dfrac{27}{1} \times \dfrac{5}{3} = \dfrac{9 \times 5}{1 \times 1} = \dfrac{45}{1} = 45$

(n) $\quad 750 \div \frac{1}{2} = \frac{750}{1} \times \frac{2}{1} = \frac{750 \times 2}{1 \times 1} = \frac{1500}{1} = 1500$

(o) $\quad 240 \div \frac{60}{5} = \frac{\overset{4}{\cancel{240}}}{1} \times \frac{5}{\underset{1}{\cancel{60}}} = \frac{4 \times 5}{1 \times 1} = \frac{20}{1} = 20$

(p) $\quad \frac{1}{500} \div 2 = \frac{1}{500} \times \frac{1}{2} = \frac{1 \times 1}{500 \times 2} = \frac{1}{1000}$

(q) $\quad \frac{2}{3} \div 200 = \frac{\overset{1}{\cancel{2}}}{3} \times \frac{1}{\underset{100}{\cancel{200}}} = \frac{1 \times 1}{3 \times 100} = \frac{1}{300}$

(r) $\quad \frac{5}{300} \div \frac{2}{150} = \frac{5}{\underset{2}{\cancel{300}}} \times \frac{\overset{1}{\cancel{150}}}{2} = \frac{5 \times 1}{2 \times 2} = \frac{5}{4}$

(s) $\quad \frac{1}{1000} \div \frac{1}{60} = \frac{1}{\underset{50}{\cancel{1000}}} \times \frac{\overset{3}{\cancel{60}}}{1} = \frac{1 \times 3}{50 \times 1} = \frac{3}{50}$

(t) $\quad \frac{3}{1000} \div \frac{1}{250} = \frac{3}{\underset{4}{\cancel{1000}}} \times \frac{\overset{1}{\cancel{250}}}{1} = \frac{3 \times 1}{4 \times 1} = \frac{3}{4}$

2.5   Simplify the following complex fractions. Give answers reduced to lowest terms.

(a) $\dfrac{\frac{1}{3}}{\frac{1}{2}}$ (f) $\dfrac{\frac{5}{1}}{\frac{1}{5}}$ (k) $\dfrac{\frac{1}{20}}{\frac{1}{60}}$ (p) $\dfrac{\frac{1}{120}}{2}$

(b) $\dfrac{\frac{1}{4}}{\frac{1}{2}}$ (g) $\dfrac{\frac{10}{2}}{\frac{2}{5}}$ (l) $\dfrac{\frac{1}{300}}{\frac{1}{200}}$ (q) $\dfrac{\frac{3}{25}}{300}$

(c) $\dfrac{\frac{2}{3}}{\frac{1}{8}}$ (h) $\dfrac{\frac{1}{4}}{2}$ (m) $\dfrac{\frac{5}{8}}{\frac{15}{100}}$ (r) $\dfrac{\frac{15}{240}}{\frac{1}{60}}$

(d) $\dfrac{\frac{1}{50}}{\frac{1}{2}}$ (i) $\dfrac{\frac{2}{3}}{2}$ (n) $\dfrac{500}{\frac{1}{2}}$ (s) $\dfrac{\frac{12}{250}}{\frac{3}{750}}$

(e) $\dfrac{\frac{3}{10}}{\frac{1}{3}}$ (j) $\dfrac{\frac{3}{8}}{3}$ (o) $\dfrac{360}{\frac{8}{5}}$ (t) $\dfrac{\frac{24}{1000}}{\frac{3}{125}}$

Solution

(a) $\dfrac{\frac{1}{3}}{\frac{1}{2}} = \dfrac{1}{3} \div \dfrac{1}{2} = \dfrac{1}{3} \times \dfrac{2}{1} = \dfrac{2}{3}$

(b) $\dfrac{\frac{1}{4}}{\frac{1}{2}} = \dfrac{1}{4} \div \dfrac{1}{2} = \dfrac{1}{\overset{}{\underset{2}{4}}} \times \dfrac{\overset{1}{2}}{1} = \dfrac{1}{2}$

(c) $\dfrac{\frac{2}{3}}{\frac{1}{8}} = \dfrac{2}{3} \div \dfrac{1}{8} = \dfrac{2}{3} \times \dfrac{8}{1} = \dfrac{16}{3}$

(d) $\dfrac{\frac{1}{50}}{\frac{1}{2}} = \dfrac{1}{50} \div \dfrac{1}{2} = \dfrac{1}{\underset{25}{50}} \times \dfrac{\overset{1}{2}}{1} = \dfrac{1}{25}$

(e) $\dfrac{\frac{3}{10}}{\frac{1}{3}} = \dfrac{3}{10} \div \dfrac{1}{3} = \dfrac{3}{10} \times \dfrac{3}{1} = \dfrac{9}{10}$

(f) $\dfrac{5}{\frac{1}{5}} = \dfrac{5}{1} \div \dfrac{1}{5} = \dfrac{5}{1} \times \dfrac{5}{1} = \dfrac{25}{1} = 25$

(g) $\dfrac{10}{\frac{2}{5}} = \dfrac{10}{1} \div \dfrac{2}{5} = \dfrac{\overset{5}{10}}{1} \times \dfrac{5}{\underset{1}{2}} = 25$

(h) $\dfrac{\frac{1}{4}}{2} = \dfrac{1}{4} \div 2 = \dfrac{1}{4} \times \dfrac{1}{2} = \dfrac{1}{8}$

(i) $\dfrac{\frac{2}{3}}{2} = \dfrac{2}{3} \div 2 = \dfrac{\overset{1}{2}}{3} \times \dfrac{1}{\underset{1}{2}} = \dfrac{1}{3}$

(j) $\dfrac{\frac{3}{8}}{3} = \dfrac{3}{8} \div 3 = \dfrac{\overset{1}{3}}{8} \times \dfrac{1}{\underset{1}{3}} = \dfrac{1}{8}$

(k) $\dfrac{\frac{1}{20}}{\frac{1}{60}} = \dfrac{1}{20} \div \dfrac{1}{60} = \dfrac{1}{\underset{1}{20}} \times \dfrac{\overset{3}{60}}{1} = \dfrac{3}{1} = 3$

(l) $\dfrac{\frac{1}{300}}{\frac{1}{200}} = \dfrac{1}{300} \div \dfrac{1}{200} = \dfrac{1}{\underset{3}{300}} \times \dfrac{\overset{2}{200}}{1} = \dfrac{2}{3}$

(m) $\dfrac{\frac{5}{8}}{\frac{15}{100}} = \dfrac{5}{8} \div \dfrac{15}{100} = \dfrac{\overset{1}{5}}{8} \times \dfrac{100}{\underset{3}{15}} = \dfrac{1}{\underset{2}{8}} \times \dfrac{\overset{25}{100}}{3} = \dfrac{25}{6}$

(n) $\dfrac{500}{\frac{1}{2}} = 500 \div \dfrac{1}{2} = \dfrac{500}{1} \times \dfrac{2}{1} = 1000$

(o) $\dfrac{360}{\frac{8}{5}} = 360 \div \dfrac{8}{5} = \dfrac{\overset{45}{\cancel{360}}}{1} \times \dfrac{5}{\underset{1}{\cancel{8}}} = \dfrac{225}{1} = 225$

(p) $\dfrac{\frac{1}{120}}{2} = \dfrac{1}{120} \div 2 = \dfrac{1}{120} \times \dfrac{1}{2} = \dfrac{1}{240}$

(q) $\dfrac{\frac{3}{25}}{300} = \dfrac{3}{25} \div 300 = \dfrac{\overset{1}{\cancel{3}}}{25} \times \dfrac{1}{\underset{100}{\cancel{300}}} = \dfrac{1}{2500}$

(r) $\dfrac{\frac{15}{240}}{\frac{1}{60}} = \dfrac{15}{240} \div \dfrac{1}{60} = \dfrac{15}{\underset{4}{\cancel{240}}} \times \dfrac{\overset{1}{\cancel{60}}}{1} = \dfrac{15}{4}$

(s) $\dfrac{\frac{12}{250}}{\frac{3}{750}} = \dfrac{12}{250} \div \dfrac{3}{750} = \dfrac{12}{\underset{1}{\cancel{250}}} \times \dfrac{\overset{3}{\cancel{750}}}{3} = \dfrac{12}{1} \times \dfrac{\overset{1}{\cancel{3}}}{\underset{1}{\cancel{3}}} = \dfrac{12}{1} = 12$

(t) $\dfrac{\frac{24}{1000}}{\frac{3}{125}} = \dfrac{24}{1000} \div \dfrac{3}{125} = \dfrac{24}{\underset{8}{\cancel{1000}}} \times \dfrac{\overset{1}{\cancel{125}}}{3} = \dfrac{\overset{3}{\cancel{24}}}{\cancel{8}} \times \dfrac{1}{3} = \dfrac{\overset{1}{\cancel{3}}}{1} \times \dfrac{1}{\cancel{3}} = \dfrac{1}{1} = 1$

2.6　Perform the following additions and subtractions. Reduce answers to lowest terms.

(a) $\dfrac{3}{8} + \dfrac{2}{8}$　　(f) $\dfrac{7}{8} + \dfrac{5}{8} + \dfrac{4}{8}$　　(k) $\dfrac{5}{6} + \dfrac{1}{8}$　　(p) $\dfrac{2}{75} - \dfrac{1}{100}$

(b) $\dfrac{1}{4} + \dfrac{1}{4}$　　(g) $\dfrac{4}{25} + \dfrac{13}{25} - \dfrac{7}{25}$　　(l) $\dfrac{3}{4} - \dfrac{1}{6}$　　(q) $\dfrac{1}{2} + \dfrac{1}{4} + \dfrac{1}{8}$

(c) $\dfrac{2}{3} + \dfrac{1}{3}$　　(h) $\dfrac{1}{2} + \dfrac{1}{3}$　　(m) $\dfrac{1}{8} - \dfrac{1}{16}$　　(r) $\dfrac{3}{8} + \dfrac{1}{5} + \dfrac{1}{10}$

(d) $\dfrac{8}{10} - \dfrac{1}{10}$　　(i) $\dfrac{1}{8} + \dfrac{2}{7}$　　(n) $\dfrac{1}{10} + \dfrac{1}{20}$　　(s) $\dfrac{4}{25} - \dfrac{1}{30} - \dfrac{1}{100}$

(e) $\dfrac{7}{12} - \dfrac{3}{12}$　　(j) $\dfrac{1}{2} + \dfrac{1}{4}$　　(o) $\dfrac{5}{16} + \dfrac{7}{12}$　　(t) $\dfrac{1}{2} - \dfrac{1}{50} - \dfrac{1}{1000}$

Solution

(a) $\dfrac{3}{8} + \dfrac{2}{8} = \dfrac{3+2}{8} = \dfrac{5}{8}$　　　　(c) $\dfrac{2}{3} + \dfrac{1}{3} = \dfrac{2+1}{3} = \dfrac{3}{3} = 1$

(b) $\dfrac{1}{4} + \dfrac{1}{4} = \dfrac{1+1}{4} = \dfrac{2}{4} = \dfrac{1}{2}$　　　　(d) $\dfrac{8}{10} - \dfrac{1}{10} = \dfrac{8-1}{10} = \dfrac{7}{10}$

(e) $\dfrac{7}{12} - \dfrac{3}{12} = \dfrac{7-3}{12} = \dfrac{4}{12} = \dfrac{1}{3}$

(l) $\dfrac{3}{4} = \dfrac{3 \times 3}{4 \times 3} = \dfrac{9}{12}$

$\dfrac{1}{6} = \dfrac{1 \times 2}{6 \times 2} = \dfrac{2}{12}$ (LCD = 12)

$\dfrac{9-2}{12} = \dfrac{7}{12}$

(f) $\dfrac{7}{8} + \dfrac{5}{8} + \dfrac{4}{8} = \dfrac{7+5+4}{8} = \dfrac{16}{8} = 2$

(m) $\dfrac{1}{8} = \dfrac{1 \times 2}{8 \times 2} = \dfrac{2}{16}$

$\dfrac{1}{16} = \dfrac{1}{16}$ (LCD = 16)

$\dfrac{2-1}{16} = \dfrac{1}{16}$

(g) $\dfrac{4}{25} + \dfrac{13}{25} - \dfrac{7}{25} = \dfrac{4+13-7}{25} = \dfrac{10}{25} = \dfrac{2}{5}$

(n) $\dfrac{1}{10} = \dfrac{1 \times 2}{10 \times 2} = \dfrac{2}{20}$

$\dfrac{1}{20} = \dfrac{1}{20}$ (LCD = 20)

$\dfrac{2+1}{20} = \dfrac{3}{20}$

(h) $\dfrac{1}{2} = \dfrac{1 \times 3}{2 \times 3} = \dfrac{3}{6}$

$\dfrac{1}{3} = \dfrac{1 \times 2}{3 \times 2} = \dfrac{2}{6}$ (LCD = 6)

$\dfrac{3+2}{6} = \dfrac{5}{6}$

(o) $\dfrac{5}{16} = \dfrac{5 \times 3}{16 \times 3} = \dfrac{15}{48}$

$\dfrac{7}{12} = \dfrac{7 \times 4}{12 \times 4} = \dfrac{28}{48}$ (LCD = 48)

$\dfrac{15+28}{48} = \dfrac{43}{48}$

(i) $\dfrac{1}{8} = \dfrac{1 \times 7}{8 \times 7} = \dfrac{7}{56}$

$\dfrac{2}{7} = \dfrac{2 \times 8}{7 \times 8} = \dfrac{16}{56}$ (LCD = 56)

$\dfrac{7+16}{56} = \dfrac{23}{56}$

(p) $\dfrac{2}{75} = \dfrac{2 \times 4}{75 \times 4} = \dfrac{8}{300}$

$\dfrac{1}{100} = \dfrac{1 \times 3}{100 \times 3} = \dfrac{3}{300}$ (LCD = 300)

$\dfrac{8-3}{300} = \dfrac{5}{300}$

$= \dfrac{1}{60}$

(j) $\dfrac{1}{2} = \dfrac{1 \times 2}{2 \times 2} = \dfrac{2}{4}$

$\dfrac{1}{4} = \dfrac{1}{4}$ (LCD = 4)

$\dfrac{2+1}{4} = \dfrac{3}{4}$

(q) $\dfrac{1}{2} = \dfrac{1 \times 4}{2 \times 4} = \dfrac{4}{8}$

$\dfrac{1}{4} = \dfrac{1 \times 2}{4 \times 2} = \dfrac{2}{8}$

$\dfrac{1}{8} = \dfrac{1}{8}$ (LCD = 8)

$\dfrac{4+2+1}{8} = \dfrac{7}{8}$

(k) $\dfrac{5}{6} = \dfrac{5 \times 4}{6 \times 4} = \dfrac{20}{24}$

$\dfrac{1}{8} = \dfrac{1 \times 3}{8 \times 3} = \dfrac{3}{24}$ (LCD = 24)

$\dfrac{20+3}{24} = \dfrac{23}{24}$

(r) $\dfrac{3}{8} = \dfrac{3 \times 5}{8 \times 5} = \dfrac{15}{40}$

$\dfrac{1}{5} = \dfrac{1 \times 8}{5 \times 8} = \dfrac{8}{40}$

$\dfrac{1}{10} = \dfrac{1 \times 4}{10 \times 4} = \dfrac{4}{40}$ (LCD = 40)

$\dfrac{15+8+4}{40} = \dfrac{27}{40}$

(s) $\dfrac{4}{25} = \dfrac{4 \times 12}{25 \times 12} = \dfrac{48}{300}$

$\dfrac{1}{30} = \dfrac{1 \times 10}{30 \times 10} = \dfrac{10}{300}$

$\dfrac{1}{100} = \dfrac{1 \times 3}{100 \times 3} = \dfrac{3}{300}$ (LCD = 300)

$\dfrac{48 - 10 - 3}{300} = \dfrac{35}{300}$

$= \dfrac{7}{60}$

(t) $\dfrac{1}{2} = \dfrac{1 \times 500}{2 \times 500} = \dfrac{500}{1000}$

$\dfrac{1}{50} = \dfrac{1 \times 20}{50 \times 20} = \dfrac{20}{1000}$

$\dfrac{1}{1000} = \dfrac{1}{1000}$ (LCD = 1000)

$\dfrac{500 - 20 - 1}{1000} = \dfrac{479}{1000}$

2.7 Write the following mixed numbers as equivalent improper fractions.

(a) $1\dfrac{1}{2}$ (d) $3\dfrac{2}{5}$ (g) $5\dfrac{7}{12}$ (j) $12\dfrac{3}{4}$

(b) $1\dfrac{2}{3}$ (e) $2\dfrac{1}{8}$ (h) $3\dfrac{1}{16}$ (k) $15\dfrac{3}{8}$

(c) $2\dfrac{1}{4}$ (f) $2\dfrac{3}{10}$ (i) $4\dfrac{7}{25}$ (l) $16\dfrac{3}{10}$

Solution

(a) $1\dfrac{1}{2} = \dfrac{1 \times 2 + 1}{2} = \dfrac{2 + 1}{2} = \dfrac{3}{2}$

(b) $1\dfrac{2}{3} = \dfrac{1 \times 3 + 2}{3} = \dfrac{3 + 2}{3} = \dfrac{5}{3}$

(c) $2\dfrac{1}{4} = \dfrac{2 \times 4 + 1}{4} = \dfrac{8 + 1}{4} = \dfrac{9}{4}$

(d) $3\dfrac{2}{5} = \dfrac{3 \times 5 + 2}{5} = \dfrac{15 + 2}{5} = \dfrac{17}{5}$

(e) $2\dfrac{1}{8} = \dfrac{2 \times 8 + 1}{8} = \dfrac{16 + 1}{8} = \dfrac{17}{8}$

(f) $2\dfrac{3}{10} = \dfrac{2 \times 10 + 3}{10} = \dfrac{20 + 3}{10} = \dfrac{23}{10}$

(g) $5\dfrac{7}{12} = \dfrac{5 \times 12 + 7}{12} = \dfrac{60 + 7}{12} = \dfrac{67}{12}$

(h) $3\dfrac{1}{16} = \dfrac{3 \times 16 + 1}{16} = \dfrac{48 + 1}{16} = \dfrac{49}{16}$

(i) $4\dfrac{7}{25} = \dfrac{4 \times 25 + 7}{25} = \dfrac{100 + 7}{25} = \dfrac{107}{25}$

(j) $12\dfrac{3}{4} = \dfrac{12 \times 4 + 3}{4} = \dfrac{48 + 3}{4} = \dfrac{51}{4}$

(k) $15\dfrac{3}{8} = \dfrac{15 \times 8 + 3}{8} = \dfrac{120 + 3}{8} = \dfrac{123}{8}$

(l) $16\dfrac{3}{10} = \dfrac{16 \times 10 + 3}{10} = \dfrac{160 + 3}{10} = \dfrac{163}{10}$

2.8 Write the following improper fractions as equivalent whole or mixed numbers.

(a) $\dfrac{3}{2}$ (d) $\dfrac{13}{5}$ (g) $\dfrac{85}{10}$ (j) $\dfrac{52}{4}$

(b) $\dfrac{8}{4}$ (e) $\dfrac{7}{1}$ (h) $\dfrac{63}{15}$ (k) $\dfrac{127}{10}$

(c) $\dfrac{5}{3}$ (f) $\dfrac{36}{8}$ (i) $\dfrac{112}{25}$ (l) $\dfrac{200}{12}$

Solution

Perform the division. The whole number part of the answer is the quotient and the fraction part is the remainder over the denominator.

(a) $\begin{array}{r} 1 \\ 2\overline{)3} \\ \underline{2} \\ 1 \end{array}$

$\dfrac{3}{2} = 1\dfrac{1}{2}$

(d) $\begin{array}{r} 2 \\ 5\overline{)13} \\ \underline{10} \\ 3 \end{array}$

$\dfrac{13}{5} = 2\dfrac{3}{5}$

(g) $\begin{array}{r} 8 \\ 10\overline{)85} \\ \underline{80} \\ 5 \end{array}$

$\dfrac{85}{10} = 8\dfrac{5}{10} = 8\dfrac{1}{2}$

(j) $\begin{array}{r} 13 \\ 4\overline{)52} \\ \underline{52} \\ 0 \end{array}$

$\dfrac{52}{4} = 13$

(b) $\begin{array}{r} 2 \\ 4\overline{)8} \\ \underline{8} \\ 0 \end{array}$

$\dfrac{8}{4} = 2$

(e) $\begin{array}{r} 7 \\ 1\overline{)7} \\ \underline{7} \\ 0 \end{array}$

$\dfrac{7}{1} = 7$

(h) $\begin{array}{r} 4 \\ 15\overline{)63} \\ \underline{60} \\ 3 \end{array}$

$\dfrac{63}{15} = 4\dfrac{3}{15} = 4\dfrac{1}{5}$

(k) $\begin{array}{r} 12 \\ 10\overline{)127} \\ \underline{10} \\ 27 \\ \underline{20} \\ 7 \end{array}$

$\dfrac{127}{10} = 12\dfrac{7}{10}$

(c) $\begin{array}{r} 1 \\ 3\overline{)5} \\ \underline{3} \\ 2 \end{array}$

$\dfrac{5}{3} = 1\dfrac{2}{3}$

(f) $\begin{array}{r} 4 \\ 8\overline{)36} \\ \underline{32} \\ 4 \end{array}$

$\dfrac{36}{8} = 4\dfrac{4}{8} = 4\dfrac{1}{2}$

(i) $\begin{array}{r} 4 \\ 25\overline{)112} \\ \underline{100} \\ 12 \end{array}$

$\dfrac{112}{25} = 4\dfrac{12}{25}$

(l) $\begin{array}{r} 16 \\ 12\overline{)200} \\ \underline{12} \\ 80 \\ \underline{72} \\ 8 \end{array}$

$\dfrac{200}{12} = 16\dfrac{8}{12} = 16\dfrac{2}{3}$

2.9   Perform the following multiplications and divisions. Give answers reduced to lowest terms.

(a) $2 \times 1\dfrac{1}{2}$ (d) $1\dfrac{1}{2} \div 3$ (g) $1\dfrac{2}{3} \div 5$ (j) $12\dfrac{1}{2} \div 4$

(b) $\dfrac{1}{2} \times 2\dfrac{1}{2}$ (e) $2\dfrac{1}{2} \div \dfrac{1}{2}$ (h) $8 \div 2\dfrac{2}{3}$ (k) $2\dfrac{2}{5} \div \dfrac{3}{100}$

(c) $1\dfrac{1}{2} \times 1\dfrac{1}{2}$ (f) $\dfrac{1}{3} \times 2\dfrac{1}{4}$ (i) $4\dfrac{1}{2} \times 3\dfrac{1}{3}$ (l) $12\dfrac{1}{2} \div \dfrac{1}{200}$

Solution

(a) $2 \times 1\dfrac{1}{2} = \dfrac{\overset{1}{\cancel{2}}}{1} \times \dfrac{3}{\underset{1}{\cancel{2}}} = \dfrac{1 \times 3}{1 \times 1} = \dfrac{3}{1} = 3$

(b) $\dfrac{1}{2} \times 2\dfrac{1}{2} = \dfrac{1}{2} \times \dfrac{5}{2} = \dfrac{1 \times 5}{2 \times 2} = \dfrac{5}{4} = 1\dfrac{1}{4}$

(c) $1\dfrac{1}{2} \times 1\dfrac{1}{2} = \dfrac{3}{2} \times \dfrac{3}{2} = \dfrac{3 \times 3}{2 \times 2} = \dfrac{9}{4} = 2\dfrac{1}{4}$

(d) $1\dfrac{1}{2} \div 3 = \dfrac{3}{2} \div \dfrac{3}{1} = \dfrac{1}{2} \times \dfrac{1}{\underset{1}{\cancel{3}}} = \dfrac{1 \times 1}{2 \times 1} = \dfrac{1}{2}$

(e) $2\dfrac{1}{2} \div \dfrac{1}{2} = \dfrac{5}{2} \div \dfrac{1}{2} = \dfrac{5}{\underset{1}{\cancel{2}}} \times \dfrac{\overset{1}{\cancel{2}}}{1} = \dfrac{5 \times 1}{1 \times 1} = \dfrac{5}{1} = 5$

(f) $\dfrac{1}{3} \times 2\dfrac{1}{4} = \dfrac{1}{\underset{1}{\cancel{3}}} \times \dfrac{\overset{3}{\cancel{9}}}{4} = \dfrac{1 \times 3}{1 \times 4} = \dfrac{3}{4}$

(g) $\quad 1\frac{2}{3} \div 5 = \frac{5}{3} \div \frac{5}{1} = \frac{\cancel{5}^{1}}{3} \times \frac{1}{\cancel{5}_{1}} = \frac{1 \times 1}{3 \times 1} = \frac{1}{3}$

(h) $\quad 8 \div 2\frac{2}{3} = \frac{8}{1} \div \frac{8}{3} = \frac{\cancel{8}^{1}}{1} \times \frac{3}{\cancel{8}_{1}} = \frac{1 \times 3}{1 \times 1} = \frac{3}{1} = 3$

(i) $\quad 4\frac{1}{2} \times 3\frac{1}{3} = \frac{\cancel{9}^{3}}{2} \times \frac{10}{\cancel{3}_{1}} = \frac{3}{\cancel{2}_{1}} \times \frac{\cancel{10}^{5}}{1} = \frac{3 \times 5}{1 \times 1} = \frac{15}{1} = 15$

(j) $\quad 12\frac{1}{2} \div 4 = \frac{25}{2} \div \frac{4}{1} = \frac{25}{2} \times \frac{1}{4} = \frac{25 \times 1}{2 \times 4} = \frac{25}{8} = 3\frac{1}{8}$

(k) $\quad 2\frac{2}{5} \div \frac{3}{100} = \frac{12}{5} \div \frac{3}{100} = \frac{12}{\cancel{5}_{1}} \times \frac{\cancel{100}^{20}}{3} = \frac{\cancel{12}^{4}}{1} \times \frac{20}{\cancel{3}_{1}} = \frac{4 \times 20}{1 \times 1} = \frac{80}{1} = 80$

(l) $\quad 12\frac{1}{2} \div \frac{1}{200} = \frac{25}{2} \div \frac{1}{200} = \frac{25}{\cancel{2}_{1}} \times \frac{\cancel{200}^{100}}{1} = \frac{25 \times 100}{1 \times 1} = \frac{2500}{1} = 2500$

2.10 Simplify the following complex fractions. Reduce answers to lowest terms.

(a) $\quad \dfrac{2\frac{1}{2}}{2}$ (c) $\quad \dfrac{2\frac{1}{2}}{1\frac{1}{4}}$ (e) $\quad \dfrac{4\frac{1}{2}}{1\frac{1}{2}}$ (g) $\quad \dfrac{\frac{1}{200}}{1\frac{2}{3}}$

(b) $\quad \dfrac{3}{1\frac{1}{2}}$ (d) $\quad \dfrac{300}{1\frac{1}{2}}$ (f) $\quad \dfrac{12\frac{1}{2}}{\frac{1}{4}}$ (h) $\quad \dfrac{3\frac{1}{3}}{\frac{1}{10}}$

Solution

(a) $\quad \dfrac{2\frac{1}{2}}{2} = 2\frac{1}{2} \div 2 = \frac{5}{2} \div \frac{2}{1} = \frac{5}{2} \times \frac{1}{2} = \frac{5 \times 1}{2 \times 2} = \frac{5}{4} = 1\frac{1}{4}$

(b) $\quad \dfrac{3}{1\frac{1}{2}} = 3 \div 1\frac{1}{2} = \frac{3}{1} \div \frac{3}{2} = \frac{\cancel{3}^{1}}{1} \times \frac{2}{\cancel{3}_{1}} = \frac{1 \times 2}{1 \times 1} = \frac{2}{1} = 2$

(c) $\quad \dfrac{2\frac{1}{2}}{1\frac{1}{4}} = 2\frac{1}{2} \div 1\frac{1}{4} = \frac{5}{2} \div \frac{5}{4} = \frac{\cancel{5}^{1}}{2} \times \frac{4}{\cancel{5}_{1}} = \frac{1}{\cancel{2}_{1}} \times \frac{\cancel{4}^{2}}{1} = \frac{1 \times 2}{1 \times 1} = \frac{2}{1} = 2$

(d) $\quad \dfrac{300}{1\frac{1}{2}} = 300 \div 1\frac{1}{2} = \frac{300}{1} \div \frac{3}{2} = \frac{\cancel{300}^{100}}{1} \times \frac{2}{\cancel{3}_{1}} = \frac{100 \times 2}{1 \times 1} = \frac{200}{1} = 200$

(e) $\quad \dfrac{4\frac{1}{2}}{1\frac{1}{2}} = 4\frac{1}{2} \div 1\frac{1}{2} = \frac{9}{2} \div \frac{3}{2} = \frac{9}{\cancel{2}_{1}} \times \frac{\cancel{2}^{1}}{3} = \frac{\cancel{9}^{3}}{1} \times \frac{1}{\cancel{3}_{1}} = \frac{3 \times 1}{1 \times 1} = \frac{3}{1} = 3$

(f) $\dfrac{12\frac{1}{2}}{\frac{1}{4}} = 12\frac{1}{2} \div \frac{1}{4} = \frac{25}{2} \div \frac{1}{4} = \frac{25}{2} \times \frac{\overset{2}{\cancel{4}}}{\underset{1}{\cancel{2}}} \times \frac{1}{1} = \frac{25 \times 2}{1 \times 1} = \frac{50}{1} = 50$

(g) $\dfrac{\frac{1}{200}}{1\frac{2}{3}} = \frac{1}{200} \div 1\frac{2}{3} = \frac{1}{200} \div \frac{5}{3} = \frac{1}{200} \times \frac{3}{5} = \frac{1 \times 3}{200 \times 5} = \frac{3}{1000}$

(h) $\dfrac{3\frac{1}{3}}{\frac{1}{10}} = 3\frac{1}{3} \div \frac{1}{10} = \frac{10}{3} \div \frac{1}{10} = \frac{10}{3} \times \frac{10}{1} = \frac{10 \times 10}{3 \times 1} = \frac{100}{3} = 33\frac{1}{3}$

2.11   Perform the following additions and subtractions.

(a) $4\frac{1}{2} + 5$ (d) $3\frac{1}{3} + 6\frac{2}{3}$ (g) $2\frac{3}{4} + \frac{1}{2}$ (j) $6\frac{2}{5} - 3\frac{1}{2}$

(b) $1\frac{1}{2} + 3\frac{1}{2}$ (e) $2\frac{1}{4} + 2\frac{1}{2}$ (h) $1\frac{1}{2} + 1\frac{2}{3}$ (k) $5\frac{1}{3} + 2\frac{1}{2} + 1\frac{1}{4}$

(c) $8\frac{1}{2} - 4\frac{1}{2}$ (f) $6\frac{1}{2} - \frac{1}{4}$ (i) $7\frac{3}{4} - 2\frac{1}{3}$ (l) $3\frac{1}{8} + 2\frac{1}{3} - 3\frac{1}{6}$

Solution

(a) $\begin{array}{r} 4\frac{1}{2} \\ +5 \\ \hline 9\frac{1}{2} \end{array}$

(d) $\begin{array}{r} 3\frac{1}{3} \\ +6\frac{2}{3} \\ \hline 9\frac{3}{3} = 9 + 1 = 10 \end{array}$

(g) $\begin{array}{r} 2\frac{3}{4} = 2\frac{3}{4} \\ +\frac{1}{2} = +\frac{2}{4} \\ \hline 2\frac{5}{4} = 2 + 1\frac{1}{4} = 3\frac{1}{4} \end{array}$

(b) $\begin{array}{r} 1\frac{1}{2} \\ +3\frac{1}{2} \\ \hline 4\frac{2}{2} = 4 + 1 = 5 \end{array}$

(e) $\begin{array}{r} 2\frac{1}{4} = 2\frac{1}{4} \\ +2\frac{1}{2} = +2\frac{2}{4} \\ \hline 4\frac{3}{4} \end{array}$

(h) $\begin{array}{r} 1\frac{1}{2} = 1\frac{3}{6} \\ +1\frac{2}{3} = +1\frac{4}{6} \\ \hline 2\frac{7}{6} \\ = 2 + 1\frac{1}{6} = 3\frac{1}{6} \end{array}$

(c) $\begin{array}{r} 8\frac{1}{2} \\ -4\frac{1}{2} \\ \hline 4 \end{array}$

(f) $\begin{array}{r} 6\frac{1}{2} = 6\frac{2}{4} \\ -\frac{1}{4} = -\frac{1}{4} \\ \hline 6\frac{1}{4} \end{array}$

(i) $\begin{array}{r} 7\frac{3}{4} = 7\frac{9}{12} \\ -2\frac{1}{3} = -2\frac{4}{12} \\ \hline 5\frac{5}{12} \end{array}$

(j)

$$6\frac{2}{5} = \ 6\frac{4}{10} = \ 5\frac{14}{10}$$
$$\underline{-3\frac{1}{2} = -3\frac{5}{10} = -3\frac{5}{10}}$$
$$2\frac{9}{10}$$

(k)

$$5\frac{1}{3} = \ 5\frac{4}{12}$$
$$+2\frac{1}{2} = +2\frac{6}{12}$$
$$\underline{+1\frac{1}{4} = +1\frac{3}{12}}$$
$$8\frac{13}{12} = 8 + 1\frac{1}{12} = 9\frac{1}{12}$$

(l)

$$3\frac{1}{8} = \ 3\frac{3}{24}$$
$$+2\frac{1}{3} = +2\frac{8}{24}$$
$$\underline{-3\frac{1}{6} = -3\frac{4}{24}}$$
$$2\frac{7}{24}$$

2.12   Insert the correct sign ($<$ or $>$ or $=$) between each pair of numbers to indicate their relationship.

(a) $\dfrac{3}{8}, \dfrac{5}{8}$ (d) $\dfrac{1}{4}, \dfrac{1}{8}$ (g) $\dfrac{7}{12}, \dfrac{2}{3}$ (j) $\dfrac{9}{10}, 1$

(b) $\dfrac{27}{100}, \dfrac{7}{100}$ (e) $\dfrac{2}{5}, \dfrac{8}{20}$ (h) $\dfrac{25}{1000}, \dfrac{1}{40}$ (k) $3\dfrac{2}{3}, \dfrac{10}{3}$

(c) $\dfrac{1}{2}, \dfrac{1}{3}$ (f) $\dfrac{3}{10}, \dfrac{1}{3}$ (i) $\dfrac{3}{100}, \dfrac{3}{1000}$ (l) $6\dfrac{1}{5}, \dfrac{94}{15}$

Solution

(a) Compare numerators: 3<5. Therefore, $\dfrac{3}{8} < \dfrac{5}{8}$.

(b) Compare numerators: 27>7. Therefore, $\dfrac{27}{100} > \dfrac{7}{100}$.

(c) Cross multiply:

$$\frac{1}{2} \ \diagup\!\!\!\!\diagdown \ \frac{1}{3}$$
$$3 > 2$$

Therefore, $\dfrac{1}{2} > \dfrac{1}{3}$.

(d) Cross multiply:

$$\frac{1}{4} \ \diagup\!\!\!\!\diagdown \ \frac{1}{8}$$
$$8 > 4$$

Therefore, $\dfrac{1}{4} > \dfrac{1}{8}$.

(e) Cross multiply:

$$\frac{2}{5} \ \diagup\!\!\!\!\diagdown \ \frac{8}{20}$$
$$40 = 40$$

Therefore, $\dfrac{2}{5} = \dfrac{8}{20}$.

(*f*) Cross multiply:

$$\frac{3}{10} \bowtie \frac{1}{3}$$
$$9 < 10$$

Therefore, $\frac{3}{10} < \frac{1}{3}$.

(*g*) Cross multiply:

$$\frac{7}{12} \bowtie \frac{2}{3}$$
$$21 < 24$$

Therefore, $\frac{7}{12} < \frac{2}{3}$.

(*h*) Cross multiply:

$$\frac{25}{1000} \bowtie \frac{1}{40}$$
$$1000 = 1000$$

Therefore, $\frac{25}{1000} = \frac{1}{40}$.

(*i*) Cross multiply:

$$\frac{3}{100} \bowtie \frac{3}{1000}$$
$$3000 > 300$$

Therefore, $\frac{3}{100} > \frac{3}{1000}$.

(*j*) Write $1 = \frac{10}{10}$; then compare the numerator with the numerator of $\frac{9}{10}$. Since $9 < 10$, $\frac{9}{10} < 1$.

(*k*) Write $\frac{10}{3} = 3\frac{1}{3}$; then compare the fractional parts:

$$\frac{2}{3} > \frac{1}{3}$$

Therefore, $3\frac{2}{3} > \frac{10}{3}$.

(*l*) Write $\frac{94}{15} = 6\frac{4}{15}$ and $6\frac{1}{5} = 6\frac{3}{15}$; then compare the fractional parts:

$$\frac{3}{15} < \frac{4}{15}$$

Therefore, $6\frac{1}{5} < \frac{94}{15}$.

Supplementary Problems

2.13   Reduce the following fractions to lowest terms.

(a) $\dfrac{9}{15}$ (f) $\dfrac{20}{20}$ (k) $\dfrac{5}{200}$ (p) $\dfrac{128}{80}$

(b) $\dfrac{25}{100}$ (g) $\dfrac{4}{64}$ (l) $\dfrac{80}{30}$ (q) $\dfrac{75}{90}$

(c) $\dfrac{24}{18}$ (h) $\dfrac{2000}{100}$ (m) $\dfrac{16}{100}$ (r) $\dfrac{54}{180}$

(d) $\dfrac{36}{9}$ (i) $\dfrac{18}{36}$ (n) $\dfrac{18}{40}$ (s) $\dfrac{48}{180}$

(e) $\dfrac{5}{60}$ (j) $\dfrac{12}{30}$ (o) $\dfrac{75}{250}$ (t) $\dfrac{48}{400}$

2.14   Build up the given fractions to have the indicated denominators.

(a) $\dfrac{2}{3}=\dfrac{?}{15}$ (f) $4=\dfrac{?}{20}$ (k) $\dfrac{1}{9}=\dfrac{?}{180}$ (p) $\dfrac{3}{16}=\dfrac{?}{240}$

(b) $\dfrac{5}{6}=\dfrac{?}{42}$ (g) $\dfrac{1}{2}=\dfrac{?}{50}$ (l) $\dfrac{9}{10}=\dfrac{?}{300}$ (q) $\dfrac{3}{25}=\dfrac{?}{125}$

(c) $\dfrac{1}{8}=\dfrac{?}{40}$ (h) $\dfrac{3}{4}=\dfrac{?}{60}$ (m) $\dfrac{3}{12}=\dfrac{?}{240}$ (r) $\dfrac{1}{36}=\dfrac{?}{540}$

(d) $\dfrac{3}{10}=\dfrac{?}{50}$ (i) $\dfrac{3}{5}=\dfrac{?}{75}$ (n) $\dfrac{5}{8}=\dfrac{?}{360}$ (s) $\dfrac{2}{75}=\dfrac{?}{300}$

(e) $4=\dfrac{?}{1}$ (j) $1=\dfrac{?}{100}$ (o) $\dfrac{7}{15}=\dfrac{?}{180}$ (t) $\dfrac{1}{150}=\dfrac{?}{900}$

2.15   Perform the following multiplications. Give answers reduced to lowest terms.

(a) $\dfrac{1}{2}\times\dfrac{1}{4}$ (f) $\dfrac{36}{10}\times\dfrac{25}{48}$ (k) $\dfrac{1}{300}\times\dfrac{200}{8}$ (p) $\dfrac{56}{100}\times\dfrac{25}{8}\times\dfrac{2}{5}$

(b) $\dfrac{3}{5}\times\dfrac{7}{2}$ (g) $8\times\dfrac{3}{16}$ (l) $\dfrac{480}{12}\times\dfrac{1}{500}$ (q) $25\times\dfrac{3}{5}\times\dfrac{4}{16}$

(c) $\dfrac{1}{3}\times\dfrac{3}{4}$ (h) $\dfrac{7}{8}\times24$ (m) $\dfrac{3000}{1500}\times250$ (r) $64\times\dfrac{1}{200}\times\dfrac{15}{4}$

(d) $\dfrac{2}{5}\times\dfrac{5}{6}$ (i) $\dfrac{3}{4}\times100$ (n) $\dfrac{480}{1600}\times360$ (s) $\dfrac{1}{60}\times\dfrac{3}{500}\times55$

(e) $\dfrac{9}{4}\times\dfrac{10}{12}$ (j) $\dfrac{16}{100}\times\dfrac{75}{32}$ (o) $\dfrac{5}{16}\times\dfrac{8}{10}\times\dfrac{1}{3}$ (t) $\dfrac{1}{150}\times350\times\dfrac{4}{2000}$

2.16 Perform the following divisions. Give answers reduced to lowest terms.

(a) $\dfrac{1}{5} \div \dfrac{1}{2}$ (f) $2 \div \dfrac{1}{4}$ (k) $\dfrac{1}{300} \div \dfrac{1}{450}$ (p) $\dfrac{8}{250} \div 2$

(b) $\dfrac{3}{5} \div \dfrac{4}{5}$ (g) $4 \div \dfrac{8}{3}$ (l) $\dfrac{6}{15} \div \dfrac{1}{300}$ (q) $\dfrac{8}{15} \div 200$

(c) $\dfrac{2}{3} \div \dfrac{1}{6}$ (h) $\dfrac{1}{60} \div 2$ (m) $\dfrac{4}{300} \div \dfrac{7}{200}$ (r) $\dfrac{36}{200} \div \dfrac{5}{100}$

(d) $\dfrac{4}{15} \div \dfrac{7}{30}$ (i) $\dfrac{3}{200} \div 30$ (n) $600 \div \dfrac{3}{2}$ (s) $\dfrac{1}{1000} \div \dfrac{3}{60}$

(e) $\dfrac{25}{8} \div \dfrac{5}{2}$ (j) $\dfrac{8}{200} \div \dfrac{1}{50}$ (o) $480 \div \dfrac{120}{3}$ (t) $\dfrac{7}{2000} \div \dfrac{1}{275}$

2.17 Simplify the following complex fractions. Give answers reduced to lowest terms.

(a) $\dfrac{\frac{1}{5}}{\frac{1}{2}}$ (f) $\dfrac{6}{\frac{1}{3}}$ (k) $\dfrac{\frac{1}{15}}{\frac{1}{45}}$ (p) $\dfrac{\frac{1}{150}}{3}$

(b) $\dfrac{\frac{1}{6}}{\frac{1}{3}}$ (g) $\dfrac{12}{\frac{2}{3}}$ (l) $\dfrac{\frac{1}{250}}{\frac{1}{300}}$ (q) $\dfrac{\frac{4}{20}}{200}$

(c) $\dfrac{\frac{3}{5}}{\frac{2}{3}}$ (h) $\dfrac{\frac{1}{5}}{2}$ (m) $\dfrac{\frac{3}{16}}{\frac{9}{20}}$ (r) $\dfrac{\frac{12}{125}}{\frac{1}{60}}$

(d) $\dfrac{\frac{1}{60}}{\frac{1}{4}}$ (i) $\dfrac{\frac{3}{4}}{3}$ (n) $\dfrac{240}{\frac{1}{2}}$ (s) $\dfrac{\frac{8}{150}}{\frac{24}{300}}$

(e) $\dfrac{\frac{3}{10}}{\frac{1}{10}}$ (j) $\dfrac{\frac{2}{5}}{4}$ (o) $\dfrac{500}{\frac{4}{3}}$ (t) $\dfrac{\frac{18}{500}}{\frac{6}{750}}$

2.18 Perform the following additions and subtractions. Reduce answers to lowest terms.

(a) $\dfrac{1}{5} + \dfrac{3}{5}$ (f) $\dfrac{1}{10} + \dfrac{4}{10} + \dfrac{2}{10}$ (k) $\dfrac{3}{4} + \dfrac{1}{6}$ (p) $\dfrac{3}{50} - \dfrac{1}{60}$

(b) $\dfrac{1}{4} + \dfrac{3}{4}$ (g) $\dfrac{7}{16} - \dfrac{3}{16} + \dfrac{5}{16}$ (l) $\dfrac{9}{10} - \dfrac{1}{4}$ (q) $\dfrac{1}{4} + \dfrac{1}{8} + \dfrac{1}{16}$

(c) $\dfrac{1}{6} + \dfrac{1}{6}$ (h) $\dfrac{1}{3} + \dfrac{1}{4}$ (m) $\dfrac{1}{5} - \dfrac{1}{10}$ (r) $\dfrac{1}{4} + \dfrac{1}{5} + \dfrac{1}{6}$

(d) $\dfrac{7}{8} - \dfrac{3}{8}$ (i) $\dfrac{2}{5} + \dfrac{1}{8}$ (n) $\dfrac{9}{10} + \dfrac{1}{100}$ (s) $\dfrac{5}{12} + \dfrac{1}{8} - \dfrac{1}{16}$

(e) $\dfrac{9}{10} - \dfrac{4}{10}$ (j) $\dfrac{1}{4} + \dfrac{1}{8}$ (o) $\dfrac{1}{15} + \dfrac{1}{12}$ (t) $\dfrac{3}{4} - \dfrac{1}{9} - \dfrac{1}{12}$

2.19 For the following problems, write the mixed numbers as improper fractions and the improper fractions as equivalent mixed or whole numbers. Reduce answers to lowest terms.

(a) $2\frac{1}{2}$ (f) $5\frac{1}{2}$ (k) $\frac{27}{12}$ (p) $15\frac{3}{4}$

(b) $1\frac{1}{4}$ (g) $\frac{12}{8}$ (l) $3\frac{1}{12}$ (q) $\frac{125}{10}$

(c) $\frac{4}{3}$ (h) $2\frac{3}{8}$ (m) $2\frac{7}{16}$ (r) $12\frac{1}{8}$

(d) $\frac{6}{2}$ (i) $3\frac{1}{10}$ (n) $\frac{48}{16}$ (s) $\frac{300}{24}$

(e) $\frac{7}{4}$ (j) $\frac{58}{10}$ (o) $\frac{65}{20}$ (t) $15\frac{6}{10}$

2.20 Perform the following multiplications and divisions. Give answers reduced to lowest terms.

(a) $2 \times 2\frac{1}{2}$ (f) $1\frac{1}{4} \div 5$ (k) $3\frac{1}{8} \div 5$ (p) $1\frac{5}{16} \div \frac{1}{8}$

(b) $\frac{1}{3} \times 1\frac{1}{2}$ (g) $6 \div 1\frac{1}{2}$ (l) $2\frac{1}{4} \times 2\frac{1}{4}$ (q) $2\frac{1}{2} \times \frac{1}{50}$

(c) $1\frac{1}{3} \times 1\frac{1}{2}$ (h) $2\frac{1}{2} \div 2\frac{1}{2}$ (m) $2\frac{1}{4} \div \frac{1}{16}$ (r) $1\frac{1}{2} \times \frac{3}{100}$

(d) $2\frac{1}{2} \div 2$ (i) $1\frac{2}{3} \div 1\frac{1}{3}$ (n) $3\frac{1}{8} \times 3\frac{1}{5}$ (s) $2\frac{1}{2} \div \frac{1}{100}$

(e) $3\frac{1}{2} \div \frac{1}{2}$ (j) $6\frac{1}{4} \times \frac{1}{5}$ (o) $10 \times 3\frac{1}{10}$ (t) $1\frac{2}{3} \div \frac{1}{300}$

2.21 Simplify the following complex fractions. Reduce answers to lowest terms.

(a) $\dfrac{1}{1\frac{1}{2}}$ (d) $\dfrac{8}{2\frac{1}{2}}$ (g) $\dfrac{7\frac{1}{2}}{2\frac{1}{2}}$ (j) $\dfrac{1\frac{1}{5}}{\frac{3}{100}}$

(b) $\dfrac{1\frac{1}{2}}{3}$ (e) $\dfrac{3\frac{1}{2}}{3\frac{1}{2}}$ (h) $\dfrac{\frac{1}{10}}{2\frac{1}{2}}$ (k) $\dfrac{\frac{1}{200}}{2\frac{1}{4}}$

(c) $\dfrac{4}{1\frac{1}{3}}$ (f) $\dfrac{\frac{1}{4}}{1\frac{1}{2}}$ (i) $\dfrac{6\frac{3}{4}}{1\frac{1}{8}}$ (l) $\dfrac{1\frac{1}{4}}{\frac{1}{100}}$

2.22   Perform the following additions and subtractions. Reduce answers to lowest terms.

(a) $2\dfrac{1}{3}+3$ (e) $3\dfrac{1}{3}+5\dfrac{2}{3}$ (i) $8-5\dfrac{7}{10}$ (m) $4\dfrac{2}{3}+1\dfrac{1}{4}$

(b) $2\dfrac{1}{2}+5\dfrac{1}{2}$ (f) $4\dfrac{1}{4}+2\dfrac{3}{4}$ (j) $12\dfrac{9}{10}-5\dfrac{3}{10}$ (n) $7-2\dfrac{1}{4}+1\dfrac{3}{8}$

(c) $7\dfrac{2}{3}-1\dfrac{1}{3}$ (g) $5-2\dfrac{1}{2}$ (k) $1\dfrac{1}{2}+2\dfrac{1}{4}$ (o) $5\dfrac{1}{2}+1\dfrac{3}{10}-2\dfrac{1}{5}$

(d) $4\dfrac{1}{3}+2\dfrac{1}{3}$ (h) $6-3\dfrac{2}{3}$ (l) $8\dfrac{1}{2}-\dfrac{1}{4}$ (p) $2\dfrac{1}{4}+3\dfrac{2}{3}-4\dfrac{3}{8}$

2.23   Insert the correct sign ($<$ or $>$ or $=$) between each pair of numbers to indicate their relationship.

(a) $\dfrac{1}{5},\dfrac{3}{5}$ (e) $\dfrac{2}{3},\dfrac{3}{4}$ (i) $\dfrac{1}{100},\dfrac{1}{50}$ (m) $2\dfrac{3}{8},2\dfrac{1}{4}$

(b) $\dfrac{7}{16},\dfrac{3}{16}$ (f) $\dfrac{5}{8},\dfrac{1}{2}$ (j) $\dfrac{1}{16},\dfrac{24}{400}$ (n) $4\dfrac{2}{3},\dfrac{13}{3}$

(c) $\dfrac{2}{3},\dfrac{1}{2}$ (g) $\dfrac{3}{10},\dfrac{9}{30}$ (k) $\dfrac{99}{100},1$ (o) $\dfrac{37}{10},3\dfrac{1}{2}$

(d) $\dfrac{1}{3},\dfrac{1}{6}$ (h) $\dfrac{1}{3},\dfrac{33}{100}$ (l) $\dfrac{36}{8},4\dfrac{1}{2}$ (p) $\dfrac{81}{16},5\dfrac{3}{16}$

Answers to Supplementary Problems

2.13   (a) $\dfrac{3}{5}$ (e) $\dfrac{1}{12}$ (i) $\dfrac{1}{2}$ (m) $\dfrac{4}{25}$ (q) $\dfrac{5}{6}$

(b) $\dfrac{1}{4}$ (f) 1 (j) $\dfrac{2}{5}$ (n) $\dfrac{9}{20}$ (r) $\dfrac{3}{10}$

(c) $\dfrac{4}{3}$ (g) $\dfrac{1}{16}$ (k) $\dfrac{1}{40}$ (o) $\dfrac{3}{10}$ (s) $\dfrac{4}{15}$

(d) 4 (h) 20 (l) $\dfrac{8}{3}$ (p) $\dfrac{8}{5}$ (t) $\dfrac{3}{25}$

2.14   (a) $\dfrac{10}{15}$ (e) $\dfrac{4}{1}$ (i) $\dfrac{45}{75}$ (m) $\dfrac{60}{240}$ (q) $\dfrac{15}{125}$

(b) $\dfrac{35}{42}$ (f) $\dfrac{80}{20}$ (j) $\dfrac{100}{100}$ (n) $\dfrac{225}{360}$ (r) $\dfrac{15}{540}$

(c) $\dfrac{5}{40}$ (g) $\dfrac{25}{50}$ (k) $\dfrac{20}{180}$ (o) $\dfrac{84}{180}$ (s) $\dfrac{8}{300}$

(d) $\dfrac{15}{50}$ (h) $\dfrac{45}{60}$ (l) $\dfrac{270}{300}$ (p) $\dfrac{45}{240}$ (t) $\dfrac{6}{900}$

2.15   (a) $\dfrac{1}{8}$ (e) $\dfrac{15}{8}$ (i) 75 (m) 500 (q) $\dfrac{15}{4}$

     (b) $\dfrac{21}{10}$ (f) $\dfrac{15}{8}$ (j) $\dfrac{3}{8}$ (n) 108 (r) $\dfrac{6}{5}$

     (c) $\dfrac{1}{4}$ (g) $\dfrac{3}{2}$ (k) $\dfrac{1}{12}$ (o) $\dfrac{1}{12}$ (s) $\dfrac{11}{2000}$

     (d) $\dfrac{1}{3}$ (h) 21 (l) $\dfrac{2}{25}$ (p) $\dfrac{7}{10}$ (t) $\dfrac{7}{1500}$

2.16   (a) $\dfrac{2}{5}$ (e) $\dfrac{5}{4}$ (i) $\dfrac{1}{2000}$ (m) $\dfrac{8}{21}$ (q) $\dfrac{1}{375}$

     (b) $\dfrac{3}{4}$ (f) 8 (j) 2 (n) 400 (r) $\dfrac{18}{5}$

     (c) 4 (g) $\dfrac{3}{2}$ (k) $\dfrac{3}{2}$ (o) 12 (s) $\dfrac{1}{50}$

     (d) $\dfrac{8}{7}$ (h) $\dfrac{1}{120}$ (l) 120 (p) $\dfrac{2}{125}$ (t) $\dfrac{77}{80}$

2.17   (a) $\dfrac{2}{5}$ (e) 3 (i) $\dfrac{1}{4}$ (m) $\dfrac{5}{12}$ (q) $\dfrac{1}{1000}$

     (b) $\dfrac{1}{2}$ (f) 18 (j) $\dfrac{1}{10}$ (n) 480 (r) $\dfrac{144}{25}$

     (c) $\dfrac{9}{10}$ (g) 18 (k) 3 (o) 375 (s) $\dfrac{2}{3}$

     (d) $\dfrac{1}{15}$ (h) $\dfrac{1}{10}$ (l) $\dfrac{6}{5}$ (p) $\dfrac{1}{450}$ (t) $\dfrac{9}{2}$

2.18   (a) $\dfrac{4}{5}$ (e) $\dfrac{1}{2}$ (i) $\dfrac{21}{40}$ (m) $\dfrac{1}{10}$ (q) $\dfrac{7}{16}$

     (b) 1 (f) $\dfrac{7}{10}$ (j) $\dfrac{3}{8}$ (n) $\dfrac{91}{100}$ (r) $\dfrac{37}{60}$

     (c) $\dfrac{1}{3}$ (g) $\dfrac{9}{16}$ (k) $\dfrac{11}{12}$ (o) $\dfrac{3}{20}$ (s) $\dfrac{23}{48}$

     (d) $\dfrac{1}{2}$ (h) $\dfrac{7}{12}$ (l) $\dfrac{13}{20}$ (p) $\dfrac{13}{300}$ (t) $\dfrac{5}{9}$

2.19   (a) $\dfrac{5}{2}$ (e) $1\dfrac{3}{4}$ (i) $\dfrac{31}{10}$ (m) $\dfrac{39}{16}$ (q) $12\dfrac{1}{2}$

     (b) $\dfrac{5}{4}$ (f) $\dfrac{11}{2}$ (j) $5\dfrac{4}{5}$ (n) 3 (r) $\dfrac{97}{8}$

     (c) $1\dfrac{1}{3}$ (g) $1\dfrac{1}{2}$ (k) $2\dfrac{1}{4}$ (o) $3\dfrac{1}{4}$ (s) $12\dfrac{1}{2}$

     (d) 3 (h) $\dfrac{19}{8}$ (l) $\dfrac{37}{12}$ (p) $\dfrac{63}{4}$ (t) $\dfrac{78}{5}$

2.20 (a) 5 (e) 7 (i) $1\frac{1}{4}$ (m) 36 (q) $\frac{1}{20}$

(b) $\frac{1}{2}$ (f) $\frac{1}{4}$ (j) $1\frac{1}{4}$ (n) 10 (r) $\frac{9}{200}$

(c) 2 (g) 4 (k) $\frac{5}{8}$ (o) 31 (s) 250

(d) $1\frac{1}{4}$ (h) 1 (l) $5\frac{1}{16}$ (p) $10\frac{1}{2}$ (t) 500

2.21 (a) $\frac{2}{3}$ (d) $3\frac{1}{5}$ (g) 3 (j) 40

(b) $\frac{1}{2}$ (e) 1 (h) $\frac{1}{25}$ (k) $\frac{1}{450}$

(c) 3 (f) $\frac{1}{6}$ (i) 6 (l) 125

2.22 (a) $5\frac{1}{3}$ (e) 9 (i) $2\frac{3}{10}$ (m) $5\frac{11}{12}$

(b) 8 (f) 7 (j) $7\frac{3}{5}$ (n) $6\frac{1}{8}$

(c) $6\frac{1}{3}$ (g) $2\frac{1}{2}$ (k) $3\frac{3}{4}$ (o) $4\frac{3}{5}$

(d) $6\frac{2}{3}$ (h) $2\frac{1}{3}$ (l) $8\frac{1}{4}$ (p) $1\frac{13}{24}$

2.23 (a) $\frac{1}{5} < \frac{3}{5}$ (e) $\frac{2}{3} < \frac{3}{4}$ (i) $\frac{1}{100} < \frac{1}{50}$ (m) $2\frac{3}{8} > 2\frac{1}{4}$

(b) $\frac{7}{16} > \frac{3}{16}$ (f) $\frac{5}{8} > \frac{1}{2}$ (j) $\frac{1}{16} > \frac{24}{400}$ (n) $4\frac{2}{3} > \frac{13}{3}$

(c) $\frac{2}{3} > \frac{1}{2}$ (g) $\frac{3}{10} = \frac{9}{30}$ (k) $\frac{99}{100} < 1$ (o) $\frac{37}{10} > 3\frac{1}{2}$

(d) $\frac{1}{3} > \frac{1}{6}$ (h) $\frac{1}{3} > \frac{33}{100}$ (l) $\frac{36}{8} = 4\frac{1}{2}$ (p) $\frac{81}{16} < 5\frac{3}{16}$

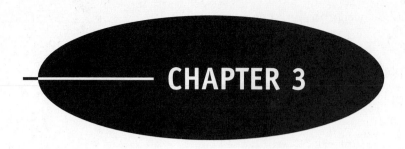

CHAPTER 3

Decimal Numerals

3.1 DECIMAL NOTATION

As was discussed in Chap. 1, a base ten numeral for a whole number tells how many ones, tens, hundreds, and so on, the number contains. For example, 364 = 3 hundreds + 6 tens + 4 ones. Similarly, a *decimal numeral* for a number which has a fractional part tells how many tenths, hundredths, thousandths, and so on, the fractional part contains. For example:

$$6.314 = 6 \text{ ones} + 3 \text{ tenths} + 1 \text{ hundredth} + 4 \text{ thousandths}$$
$$= 6 + \frac{3}{10} + \frac{1}{100} + \frac{4}{1000}$$
$$= 6\frac{314}{1000}$$

The period or dot in a decimal numeral is called a *decimal point*. It serves to separate the whole number part (on the left) from the fractional part (on the right). The digits to the right of the decimal point have *fractional place values*. The first digit to the right of the decimal point has place value *one-tenth*; it tells how many tenths the number has. The second digit to the right has place value *one-hundredth*; it tells how many hundredths the number has. The third digit to the right has place value *one-thousandth*; it tells how many thousandths the number has, and so on. Note that the ending *th* as used here indicates a fractional value. Figure 3-1 gives the general scheme of place values in decimal notation. Compare this with Fig. 1-3.

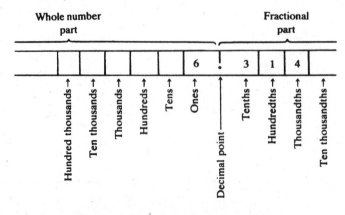

Fig. 3-1 Place values of decimal digits.

Changing Decimal Numerals to Fractional Form.   Compare the decimal form of a number to the fractional form:

$$6.314 = 6\frac{314}{1000}$$

This illustrates the following rule: *To convert a decimal numeral into fractional form, use the digits after the decimal point as the numerator of the fraction; the denominator is the digit 1 followed by as many zeros as there are places after the decimal point.*

EXAMPLE 3.1   Write the following decimal numerals in fractional form. Reduce the fraction to lowest terms. (*a*) 3.4; (*b*) 0.28; (*c*) 5.250.

   Follow the rule stated above.

(*a*) $3.4 = 3\frac{4}{10} = 3\frac{2}{5}$

(*b*) $0.28 = .28 = \frac{28}{100} = \frac{7}{25}$ (When the whole number part is 0 it need not be written in the decimal form, but the 0 is often used to call attention to the decimal point)

(*c*) $5.250 = 5\frac{250}{1000} = 5\frac{1}{4}$

EXAMPLE 3.2   Write the following decimal numerals in fractional form. Reduce the fraction to lowest terms. (*a*) 3.500; (*b*) 3.050; (*c*) 3.005.

(*a*) $3.500 = 3\frac{500}{1000} = 3\frac{1}{2}$

(*b*) $3.050 = 3\frac{50}{1000} = 3\frac{1}{20}$

(*c*) $3.005 = 3\frac{5}{1000} = 3\frac{1}{200}$

Observe that in writing the numerator of the fractional part, the zeros *before* the first nonzero digit are *not* written. Thus, for 3.050 we wrote $3\frac{50}{1000}$, and *not* $3\frac{050}{1000}$.

Reading Decimal Numerals.   When reading or writing a decimal numeral in words, use the word "and" to show the location of the decimal point.

EXAMPLE 3.3   Write the following decimal numerals in fractional form. Then write the number in words. (*a*) 5.13; (*b*) 72.503; (*c*) 18.084.

(*a*) $5.13 = 5\frac{13}{100}$ = five and thirteen hundredths

(*b*) $72.503 = 72\frac{503}{1000}$ = seventy-two and five hundred three thousandths

(*c*) $18.084 = 18\frac{84}{1000}$ = eighteen and eighty-four thousandths

3.2   ROUNDING DECIMAL NUMERALS

   The process of *rounding* a number is one of giving its approximate value to a specified level of accuracy. For example, when we say that $12.18 is approximately equal to $12, we are rounding $12.18 to the nearest whole dollar. On the other hand, when we say that $12.18 is approximately equal to $12.20, we are rounding $12.18 to the nearest dime or tenth of a dollar.

In rounding a decimal numeral, we always specify to which decimal position we are rounding. This is called the *round-off position*. The digits which follow the round-off position are said to be *rounded off*, that is, either discarded or changed to zero. Both cases will be discussed below.

Rounding to a Nearest One or Fraction.   When the round-off position is either the units position or to the right of the decimal point, the procedure for rounding is as follows.

1. Locate the round-off position and note the digit in the next place to the right.
2. If this digit is less than 5, all the digits after the round-off position are dropped.
3. If this digit is 5 or greater, the digit in the round-off place is increased by 1, and all the digits after the round-off position are dropped.

EXAMPLE 3.4   Round the following numbers as indicated.

(*a*) Round 15.4 to the nearest one.
(*b*) Round 2.417 to the nearest tenth.
(*c*) Round 0.374 to the nearest tenth.
(*d*) Round 72.2082 to the nearest hundredth.
(*e*) Round 0.6325 to the nearest thousandth.
(*f*) Round 23.96 to the nearest tenth.
(*g*) Round 29.50 to the nearest one.

Follow the rounding procedure outlined above.

(*a*) Locate the round-off place and note the next digit to the right:

round-off place (ones)

15.4

next digit

Since 4 is less than 5, we drop the 4 to obtain the answer: 15.

(*b*) Locate the round-off place and note the next digit to the right:

round-off place (tenths)

2.417

next digit

Since 1 is less than 5, we drop the 17 to obtain the answer: 2.4.

(*c*) Locate the round-off place and note the next digit to the right:

round-off place (tenths)

0.374

next digit

Since 7 is greater than 5, we raise the digit 3 to 4 and drop the 74 to obtain the answer: 0.4.

(*d*) Locate the round-off place and note the next digit to the right:

round-off place (hundredths)

72.2082

next digit

Since 8 is greater than 5, we raise the digit 0 to 1 and drop the 82 to obtain the answer: 72.21.

(*e*) Locate the round-off place and note the next digit to the right:

round-off place (thousandths)

0.6325

next digit

Since the next digit is 5, we raise the digit 2 to 3 and drop the 5 to obtain the answer: 0.633.

(*f*) Locate the round-off place and note the next digit to the right:

round-off place (tenths)

23.96

next digit

Since 6 is greater than 5, we raise the 9 to 10. Write the 0 and carry the 1 to the 3, which raises it to 4. Drop the 6 to obtain the answer: 24.0.

(*g*) Locate the round-off place and note the next digit to the right:

round-off place (ones)

29.50

next digit

Since the next digit is 5, we raise the 9 to 10. Write the 0 and carry the 1 to the 2, which raises it to 3. Drop the 50 to obtain the answer: 30.

Rounding to a Nearest Ten or Greater.   When the round-off position is the tens position or greater, the procedure is the same except that the digits between the round-off position and the decimal point become 0 instead of being discarded. The digits to the right of the decimal point are discarded as before.

EXAMPLE 3.5   Round the following numbers as indicated.

(*a*) Round 42 to the nearest ten.
(*b*) Round 738 to the nearest hundred.
(*c*) Round 38 to the nearest ten.
(*d*) Round 2651.3 to the nearest hundred.
(*e*) Round 396.82 to the nearest ten.
(*f*) Round 36,495.7 to the nearest thousand.

Follow the procedure for rounding indicated above.

(*a*) Locate the round-off place and note the next digit to the right:

round-off place (tens)

42

next digit

Since 2 is less than 5, the 2 becomes 0 to obtain the answer: 40.

(*b*) Locate the round-off place and note the next digit to the right:

round-off place (hundreds)

738

next digit

Since 3 is less than 5, the 38 becomes 00 to obtain the answer: 700.

(*c*) Locate the round-off place and note the next digit to the right:

round-off place (tens)

38

next digit

Since 8 is greater than 5, we raise the 3 to 4. The 8 becomes 0 to obtain the answer: 40.

(*d*) Locate the round-off place and note the next digit to the right:

round-off place (hundreds)

2651.3

next digit

Since the next digit is 5, we raise the 6 to 7. The 51 becomes 00, and the .3 is dropped to obtain the answer: 2700.

(*e*) Locate the round-off place and note the next digit to the right:

round-off place (tens)

396.82

next digit

Since 6 is greater than 5, we raise the 9 to 10. Write the 0 and carry the 1 to the 3, which raises it to 4. The 6 becomes 0 and the .82 is dropped to obtain the answer: 400.

(*f*) Locate the round-off place and note the next digit to the right:

round-off place (thousands)

36,495.7

next digit

Since 4 is less than 5, we drop the .7 and the 495 becomes 000 to obtain the answer: 36,000.

Understanding the Rounding Procedure.   To understand the concept of rounding, consider Fig. 3-2, which shows a part of a scale, such as the markings on a ruler or the markings on a syringe, marked off in tenths and hundredths. As the figure shows, rounding is used to find the nearest approximate value of a given number. Note that 4.38 is rounded to 4.4 because it is closer to 4.4 than to 4.3, but that 4.32 is rounded to 4.3 because it is closer to 4.3 than to 4.4. A number such as 4.45 which is exactly halfway between is usually rounded *up* to the next higher, which in this case is 4.5.

3.3   ADDITION AND SUBTRACTION OF DECIMALS

Addition and subtraction of decimal numerals are similar to addition and subtraction of whole numbers. That is, when setting up an addition vertically by columns, *align digits with the same place value in the same vertical column*—not only the digits to the left of the decimal point, but also the digits to the right of the point. This means, therefore, that *the decimal points in the numerals must also be aligned*. It is sometimes helpful to add zeros to fill in the columns on the right-hand side of the computation.

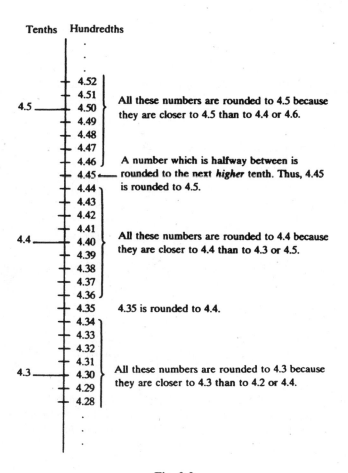

Fig. 3-2

EXAMPLE 3.6   Perform the addition $36.8 + 9.67 + 472 + 0.76$.

Line up the decimal points

36.80 ←— Add as many zeros as necessary to fill in the columns
9.67
472.00 In a whole number, the decimal point comes to the
$+0.76$ right of the last digit
$\overline{519.23}$

‾‾‾ The decimal point in the answer goes under the column of decimal points

After the problem has been set up correctly, addition of the digits is carried out exactly as with the whole numbers.

The procedures given for performing an addition also hold true for subtraction of decimal numerals.

EXAMPLE 3.7   Perform the subtraction $235.4 - 87.92$.

Line up the decimal points

235.40 ←— Fill in with a zero when necessary
-87.92
$\overline{147.48}$

‾‾‾ The decimal point in the answer goes
under the column of decimal points

Subtraction of the digits is carried out exactly as with whole numbers.

3.4 MULTIPLICATION OF DECIMALS

When multiplying decimal numerals, write the problem the same way as when multiplying whole numbers. Then perform the multiplication of the digits *without regard to the decimal points*. Only *after* the multiplication of the digits is performed is the decimal point in the answer located. This is done as follows. *To find the number of places to the right of the decimal point in the answer, add the number of places to the right of the decimal point in each of the factors.*

EXAMPLE 3.8 Perform the multiplication 43.6×0.83.

$$
\begin{array}{r}
43.6 \leftarrow 1 \text{ place to the right of the decimal point} \\
\times 0.83 \leftarrow 2 \text{ places to the right of the decimal point} \\
\hline
1\,308 \\
34\,88 \\
\hline
36.188 \leftarrow 1 + 2 = 3 \text{ places to the right of the decimal point}
\end{array}
$$

Because there is a total of 3 places to the right of the decimal point in the two factors, there are 3 places to the right of the decimal point in the answer.

EXAMPLE 3.9 Perform the multiplication 0.021×0.0053.

$$
\begin{array}{r}
0.021 \leftarrow 3 \text{ places to the right of the decimal point} \\
\times 0.0053 \leftarrow 4 \text{ places to the right of the decimal point} \\
\hline
63 \\
105 \\
\hline
0.0001113 \leftarrow 3 + 4 = 7 \text{ places to the right of the decimal point}
\end{array}
$$

Note that extra zeros must be added *in front* to provide a total of 7 places to the right of the decimal point in the answer.

3.5 DIVISION OF DECIMALS

Dividing by a Whole Number.   To understand the procedure for division of decimals, consider a problem in dividing one whole number by another: $17 \div 8$. Writing the dividend with a decimal point, the division begins as below:

$$
\begin{array}{r}
2. \\
8\overline{)17.} \\
16 \\
\hline
1
\end{array}
$$

The division up to this point is ordinary division of whole numbers; it shows that $\dfrac{17}{8} = 2\dfrac{1}{8}$. The division proceeds past the decimal point as follows: *Whenever the remainder is zero, the division ends. If the remainder is not zero, more zeros may be added to the dividend and the division carried on.* Since the remainder in this problem is not zero, we add a zero to the right of the decimal point in the dividend, bring it down, and carry on the division.

$$
\begin{array}{r}
2.1 \\
8\overline{)17.0} \\
16 \\
\hline
1\,0 \\
8 \\
\hline
2
\end{array}
$$

The remainder is not zero, so add another zero to the dividend, bring it down, and continue the division.

$$
\begin{array}{r}
2.12 \\
8{\overline{)17.00}} \\
16 \\
\hline
1\ 0 \\
8 \\
\hline
20 \\
16 \\
\hline
4
\end{array}
$$

The remainder is still not zero, so we add another zero to the dividend, bring it down, and continue the division.

$$
\begin{array}{r}
2.125 \\
8{\overline{)17.000}} \\
16 \\
\hline
1\ 0 \\
8 \\
\hline
20 \\
16 \\
\hline
40 \\
40 \\
\hline
0
\end{array}
$$

The remainder is now zero, so the division ends. The answer is 2.125. That is, $\dfrac{17}{8} = 2\dfrac{1}{8} = 2.125$.

The above discussion has illustrated the following division procedure for whole number divisors:

1. Set up the division in the same way as with whole numbers.
2. Locate the decimal point of the quotient directly above the decimal point in the dividend.
3. Proceed with the division in the same way as with whole numbers, adding zeros to the dividend whenever the remainder is not zero.

The next example illustrates the procedure in abbreviated form.

EXAMPLE 3.10 Perform the division $147 \div 12$.

1. Set up the division.
$$12{\overline{)147.}}$$

2. Locate the decimal point of the quotient directly above the decimal point in the dividend.
$$12{\overline{)147.}}$$

3. Proceed with the division.
$$
\begin{array}{r}
12. \\
12{\overline{)147.}} \\
12 \\
\hline
27 \\
24 \\
\hline
3
\end{array}
$$

4. The division is now carried beyond the decimal
    point by adding zeros to the dividend and
    bringing them down until the remainder is zero.

$$
\begin{array}{r}
12.25 \\
12\overline{)147.00} \\
\underline{12} \\
27 \\
\underline{24} \\
3\,0 \\
\underline{2\,4} \\
60 \\
\underline{60} \\
0 \\
\end{array}
$$

This division shows that $\dfrac{147}{12} = 12\dfrac{1}{4} = 12.25$.

EXAMPLE 3.11 Perform the division $4 \div 25$.

1. Set up the division.

$$25\overline{)4.}$$

2. Locate the decimal point of the quotient.

$$25\overline{)\overset{.}{4.}}$$

3. We cannot begin this division until we add a zero
    to the dividend, since the divisor is larger than
    the dividend. Perform the division, adding zeros
    when necessary.

$$
\begin{array}{r}
.16 \\
25\overline{)4.00} \\
\underline{2\,5} \\
1\,50 \\
\underline{1\,50} \\
\end{array}
$$

In Examples 3.10 and 3.11, the division stopped when the remainder was zero. This does not always happen. In some divisions, there is a remainder at every step. Therefore, the division will go on indefinitely unless it is terminated in some way. In such cases we cannot find an exact answer, and thus we will find the answer only to some prescribed level of accuracy—for example, to the nearest whole or to the nearest tenth. This is a problem in rounding. The procedure is as follows: *To carry out a division to a prescribed level of accuracy, carry it out to one place beyond the round-off place. Then round the answer.*

EXAMPLE 3.12 Perform the division $2 \div 3$ and find the answer to the nearest hundredth.

1. Set up the division as usual. Since you are to find
    the answer to the nearest hundredth, add enough
    zeros to the right of the decimal point in the
    dividend to carry out the answer to the
    thousandths place, one place beyond the
    hundredths.

$$3\overline{)\overset{.}{2.000}}$$

2. Carry out the division.

$$
\begin{array}{r}
.666 \\
3\overline{)2.000} \\
\underline{1\,8} \\
20 \\
\underline{18} \\
20 \\
\underline{18} \\
2 \\
\end{array}
$$

3. Round the quotient to the nearest hundredth.

$$0.666 \rightarrow 0.67$$

This division shows that $\frac{2}{3} = 0.67$ to the nearest hundredth. Note that this does *not* mean that $\frac{2}{3}$ is exactly equal to 0.67. This is only an approximation.

EXAMPLE 3.13   Perform the division $253.9 \div 62$ and find the answer to the nearest tenth.

1. Set up the division, adding as many zeros as necessary to the right of the decimal point in the dividend to carry the answer to the hundredths place.

$$62\overline{)253.90} \leftarrow \text{one zero added for the hundredths place}$$

2. Perform the division.

$$\begin{array}{r} 4.09 \\ 62\overline{)253.90} \\ \underline{248} \\ 5\ 90 \\ \underline{5\ 58} \\ 32 \end{array}$$

3. Round the quotient to the nearest tenth.

$$4.09 \rightarrow 4.1$$

Dividing by a Decimal Number.   Any division of one decimal number by another can be changed to an equivalent division of a decimal number by a whole number. For example, consider the division $368.45 \div 2.3$, which, in fractional form, is $\frac{368.45}{2.3}$. This fraction can be changed to an equivalent fraction with a whole denominator by building up by the factor 10:

$$\frac{368.45}{2.3} = \frac{368.45 \times 10}{2.3 \times 10} = \frac{3684.5}{23}$$

Thus, *to divide one decimal number by another, change the problem into a division of a decimal by a whole number* by moving the decimal point in the divisor to the right to make it into a whole number, and then moving the decimal point in the dividend an equal number of places to the right:

$$2.3{,}\overline{)368.4{,}5}$$

Moving the decimal points as needed to change the divisor to a whole number is the first step in dividing by a decimal number.

EXAMPLE 3.14   Perform the division $368.45 \div 2.3$ and find the answer to the nearest tenth.

1. Set up the division.

$$2.3\overline{)368.45}$$

2. Move the decimal point in the divisor to the right of the last digit. Then move the decimal point in the dividend the same number of places to the right.

$$2.3{,}\overline{)368.4{,}5}$$

3. Now place the decimal point of the quotient directly over the new decimal point in the dividend.

$$23\overline{)3684.5}$$

4. Now perform the division.

$$\begin{array}{r} 160.19 \\ 23\overline{)3684.50} \\ \underline{23} \\ 138 \\ \underline{138} \\ 04\ 5 \\ \underline{2\ 3} \\ 2\ 20 \\ \underline{2\ 07} \\ 13 \end{array}$$

5. Round the quotient. $160.19 \rightarrow 160.2$ (Nearest tenth)

EXAMPLE 3.15   Perform the division $0.35 \div 0.829$ and find the answer to the nearest thousandth.

1. Set up the division. $0.829\overline{)0.35}$

2. Move the decimal point 3 places to the right. $0.829,\overline{)0.350,}$ Note the extra zero needed to move the decmal point 3 places to the right.

3. Place the decimal point of the quotient directly above the new decimal point in the dividend. $829\overline{)350.}$

4. Add 4 zeros to the dividend to carry the division to the ten-thousandths place. Then perform the division.

$$\begin{array}{r} .4221 \\ 829\overline{)350.0000} \\ \underline{331\ 6} \\ 18\ 40 \\ \underline{16\ 58} \\ 1\ 820 \\ \underline{1\ 658} \\ 1620 \\ \underline{829} \\ 791 \end{array}$$

5. Round the quotient. $.4221 \rightarrow .422$ (Nearest thousandth)

3.6   MULTIPLYING AND DIVIDING BY POWERS OF TEN

There are some especially useful shortcuts for multiplying or dividing by the numbers 10, 100, 1000, etc., in decimal numerals. Suppose, for example, you were to multiply 3.268 by 10, 100, 1000, and 10,000. You would obtain:

$$3.268 \times 10 \quad\ \ = 32.68$$
$$3.268 \times 100 \quad = 326.8$$
$$3.268 \times 1000 \ \ = 3268.$$
$$3.268 \times 10,000 = 32,680.$$

The effect of multiplying 3.268 by these numbers is to move the decimal point only, leaving the digits unchanged. This illustrates the following rule: *To multiply a decimal numeral by a power of ten* (10, 100, 1000, etc.), *move the decimal point to the right as many places as there are zeros in the power of ten.*

EXAMPLE 3.16   Multiply 0.095 by the following: (*a*) 10; (*b*) 100; (*c*) 1000; (*d*) 10,000.
According to the above rule:

(*a*) $0.095 \times 10 = 0.0,95 = 0.95$ (1 place to the right)

(b) $0.095 \times 100 = 0.09\underset{\smile}{,}5 = 9.5$ (2 places to the right)

(c) $0.095 \times 1000 = 0.095\underset{\smile}{,} = 95$ (3 places to the right)

(d) $0.095 \times 10,000 = 0.0950\underset{\smile}{,} = 950$ (4 places to the right; add a zero)

Since division is the inverse of multiplication, there is a corresponding inverse rule for division: *To divide a decimal numeral by a power of ten* (10, 100, 1000, etc.), *move the decimal point to the left as many places as there are zeros in the power of ten.*

EXAMPLE 3.17 Divide 51.7 by the following: (*a*) 10; (*b*) 100; (*c*) 1000; (*d*) 10,000.

According to the above rule:

(a) $\dfrac{51.7}{10} = 5\underset{\smile}{.}1.7 = 5.17$ (1 place to the left)

(b) $\dfrac{51.7}{100} = \underset{\smile}{.}51.7 = .517$ (2 places to the left)

(c) $\dfrac{51.7}{1000} = \underset{\smile}{.}051.7 = .0517$ (3 places to the left; add a zero)

(d) $\dfrac{51.7}{10,000} = \underset{\smile}{.}0051.7 = .00517$ (4 places to the left; add two zeros)

3.7   PROBLEMS INVOLVING DECIMALS AND FRACTIONS

A fraction can be expressed as an equivalent decimal numeral to any given degree of accuracy by performing the indicated division.

EXAMPLE 3.18 Express the fraction $\dfrac{55}{13}$ as a decimal to the nearest thousandth.

1. The indicated division is $13\overline{)55}$. Perform the
    division to the ten-thousandths place.

$$\begin{array}{r} 4.2307 \\ 13\overline{)55.0000} \\ \underline{52} \\ 3\;0 \\ \underline{2\;6} \\ 40 \\ \underline{39} \\ 100 \\ \underline{91} \\ 9 \end{array}$$

2. Round the quotient. $4.2307 \rightarrow 4.231$ (Nearest thousandth)

EXAMPLE 3.19 Express the mixed number $8\dfrac{5}{12}$ as a decimal to the nearest hundredth.

1. We already know that the whole number part is
    8. Thus, we need only calculate the fractional
    part $\dfrac{5}{12}$.

$$\begin{array}{r} .416 \\ 12\overline{)5.000} \\ \underline{4\;8} \\ 20 \\ \underline{12} \\ 80 \\ \underline{72} \\ 8 \end{array}$$

2. Round the quotient. $.416 \rightarrow .42$ (Nearest hundredth)

Thus, the answer is $8\dfrac{5}{12} = 8.42$ to the nearest hundredth.

EXAMPLE 3.20   Calculate $2\dfrac{1}{3} \times 4.75$ as a decimal to the nearest hundredth.

1. Change $2\dfrac{1}{3}$ to an improper fraction. $2\dfrac{1}{3} \times 4.75 = \dfrac{7}{3} \times 4.75$

2. Perform the multiplication. $= \dfrac{7 \times 4.75}{3}$

                                                            $= \dfrac{33.25}{3}$

3. Perform the division.

$$
\begin{array}{r}
11.083 \\
3\overline{)33.250} \\
\underline{3} \\
3 \\
\underline{3} \\
2\,5 \\
\underline{2\,4} \\
10 \\
\underline{9} \\
1
\end{array}
$$

4. Round the quotient. $11.083 \rightarrow 11.08$ (Nearest hundredth)

EXAMPLE 3.21   Express $\dfrac{0.005}{\dfrac{1}{60}}$ as a simple fraction.

1. Invert the divisor and multiply. $\dfrac{0.005}{\dfrac{1}{60}} = 0.005 \times \dfrac{60}{1}$

                                                            $= 0.3$

2. Express the answer as a fraction. $= \dfrac{3}{10}$

EXAMPLE 3.22   Calculate $2.5 \times 0.80 \times \dfrac{1}{300}$ and give the answer as a fraction.

1. Write the decimals as fractions. $2.5 \times 0.80 \times \dfrac{1}{300}$

                                                            $= \dfrac{5}{2} \times \dfrac{8}{10} \times \dfrac{1}{300}$

2. Reduce and multiply. $= \dfrac{\overset{1}{\cancel{5}}}{2} \times \dfrac{\overset{4}{\cancel{8}}}{\underset{2}{\cancel{10}}} \times \dfrac{1}{300}$

                                                            $= \dfrac{1}{1} \times \dfrac{\overset{1}{\cancel{4}}}{2} \times \dfrac{1}{\underset{75}{\cancel{300}}} = \dfrac{1}{150}$

EXAMPLE 3.23   Calculate $\dfrac{1}{2.2} \times \dfrac{1.35}{\dfrac{1}{120}} \times \dfrac{1}{60}$ and express the answer as a decimal to the nearest hundredth.

1.   Invert the $\dfrac{1}{120}$.

$$\dfrac{1}{2.2} \times \dfrac{1.35}{1} \times \dfrac{120}{1} \times \dfrac{1}{60}$$

2.   Reduce and multiply.

$$= \dfrac{1}{2.2} \times \dfrac{1.35}{1} \times \dfrac{\overset{2}{\cancel{120}}}{1} \times \dfrac{1}{\underset{1}{\cancel{60}}}$$

$$= \dfrac{1 \times 1.35 \times 2 \times 1}{2.2 \times 1 \times 1 \times 1}$$

$$= \dfrac{2.70}{2.2}$$

3.   Perform the division.

$$\begin{array}{r} 1.227 \\ 2\,2\,)\overline{2\,7.000} \\ \underline{2\,2} \\ 5\,0 \\ \underline{4\,4} \\ 60 \\ \underline{44} \\ 160 \\ \underline{154} \\ 6 \end{array}$$

4.   Round the quotient.

$1.227 \to 1.23$ (Nearest hundredth)

3.8   COMPARING DECIMAL NUMERALS

When comparing whole numbers, the number with fewer digits is the smaller number. For example, $864 < 2104$ simply because 864 has fewer digits than 2104. To compare numbers with the same number of digits, compare digits in corresponding positions (starting from the left) until we find a pair of digits that are different; the number with the smaller digit is then the smaller number. For example, $8317 < 8342$, since the first two digits (8 and 3) are identical in the two numbers, but the third digits are different ($1 < 4$). That is, both numbers contain 8 thousands and 3 hundreds, but 8317 has only 1 ten while 8342 has 4 tens.

Comparing Decimal Numerals.   To compare decimal numerals, first compare the whole number parts. The number with the smaller whole is the smaller number. If the whole number parts are equal, the fractional parts are compared by comparing digits in corresponding positions—starting with the tenths position, then the hundredths position, and so on. The fractional parts should have the same number of places after the decimal point—add zeros at the end if necessary. For example, 0.32 and 0.3 are compared by changing 0.3 to 0.30.

EXAMPLE 3.24   Compare the numbers 5.048 and 5.029.

1.   Compare the digits starting from the left. They
are the same until we come to the hundredths
position.

5.048
$\updownarrow$
5.029

2.   Since $2 < 4$, it follows that

$5.029 < 5.048$

EXAMPLE 3.25   Compare 52.416 and 52.4.

1. Add zeros to 52.4 so that the numbers contain the
    same number of places to the right of the decimal
    point. Compare the digits, starting from the left.   52.400

                                                               ↑
                                                               ↓

                                                             52.416

2. Since 0 < 1, it follows that   52.400 < 52.416

EXAMPLE 3.26   Compare 0.0012 and 0.00095.

1. Add a zero to 0.0012 so that the numbers contain
    the same number of places to the right of the
    decimal point. Compare the digits, starting from
    the left.   0.00120

                                                               ↑
                                                               ↓

                                                             0.00095

2. Since 0 < 1, it follows that   0.00095 < 0.0012

Comparing Fractions with Decimals.   To compare two numbers in different forms, put them into the same form. For example, when comparing $3\frac{1}{8}$ and 3.2, put both into either fractional form or decimal form.

EXAMPLE 3.27   Compare $3\frac{1}{8}$ with 3.2.

First method. Write both numbers in fractional form.

1. Write 3.2 as an equivalent mixed number. $3.2 = 3\frac{2}{10} = 3\frac{1}{5}$

2. Compare the fractional parts. $\frac{1}{8} < \frac{1}{5}$

3. Therefore: $3\frac{1}{8} < 3\frac{1}{5}$. That is, $3\frac{1}{8} < 3.2$.

Second method. Write both numbers in decimal form.

1. Write $3\frac{1}{8}$ in decimal form.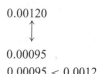

2. Compare the two.   3.200

                                                      ↑
                                                      ↓

                                                    3.125

3. 1 < 2, therefore: $3.125 < 3.200$. That is, $3\frac{1}{8} < 3.2$.

EXAMPLE 3.28 Compare $\frac{1}{3}$ with 0.333.

First method. Write both numbers in fractional form.

1. Write 0.333 as a fraction. $0.333 = \frac{333}{1000}$

2. Compare with $\frac{1}{3}$. $\frac{333}{1000} \bowtie \frac{1}{3}$ (Cross multiply)

                                                              $999 < 1000$

                                                              $\frac{333}{1000} < \frac{1}{3}$

3. Therefore: $0.333 < \frac{1}{3}$

Second method. Write both numbers in decimal form.

1. Write $\frac{1}{3}$ as a decimal. $3)\overline{1.0000}$ .3333

Note that the first three digits in the above division are the same as those in the given decimal 0.333. Since the division does not terminate there, the division was carried out one more place. Now compare the decimals.

2. Write 0.333 as 0.3330 and compare the decimals. $0.3330 < 0.3333$

3. Therefore: $0.333 < \frac{1}{3}$

As Example 3.28 shows, 0.333 is not precisely equal to $\frac{1}{3}$. However, in most practical situations they may be treated as being the same. The error introduced, being equal to $\frac{1}{3000}$, is very small.

Solved Problems

3.1 Write the following decimal numerals as equivalent mixed numbers or fractions, reduced to lowest terms.

(a)	0.1	(f)	0.25	(k)	0.01	(p)	0.550
(b)	0.5	(g)	0.30	(l)	0.06	(q)	0.055
(c)	0.2	(h)	0.33	(m)	0.15	(r)	0.400
(d)	2.7	(i)	3.40	(n)	12.45	(s)	0.004
(e)	95.6	(j)	2.75	(o)	0.333	(t)	16.750

Solution

(a) $0.1 = \frac{1}{10}$ (c) $0.2 = \frac{2}{10} = \frac{1}{5}$

(b) $0.5 = \frac{5}{10} = \frac{1}{2}$ (d) $2.7 = 2\frac{7}{10}$

(e) $95.6 = 95\dfrac{6}{10} = 95\dfrac{3}{5}$ (m) $0.15 = \dfrac{15}{100} = \dfrac{3}{20}$

(f) $0.25 = \dfrac{25}{100} = \dfrac{1}{4}$ (n) $12.45 = 12\dfrac{45}{100} = 12\dfrac{9}{20}$

(g) $0.30 = \dfrac{30}{100} = \dfrac{3}{10}$ (o) $0.333 = \dfrac{333}{1000}$

(h) $0.33 = \dfrac{33}{100}$ (p) $0.550 = \dfrac{550}{1000} = \dfrac{11}{20}$

(i) $3.40 = 3\dfrac{40}{100} = 3\dfrac{2}{5}$ (q) $0.055 = \dfrac{55}{1000} = \dfrac{11}{200}$

(j) $2.75 = 2\dfrac{75}{100} = 2\dfrac{3}{4}$ (r) $0.400 = \dfrac{400}{1000} = \dfrac{2}{5}$

(k) $0.01 = \dfrac{1}{100}$ (s) $0.004 = \dfrac{4}{1000} = \dfrac{1}{250}$

(l) $0.06 = \dfrac{6}{100} = \dfrac{3}{50}$ (t) $16.750 = 16\dfrac{750}{1000} = 16\dfrac{3}{4}$

3.2   Round the following numbers to the indicated degree of accuracy.

(a) 0.32 (nearest tenth)   (k) 0.998 (nearest hundredth)
(b) 5.046 (nearest tenth)   (l) 5.6123 (nearest thousandth)
(c) 0.27 (nearest tenth)   (m) 0.47181 (nearest thousandth)
(d) 8.251 (nearest tenth)   (n) 0.4995 (nearest thousandth)
(e) 4.96 (nearest tenth)   (o) 6.1 (nearest one)
(f) 9.95 (nearest tenth)   (p) 3.67 (nearest one)
(g) 0.043 (nearest hundredth)   (q) 0.95 (nearest one)
(h) 0.117 (nearest hundredth)   (r) 6.52 (nearest one)
(i) 7.5653 (nearest hundredth) (s) 18 (nearest ten)
(j) 8.396 (nearest hundredth)   (t) 237 (nearest ten)

Solution

(a) $0.32 \rightarrow 0.3$ (Discard the 2. Do nothing else since the discarded digit 2 is less than 5.)
(b) $5.046 \rightarrow 5.0$ (Discard the 46. Do nothing else since the first discarded digit 4 is less than 5.)
(c) $0.27 \rightarrow 0.3$ (Discard the 7 and raise the .2 to .3 since the first discarded digit 7 is greater than 5.)
(d) $8.251 \rightarrow 8.3$ (Discard the 51 and raise the 8.2 to 8.3 since the first discarded digit is equal to 5.)
(e) $4.96 \rightarrow 5.0$ (Discard the 6 and raise the 4.9 to 5.0 since the first discarded digit 6 is greater than 5.)
(f) $9.95 \rightarrow 10.0$ (Discard the 5 and raise the 9.9 to 10.0 since the discarded digit is equal to 5.)
(g) $0.043 \rightarrow 0.04$ (Discard the 3. Do nothing else since the discarded digit 3 is less than 5.)
(h) $0.117 \rightarrow 0.12$ (Discard the 7 and raise the 0.11 to 0.12 since the discarded digit 7 is greater than 5.)
(i) $7.5653 \rightarrow 7.57$ (Discard the 53 and raise 7.56 to 7.57 since the first discarded digit is equal to 5.)
(j) $8.396 \rightarrow 8.40$ (Discard the 6 and raise 8.39 to 8.40 since the discarded digit 6 is greater than 5.)
(k) $0.998 \rightarrow 1.00$ (Discard the 8 and raise 0.99 to 1.00 since the discarded digit 8 is greater than 5.)
(l) $5.6123 \rightarrow 5.162$ (Discard the 3. Do nothing else since the discarded digit 3 is less than 5.)
(m) $0.47181 \rightarrow 0.472$ (Discard the 81 and raise 0.471 to 0.472 since the first discarded digit 8 is greater than 5.)

(n) 0.4995 → 0.500 (Discard the 5 and raise 0.499 to 0.500 since the discarded digit is equal to 5.)

(o) 6.1 → 6 (Discard the .1. Do nothing else since the discarded digit 1 is less than 5.)

(p) 3.67 → 4 (Discard the .67 and raise the 3 to 4 since the first discarded digit 6 is greater than 5.)

(q) 0.95 → 1 (Discard the .95 and raise the 0 to 1 since the first discarded digit 9 is greater than 5.)

(r) 6.52 → 7 (Discard the .52 and raise the 6 to 7 since the first discarded digit is equal to 5.)

(s) 18 → 20 (*Change* the 8 to 0. Do *not* discard it. Raise the 1 to 2 since the digit 8 is greater than 5.)

(t) 237 → 240 (*Change* the 7 to 0. Do *not* discard it. Raise the 3 to 4 since 7 is greater than 5.)

3.3   Perform the following additions and subtractions.

(a) 6.3 + 4.9   (k) 6.89 − 3.47

(b) 5.7 + 9.3 + 2.1   (l) 7.2 − 4.8

(c) 3.67 + 4.20   (m) 9.12 − 6.77

(d) 8.9 + 5.07   (n) 48 − 12.6

(e) 8.15 + 7.34 + 9.05   (o) 301 − 162.84

(f) 13.9 + 6.11 + 0.8   (p) 46.7 + 19.8 − 36.4

(g) 13.7 + 24 + 1.23   (q) 31.6 − 12.3 + 6.5

(h) 45.92 + 136 + 8.1   (r) 93.65 + 17.8 − 73.46

(i) 0.512 + 61.7 + 18   (s) 127.6 − 93.4 + 13.78

(j) 5.8 − 2.6   (t) 317 − 138.99 + 58.7

Solution

(a)   6.3   (f)   13.90   (k)   6.89   (p)   46.7
      +4.9   6.11   −3.47   +19.8
      11.2   +0.80   3.42   66.5
                       20.81   −36.4
                                                          30.1

(b)   5.7   (g)   13.70   (l)   7.2   (q)   31.6
       9.3   24.00   −4.8   −12.3
      +2.1   +1.23   2.4   19.3
      17.1   38.93   +6.5
                                                          25.8

(c)   3.67   (h)   45.92   (m)   9.12   (r)   93.65
      +4.20   136.00   −6.77   +17.80
       7.87   +8.10   2.35   111.45
                      190.02   −73.46
                                                          37.99

(d)   8.90   (i)   0.512   (n)   48.0   (s)   127.6
      +5.07   61.700   −12.6   −93.4
      13.97   +18.000   35.4   34.20
                      80.212   +13.78
                                                          47.98

(e)   8.15   (j)   5.8   (o)   301.00   (t)   317.00
       7.34   −2.6   −162.84   −138.99
      +9.05   3.2   138.16   178.01
      24.54   +58.70
                                                          236.71

3.4   Perform the following multiplications.

(a)	3.4×2	(f)	2.25×72	(k)	327×0.034	(p)	34.26×15.03
(b)	5.63×3	(g)	0.63×2.6	(l)	0.21×0.89	(q)	24×0.0037
(c)	4.7×9.2	(h)	31.7×4.81	(m)	3.87×1.56	(r)	14×0.0005
(d)	0.8×8.6	(i)	30.5×28.9	(n)	3400×0.075	(s)	0.0027×3.7
(e)	64×0.75	(j)	37.2×0.06	(o)	8.03×3.02	(t)	0.26×0.0038

Solution

(a) 3.4
     ×2
     6.8

(f)   2.25
      ×72
      4 50
      157 5
      162.00

(k)   327
      ×0.034
      1 308
      9 81
      11.118

(p)   34.26
      ×15.03
      1 0278
      171 300
      342 6
      514.9278

(b) 5.63
     ×3
     16.89

(g)   0.63
      ×2.6
      378
      1 26
      1.638

(l)   0.89
      ×0.21
      89
      178
      .1869

(q)   0.0037
      ×24
      148
      74
      .0888

(c) 4.7
     ×9.2
     94
     42 3
     43.24

(h)   31.7
      × 4.81
      317
      25 36
      126 8
      152.477

(m)   3.87
      ×1.56
      2322
      1 935
      3 87
      6.0372

(r)   14
      ×0.0005
      .0070

(d) 8.6
     ×0.8
     6.88

(i)   28.9
      ×30.5
      14 45
      867 0
      881.45

(n)   3400
      ×0.075
      17 000
      238 00
      255.000

(s)   0.0027
      ×3.7
      189
      81
      .00999

(e) 0.75
     ×64
     3 00
     45 0
     48.00

(j)   37.2
      ×0.06
      2.232

(o)   8.03
      ×3.02
      1606
      24 090
      24.2506

(t)   0.0038
      ×0.26
      228
      76
      .000988

3.5   Perform the following divisions to the indicated degree of accuracy.

(a)	$48 \div 5$ (exactly)	(k)	$0.06 \div 30$ (exactly)
(b)	$37 \div 3$ (nearest tenth)	(l)	$3.6 \div 1.8$ (exactly)
(c)	$64 \div 7$ (nearest hundredth)	(m)	$2.7 \div 5.4$ (exactly)
(d)	$745 \div 9$ (nearest tenth)	(n)	$1.25 \div 3.4$ (nearest tenth)
(e)	$7 \div 20$ (exactly)	(o)	$0.4 \div 1.25$ (nearest tenth)
(f)	$1 \div 30$ (nearest hundredth)	(p)	$78 \div 2.2$ (nearest tenth)
(g)	$2 \div 30$ (nearest hundredth)	(q)	$0.6 \div 0.25$ (exactly)
(h)	$5 \div 16$ (exactly)	(r)	$10 \div 0.35$ (nearest hundredth)
(i)	$9.25 \div 12$ (nearest tenth)	(s)	$4.2 \div 0.033$ (nearest unit)
(j)	$4.8 \div 200$ (exactly)	(t)	$25 \div 0.024$ (nearest unit)

Solution

(a)
```
      9.6
  5)48.0
    45
     3 0
     3 0
```

(g)
```
          .066 → .07
    30)2.000
       1 80
        200
        180
```

(m)
```
            .5
   5 4,)2 7,0
         2 7 0
```

(b)
```
      12.33 → 12.3
  3)37.00
    3
    7
    6
    1 0
     9
     10
      9
```

(h)
```
        .3125
   16)5.0000
      4 8
       20
       16
       40
       32
       80
       80
```

(n)
```
         .36 → 0.4
   3 4,)1 2,50
          1 0 2
           230
           204
```

(c)
```
      9.142 → 9.14
  7)64.000
    63
    1 0
     7
     30
     28
     20
     14
```

(i)
```
        .77 → 0.8
   12)9.25
      8 4
       85
       84
        1
```

(o)
```
            .32 → 0.3
   1 25,)0 40,00
           37 5
           2 50
           2 50
```

(d)
```
      82.77 → 82.8
  9)745.00
    72
    25
    18
     7 0
     6 3
      70
      63
```

(j)
```
          .024
   200)4.800
       4 00
        800
        800
```

(p)
```
        3 5.45 → 35.5
   2 2,)78 0,00
          66
          12 0
          11 0
           1 0 0
             8 8
             1 20
             1 10
```

(e)
```
        .35
   20)7.00
      6 0
      1 00
      1 00
```

(k)
```
         .002
   30)0.060
       60
```

(q)
```
           2.4
   0 25,)0 60,0
            50
            100
            10 0
```

(f)
```
        .033 → .03
   30)1.000
       90
       100
        90
        10
```

(l)
```
        2.
   1 8,)3 6,
         3 6
```

(r)
```
        2 8.571 → 28.57
   0 35,)10 00,000
           7 0
           3 00
           2 8 0
            2 00
            1 7 5
             2 50
             2 45
              50
              35
```

$$(s) \quad \begin{array}{r} 127.2 \rightarrow 127 \\ 033\,)\overline{4\,200.0} \\ \underline{3\,3} \\ 90 \\ \underline{66} \\ 240 \\ \underline{231} \\ 9\,0 \\ \underline{6\,6} \end{array}$$

$$(t) \quad \begin{array}{r} 1\,041.6 \rightarrow 1042 \\ 024\,)\overline{25\,000.0} \\ \underline{24} \\ 1\,00 \\ \underline{96} \\ 40 \\ \underline{24} \\ 16\,0 \\ \underline{14\,4} \end{array}$$

3.6 Express the following fractions and mixed numbers as equivalent decimals to the indicated degree of accuracy.

(a) $\frac{1}{4}$ (exactly)

(g) $\frac{1}{6}$ (nearest hundredth)

(b) $\frac{1}{3}$ (nearest hundredth)

(h) $5\frac{1}{12}$ (nearest hundredth)

(c) $\frac{2}{3}$ (nearest hundredth)

(i) $\frac{1}{200}$ (exactly)

(d) $2\frac{3}{5}$ (exactly)

(j) $\frac{1}{30}$ (nearest hundredth)

(e) $3\frac{3}{4}$ (exactly)

(k) $\frac{1}{60}$ (nearest hundredth)

(f) $\frac{3}{8}$ (exactly)

(l) $4\frac{7}{16}$ (exactly)

Solution

(a) $\frac{1}{4} = 4)\overline{1.00}^{.25}$

(g) $\frac{1}{6} = 6)\overline{1.000}^{.166 \rightarrow 0.17}$

(b) $\frac{1}{3} = 3)\overline{1.000}^{.333 \rightarrow 0.33}$

(h) $5\frac{1}{12} = \frac{61}{12} = 12)\overline{61.000}^{5.083 \rightarrow 5.08}$

(c) $\frac{2}{3} = 3)\overline{2.000}^{.666 \rightarrow 0.67}$

(i) $\frac{1}{200} = 200)\overline{1.000}^{.005}$

(d) $2\frac{3}{5} = \frac{13}{5} = 5)\overline{13.0}^{2.6}$

(j) $\frac{1}{30} = 30)\overline{1.000}^{.033 \rightarrow 0.03}$

(e) $3\frac{3}{4} = \frac{15}{4} = 4)\overline{15.00}^{3.75}$

(k) $\frac{1}{60} = 60)\overline{1.000}^{.016 \rightarrow 0.02}$

(f) $\frac{3}{8} = 8)\overline{3.000}^{.375}$

(l) $4\frac{7}{16} = \frac{71}{16} = 16)\overline{71.0000}^{4.4375}$

3.7 Perform the following operations.

(a) 4.9×10 (e) $.0017 \times 100$ (i) $33.1 \div 100$

(b) 0.8×10 (f) 3.3×1000 (j) $1.2 \div 100$

(c) $.056 \times 10$ (g) $4.2 \div 10$ (k) $986.2 \div 1000$

(d) 7.6×100 (h) $.05 \div 10$ (l) $6.7 \div 1000$

Solution

(a) $4.9 \times 10 = 4\,9. = 49$

(b) $0.8 \times 10 = 0\,8. = 8$

(c) $.056 \times 10 = 0.56 = 0.56$

(d) $7.6 \times 100 = 7\,60. = 760$

(e) $.0017 \times 100 = 00.17 = 0.17$

(f) $3.3 \times 1000 = 3\,300. = 3300$

(g) $4.2 \div 10 = .4\,2 = 0.42$

(h) $.05 \div 10 = .0\,05 = 0.005$

(i) $33.1 \div 100 = .33\,1 = 0.331$

(j) $1.2 \div 100 = .01\,2 = 0.012$

(k) $986.2 \div 1000 = .986\,2 = 0.9862$

(l) $6.7 \div 1000 = .006\,7 = 0.0067$

3.8 Perform the following calculations and write the answer as indicated.

(a) $\frac{1}{2} \times 7.5$ (decimal, exactly)

(b) $\frac{3}{4} \times 15.5$ (decimal, nearest tenth)

(c) $1\frac{1}{2} \times 4.8$ (decimal, exactly)

(d) $2\frac{1}{2} \times 3.75$ (decimal, nearest hundredth)

(e) $0.2 \times \frac{1}{60}$ (simple fraction)

(f) $\frac{1}{500} \times 2.5$ (simple fraction)

(g) $6.25 \times \frac{1}{250}$ (simple fraction)

(h) $0.125 \times \frac{1}{60}$ (decimal, nearest thousandth)

(i) $\dfrac{2.5}{\frac{1}{3}}$ (decimal, exactly)

(j) $\dfrac{0.4}{\frac{1}{4}}$ (decimal, exactly)

(k) $\dfrac{2.5}{\frac{1}{60}}$ (decimal, exactly)

(l) $\dfrac{1.5}{\frac{1}{200}}$ (decimal, exactly)

(m) $\dfrac{4.5}{1\frac{1}{2}}$ (decimal, exactly)

(n) $0.1 \times 5 \times \dfrac{1}{25}$ (decimal, exactly)

(o) $0.25 \times 1000 \times \dfrac{1}{500}$ (simple fraction)

(p) $45 \times 0.25 \times \dfrac{1}{150}$ (decimal, nearest hundredth)

(q) $0.2 \times \dfrac{1}{1000} \times \dfrac{1}{0.008}$ (simple fraction)

(r) $2\frac{1}{2} \times 0.75 \times \dfrac{4}{\frac{1}{150}}$ (whole number)

(s) $24 \times \dfrac{15}{4} \times \dfrac{1}{\frac{1}{60}}$ (whole number)

(t) $75 \times \dfrac{1}{2.2} \times \dfrac{1}{24} \times 60$ (decimal, nearest whole)

Solution

(a) $\dfrac{1}{2} \times 7.5 = \dfrac{7.5}{2} = 2\overline{)7.50}^{\,3.75}$

(b) $\dfrac{3}{4} \times 15.5 = .75 \times 15.5 = 11.625 \to 11.6$

(c) $1\dfrac{1}{2} \times 4.8 = 1.5 \times 4.8 = 7.2$

(d) $2\dfrac{1}{2} \times 3.75 = 2.5 \times 3.75 = 9.375 \to 9.38$

(e) $0.2 \times \dfrac{1}{60} = \dfrac{\overset{1}{\cancel{2}}}{\underset{5}{\cancel{10}}} \times \dfrac{1}{60} = \dfrac{1}{300}$

(f) $\dfrac{1}{500} \times 2.5 = \dfrac{1}{500} \times 2\dfrac{1}{2} = \dfrac{1}{\underset{100}{\cancel{500}}} \times \dfrac{\overset{1}{\cancel{5}}}{2} = \dfrac{1}{200}$

(g) $6.25 \times \dfrac{1}{250} = 6\dfrac{1}{4} \times \dfrac{1}{250} = \dfrac{\overset{1}{\cancel{25}}}{4} \times \dfrac{1}{\underset{10}{\cancel{250}}} = \dfrac{1}{40}$

(h) $0.125 \times \dfrac{1}{60} = \dfrac{0.125}{60} = 60\overline{)0.1250}^{\,.0020} \to 0.002$

(i) $\dfrac{2.5}{\frac{1}{3}} = 2.5 \times \dfrac{3}{1} = 7.5$

(j) $\dfrac{0.4}{\dfrac{1}{4}} = 0.4 \times \dfrac{4}{1} = 1.6$

(k) $\dfrac{2.5}{\dfrac{1}{60}} = 2.5 \times \dfrac{60}{1} = 150$

(l) $\dfrac{1.5}{\dfrac{1}{200}} = 1.5 \times \dfrac{200}{1} = 300$

(m) $\dfrac{4.5}{1\frac{1}{2}} = \dfrac{4.5}{1.5} = 1.5,\ 1.5\overline{)4.5}$

(n) $0.1 \times \overset{1}{5} \times \dfrac{1}{\underset{5}{25}} = \dfrac{0.1}{5} = \dfrac{.02}{5\overline{)0.10}}$

(o) $0.25 \times 1000 \times \dfrac{1}{500} = \dfrac{1}{4} \times \overset{2}{1000} \times \dfrac{1}{\underset{1}{500}} = \dfrac{\overset{1}{2}}{\underset{2}{4}} = \dfrac{1}{2}$

(p) $45 \times 0.25 \times \dfrac{1}{150} = \overset{3}{45} \times 0.25 \times \dfrac{1}{\underset{10}{150}} = \dfrac{0.75}{10} = \dfrac{.075}{10\overline{)0.750}} \to 0.08$

(q) $0.2 \times \dfrac{1}{1000} \times \dfrac{1}{0.008} = \dfrac{0.2}{1000 \times 0.008} = \dfrac{0.2}{8} = \dfrac{\overset{1}{2}}{10} \times \dfrac{1}{\underset{4}{8}} = \dfrac{1}{40}$

(r) $2\frac{1}{2} \times 0.75 \times \dfrac{4}{\dfrac{1}{150}} = \dfrac{5}{2} \times \dfrac{3}{\underset{1}{4}} \times \overset{1}{4} \times \dfrac{150}{1} = \dfrac{5 \times 3 \times \overset{75}{150}}{\underset{1}{2}} = 1125$

(s) $24 \times \dfrac{15}{4} \times \dfrac{1}{\dfrac{1}{60}} = 24 \times \dfrac{15}{\underset{1}{4}} \times \dfrac{\overset{15}{60}}{1} = 5400$

(t) $75 \times \dfrac{1}{2.2} \times \dfrac{1}{24} \times 60 = \dfrac{75 \times \overset{5}{60}}{2.2 \times \underset{2}{24}} = \dfrac{375}{4.4} = 4.4\overline{)375.0,0}\ \ \dfrac{8\ 5.2}{} \to 85$

3.9 Insert the proper symbol ($<$ or $>$ or $=$) between each pair of numbers to indicate their relationship.

(a) 0.56 and 0.50

(b) 2.394 and 2.40

(c) 0.0095 and 0.1

(d) 0.014 and 0.0087

(e) 8.005 and 8.0049

(f) 0.05 and 0.050

(g) 5.03 and 5.30

(h) 0.099 and 0.1

(i) 0.6 and $\dfrac{7}{10}$

(j) 0.75 and $\dfrac{3}{4}$

(k) $\dfrac{1}{3}$ and 0.33

(l) 1.65 and $\dfrac{33}{20}$

(m) 0.66 and $\dfrac{2}{3}$

(n) 0.67 and $\dfrac{2}{3}$

(o) $\dfrac{1}{16}$ and 0.0625

Solution

$$
\begin{array}{c} 0.56 \\ \uparrow \\ 0.50 \end{array}
$$

(a) Compare $\quad\updownarrow\quad$ $0 < 6$; therefore, $0.50 < 0.56$.

(b) Compare $\quad\updownarrow\quad$ $3 < 4$; therefore, $2.394 < 2.4$.

$$
\begin{array}{c} 2.394 \\ \uparrow \\ 2.400 \end{array}
$$

(c) Compare $\quad\updownarrow\quad$ $0 < 1$; therefore, $0.0095 < 0.1$.

$$
\begin{array}{c} 0.0095 \\ \uparrow \\ 0.1000 \end{array}
$$

(d) Compare $\quad\updownarrow\quad$ $0 < 1$; therefore $0.0087 < 0.014$.

$$
\begin{array}{c} 0.0140 \\ \uparrow \\ 0.0087 \end{array}
$$

(e) Compare $\quad\updownarrow\quad$ $4 < 5$; therefore, $8.0049 < 8.005$.

$$
\begin{array}{c} 8.0050 \\ \uparrow \\ 8.0049 \end{array}
$$

(f) Compare 0.050 and 0.050. They are equal: $0.050 = 0.05$.

(g) Compare $\quad\updownarrow\quad$ $0 < 3$; therefore, $5.03 < 5.30$.

$$
\begin{array}{c} 5.03 \\ \uparrow \\ 5.30 \end{array}
$$

(h) Compare $\quad\updownarrow\quad$ $0 < 1$; therefore, $0.099 < 0.1$.

$$
\begin{array}{c} 0.099 \\ \uparrow \\ 0.100 \end{array}
$$

(i) $0.6 = \dfrac{6}{10} < \dfrac{7}{10}$.

(j) $.75 = \dfrac{75}{100} = \dfrac{3}{4}$.

(k) $0.33 = \dfrac{33}{100} \bowtie \dfrac{1}{3}$ (Cross multiply and compare)

  $99 < 100$

  Therefore, $0.33 < \dfrac{1}{3}$.

(l) $1.65 = 1\dfrac{65}{100} = 1\dfrac{13}{20} = \dfrac{33}{20}$.

(m) $0.66 = \dfrac{66}{100} = \dfrac{33}{50} \bowtie \dfrac{2}{3}$ (Cross multiply and compare)

  $99 < 100$

  Therefore, $0.66 < \dfrac{2}{3}$.

(n) $0.67 = \dfrac{67}{100} \bowtie \dfrac{2}{3}$ (Cross multiply and compare)

  $201 > 200$

  Therefore, $0.67 > \dfrac{2}{3}$.

(o) $0.0625 = \dfrac{625}{10,000} = \dfrac{1}{16}$.

Supplementary Problems

3.10 Write the following decimal numerals as equivalent mixed numbers or fractions, reduced to lowest terms.

(a)	0.3	(f)	0.75	(k)	0.03	(p)	0.450
(b)	0.8	(g)	0.60	(l)	0.04	(q)	0.045
(c)	0.4	(h)	0.67	(m)	0.35	(r)	0.600
(d)	3.1	(i)	4.60	(n)	15.65	(s)	0.006
(e)	15.2	(j)	5.25	(o)	0.667	(t)	20.250

3.11 Round the following numbers to the indicated degree of accuracy.

(a)	0.61 (nearest tenth)	(k)	9.995 (nearest hundredth)
(b)	6.139 (nearest tenth)	(l)	5.2052 (nearest thousandth)
(c)	1.38 (nearest tenth)	(m)	8.00692 (nearest thousandth)
(d)	0.050 (nearest tenth)	(n)	0.6998 (nearest thousandth)
(e)	8.97 (nearest tenth)	(o)	11.2 (nearest one)
(f)	9.98 (nearest tenth)	(p)	0.82 (nearest one)
(g)	1.152 (nearest hundredth)	(q)	8.92 (nearest one)
(h)	0.125 (nearest hundredth)	(r)	2.5 (nearest one)
(i)	0.05052 (nearest hundredth)	(s)	25.1 (nearest ten)
(j)	16.795 (nearest hundredth)	(t)	156 (nearest ten)

3.12 Perform the following additions and subtractions.

(a)	$5.7 + 7.6$	(k)	$8.46 - 5.98$
(b)	$4.8 + 0.9 + 6.6$	(l)	$6.2 - 5.07$
(c)	$2.83 + 6.58$	(m)	$13.15 - 8.974$
(d)	$4.58 + 7.23 + 6.99$	(n)	$56 - 18.24$
(e)	$14.6 + 8.19$	(o)	$523 - 97.61$
(f)	$0.67 + 9.8 + 21.6$	(p)	$5.8 + 37.4 - 18.7$
(g)	$8.94 + 16 + 12.6$	(q)	$19.4 - 16.8 + 0.42$
(h)	$12.08 + 207 + 0.87$	(r)	$42.8 + 13.9 - 41.73$
(i)	$38.9 + 6.623 + 14$	(s)	$163.4 - 33.4 - 70.8$
(j)	$9.6 - 4.7$	(t)	$423 - 256.87 + 19.6$

3.13 Perform the following multiplications.

(a)	4×2.3	(h)	7.4×0.77	(o)	6.35×1.07
(b)	2.97×3	(i)	46.2×1.89	(p)	10.65×23.17
(c)	5.6×4.6	(j)	22.4×3.65	(q)	0.0025×36
(d)	7.2×1.5	(k)	0.028×518	(r)	0.0004×20
(e)	0.35×59	(l)	0.65×0.73	(s)	4.2×0.0021
(f)	7.02×33	(m)	6.03×0.78	(t)	0.0029×0.17
(g)	0.08×67.9	(n)	0.064×7200		

3.14   Perform the following divisions to the indicated degree of accuracy.

(a) $62 \div 5$ (exactly)   (k) $0.08 \div 12$ (nearest hundredth)

(b) $25 \div 3$ (nearest tenth)   (l) $5.7 \div 2.4$ (exactly)

(c) $71 \div 7$ (nearest hundredth)   (m) $0.6 \div 9.2$ (nearest tenth)

(d) $165 \div 8$ (nearest hundredth)   (n) $3.66 \div 4.8$ (nearest tenth)

(e) $9 \div 20$ (exactly)   (o) $0.1 \div 10.25$ (nearest hundredth)

(f) $2 \div 15$ (nearest hundredth)   (p) $63 \div 4.5$ (exactly)

(g) $1 \div 15$ (nearest hundredth)   (q) $0.9 \div 0.75$ (exactly)

(h) $14 \div 16$ (exactly)   (r) $16 \div 0.45$ (nearest hundredth)

(i) $3.41 \div 12$ (nearest tenth)   (s) $6.5 \div 0.024$ (nearest one)

(j) $5.6 \div 150$ (nearest hundredth)   (t) $16 \div 0.085$ (nearest one)

3.15   Express the following fractions and mixed numbers as equivalent decimals to the indicated degree of accuracy.

(a) $\frac{2}{5}$ (exactly)   (k) $\frac{1}{25}$ (exactly)

(b) $\frac{3}{4}$ (exactly)   (l) $\frac{1}{50}$ (exactly)

(c) $\frac{1}{8}$ (exactly)   (m) $\frac{1}{15}$ (nearest hundredth)

(d) $3\frac{1}{4}$ (exactly)   (n) $\frac{5}{12}$ (nearest hundredth)

(e) $2\frac{1}{3}$ (nearest hundredth)   (o) $\frac{1}{24}$ (nearest hundredth)

(f) $2\frac{2}{3}$ (nearest hundredth)   (p) $\frac{1}{250}$ (exactly)

(g) $\frac{5}{6}$ (nearest hundredth)   (q) $\frac{1}{500}$ (exactly)

(h) $3\frac{7}{8}$ (nearest hundredth)   (r) $\frac{1}{120}$ (nearest thousandth)

(i) $\frac{1}{9}$ (nearest hundredth)   (s) $\frac{1}{300}$ (nearest thousandth)

(j) $\frac{1}{20}$ (exactly)   (t) $\frac{1}{150}$ (nearest thousandth)

3.16   Perform the following calculations and write each answer in decimal form.

(a) 5.8×10 (h) 0.4×1000 (o) $4.2 \div 100$

(b) 0.7×10 (i) 0.0026×1000 (p) $0.8 \div 100$

(c) 0.008×10 (j) $62 \div 10$ (q) $634 \div 1000$

(d) 6.2×100 (k) $3.3 \div 10$ (r) $72 \div 1000$

(e) 0.9×100 (l) $0.7 \div 10$ (s) $3.5 \div 1000$

(f) 0.035×100 (m) $0.05 \div 10$ (t) $0.41 \div 1000$

(g) 8.8×1000 (n) $73 \div 100$

3.17 Perform the following calculations and write each answer as indicated.

(a) $\frac{1}{3} \times 3.6$ (decimal, exactly)

(b) $4.8 \times \frac{2}{3}$ (decimal, exactly)

(c) $1\frac{1}{4} \times 3.8$ (decimal, nearest tenth)

(d) $4.65 \times 2\frac{1}{2}$ (decimal, nearest hundredth)

(e) $\frac{1}{60} \times 3.6$ (simple fraction)

(f) $\frac{1}{200} \times 0.8$ (simple fraction)

(g) $125 \times \frac{1}{240}$ (decimal, nearest hundredth)

(h) $8\frac{1}{4} \times \frac{1}{2.2}$ (decimal, exactly)

(i) $\frac{7.5}{\frac{1}{2}}$ (decimal, exactly)

(j) $\frac{6.5}{\frac{2}{3}}$ (decimal, nearest tenth)

(k) $\frac{1.25}{\frac{1}{60}}$ (decimal, exactly)

(l) $\frac{0.75}{\frac{1}{200}}$ (decimal, exactly)

(m) $\frac{250}{1\frac{1}{2}}$ (decimal, nearest tenth)

(n) $0.6 \times 8 \times \frac{1}{24}$ (decimal, exactly)

(o) $1500 \times 0.75 \times \frac{1}{240}$ (decimal, nearest tenth)

(p) $120 \times 0.25 \times \frac{1}{500}$ (simple fraction)

(q) $\frac{1}{1000} \times \frac{1}{0.001} \times 0.75$ (simple fraction)

(r) $\frac{1}{30} \times 0.25 \times \frac{1}{\frac{1}{60}}$ (simple fraction)

(s) $1.25 \times \frac{1}{60} \times \frac{1000}{\frac{1}{60}}$ (nearest one)

(t) $0.6 \times \frac{60}{2.2} \times \frac{1}{\frac{1}{6}}$ (decimal, nearest tenth)

3.18 Insert the proper symbol ($<$ or $>$ or $=$) between the following pairs of numbers to indicate their relationships.

(a) 0.34 and 0.32

(b) 0.56 and 0.6

(c) 0.3 and 0.42

(d) 3.1 and 3.09

(e) 10.02 and 10.019

(f) 0.0017 and 0.002

(g) 0.0015 and 0.003

(h) 0.36 and 0.360

(i) 6.40 and 6.04

(j) $\frac{3}{10}$ and 0.3

(k) 0.3 and $\frac{1}{3}$

(l) 1.20 and $1\frac{1}{4}$

(m) 0.125 and $\frac{1}{8}$

(n) $\frac{2}{3}$ and 0.7

(o) $\frac{1}{20}$ and 0.05

(p) 0.666 and $\frac{2}{3}$

(q) 0.667 and $\frac{2}{3}$

(r) $\frac{1}{24}$ and 0.04

(s) $\frac{1}{30}$ and 0.03

(t) $\frac{1}{240}$ and 0.004

Answers to Supplementary Problems

3.10 (a) $\dfrac{3}{10}$ (e) $15\dfrac{1}{5}$ (i) $4\dfrac{3}{5}$ (m) $\dfrac{7}{20}$ (q) $\dfrac{9}{200}$

(b) $\dfrac{4}{5}$ (f) $\dfrac{3}{4}$ (j) $5\dfrac{1}{4}$ (n) $15\dfrac{13}{20}$ (r) $\dfrac{3}{5}$

(c) $\dfrac{2}{5}$ (g) $\dfrac{3}{5}$ (k) $\dfrac{3}{100}$ (o) $\dfrac{667}{1000}$ (s) $\dfrac{3}{500}$

(d) $3\dfrac{1}{10}$ (h) $\dfrac{67}{100}$ (l) $\dfrac{1}{25}$ (p) $\dfrac{9}{20}$ (t) $20\dfrac{1}{4}$

3.11 (a) 0.6 (e) 9.0 (i) 0.05 (m) 8.007 (q) 9
(b) 6.1 (f) 10.0 (j) 16.80 (n) 0.700 (r) 3
(c) 1.4 (g) 1.15 (k) 10.00 (o) 11 (s) 30
(d) 0.1 (h) 0.13 (l) 5.205 (p) 1 (t) 160

3.12 (a) 13.3 (e) 22.79 (i) 59.523 (m) 4.176 (q) 3.02
(b) 12.3 (f) 32.07 (j) 4.9 (n) 37.76 (r) 14.97
(c) 9.41 (g) 37.54 (k) 2.48 (o) 425.39 (s) 59.2
(d) 18.8 (h) 219.95 (l) 1.13 (p) 24.5 (t) 185.73

3.13 (a) 9.2 (e) 20.65 (i) 87.318 (m) 4.7034 (q) 0.09
(b) 8.91 (f) 231.66 (j) 81.76 (n) 460.8 (r) 0.008
(c) 25.76 (g) 5.432 (k) 14.504 (o) 6.7945 (s) 0.00882
(d) 10.80 (h) 5.698 (l) 0.4745 (p) 246.7605 (t) 0.000493

3.14 (a) 12.4 (e) 0.45 (i) 0.3 (m) 0.1 (q) 1.2
(b) 8.3 (f) 0.13 (j) 0.04 (n) 0.8 (r) 35.56
(c) 10.14 (g) 0.07 (k) 0.01 (o) 0.01 (s) 271
(d) 20.63 (h) 0.875 (l) 2.375 (p) 14 (t) 188

3.15 (a) 0.4 (e) 2.33 (i) 0.11 (m) 0.07 (q) 0.002
(b) 0.75 (f) 2.67 (j) 0.05 (n) 0.42 (r) 0.008
(c) 0.125 (g) 0.83 (k) 0.04 (o) 0.04 (s) 0.003
(d) 3.25 (h) 3.88 (l) 0.02 (p) 0.004 (t) 0.007

3.16 (a) 58 (e) 90 (i) 2.6 (m) 0.005 (q) 0.634
(b) 7 (f) 3.5 (j) 6.2 (n) 0.73 (r) 0.072
(c) 0.08 (g) 8800 (k) 0.33 (o) 0.042 (s) 0.0035
(d) 620 (h) 400 (l) 0.07 (p) 0.008 (t) 0.00041

3.17 (a) 1.2 (e) $\dfrac{3}{50}$ (i) 15 (m) 166.7 (q) $\dfrac{3}{4}$

(b) 3.2 (f) $\dfrac{1}{250}$ (j) 9.8 (n) 0.2 (r) $\dfrac{1}{2}$

(c) 4.8 (g) 0.52 (k) 75 (o) 4.7 (s) 1250

(d) 11.63 (h) 3.75 (l) 150 (p) $\dfrac{3}{50}$ (t) 98.2

3.18   (a) $0.34 > 0.32$ (h) $0.36 = 0.360$ (o) $\dfrac{1}{20} = 0.05$

(b) $0.56 < 0.6$ (i) $6.40 > 6.04$ (p) $0.666 < \dfrac{2}{3}$

(c) $0.3 < 0.42$ (j) $\dfrac{3}{10} = 0.3$ (q) $0.667 > \dfrac{2}{3}$

(d) $3.1 > 3.09$ (k) $0.3 < \dfrac{1}{3}$ (r) $\dfrac{1}{24} > 0.04$

(e) $10.02 > 10.019$ (l) $1.20 < 1\dfrac{1}{4}$ (s) $\dfrac{1}{30} > 0.03$

(f) $0.0017 < 0.002$ (m) $0.125 = \dfrac{1}{8}$ (t) $\dfrac{1}{240} > 0.004$

(g) $0.0015 < 0.003$ (n) $\dfrac{2}{3} < 0.7$

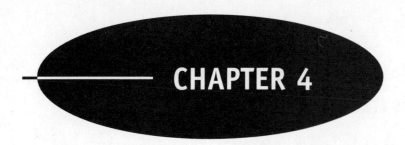

CHAPTER 4

Metric, Apothecary, and Household Measurements— Dimensional Analysis

4.1 WEIGHT AND VOLUME

Most medications come either in solid (dry) form, such as powders or tablets, or in liquid form, such as solutions or suspensions. Medications in solid form are usually measured by weight; medications in liquid form are usually measured by volume.

Drugs are also measured in terms of chemical or therapeutic activity. For example, electrolytic compounds such as potassium chloride are measured in terms of their ability to combine chemically using units called *milliequivalents* (mEq), and drugs such as the penicillins are measured in USP (United States Pharmacopeia) units, which measure the therapeutic activity of the drug. This chapter is concerned with measurements of weight and volume.

Volume or *capacity* is a measure of the space occupied by some substance and is independent of the substance occupying that space. A liter of water has the same volume as a liter of ethyl alcohol. On the other hand, *weight* is a property which depends not only on the volume a substance occupies but also on the nature of the substance. For example, a liter of water weighs 1000 grams (g), while the same volume of ethyl alcohol weighs 810 g.

There are three systems of measuring weight and volume for medications: the metric system, the apothecary system, and the household system.

4.2 THE METRIC SYSTEM

The *metric system* is a system of measurement which was devised to be easily used with decimal numerals. The units and their subdivisions are based on the powers of ten, i.e., 10, 100, 1000, etc.

Length in the Metric System.   The basic unit of length in the metric system is the *meter* (m). The meter is slightly longer than a yard. More precisely, to the nearest hundredth of an inch, it is 39.37 inches (in) (see Fig. 4-1).

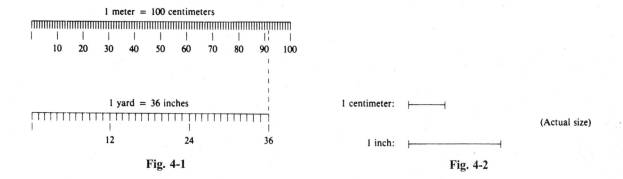

Fig. 4-1   **Fig. 4-2**

Just as a yard is divided into smaller subunits [1 yard (yd) = 36 in], the meter is divided into 100 equal subunits called *centimeters* (cm) as illustrated in Fig. 4-1. The prefix *centi-* means "one hundredth." Thus, the centimeter is a hundredth of a meter. Figure 4-2 shows the actual size of the centimeter and the inch for comparison. One inch is equal to about 2.54 cm.

The centimeter is further divided into 10 equal subunits called *millimeters* (mm). Since there are 100 cm in 1 m, and each centimeter contains 10 mm, then 1 m contains $10 \times 100 = 1000$ mm. Thus, the millimeter is a thousandth of a meter. The prefix *milli-* means "one thousandth."

Volume in the Metric System.   The basic unit of volume in the metric system is the *liter* (L), which is the volume contained in a cube 10 cm on each side (see Fig. 4-3). This is equal to slightly more than a quart. Another unit of volume used in the metric system is the *cubic centimeter* (cc), which is the volume contained in a cube 1 cm on each side (see Fig. 4-3). Figure 4-3 shows 1 L divided into smaller units, each equal to 1 cc. There are 10 layers, each of which is divided into $10 \times 10 = 100$ cc. Thus, there are altogether $10 \times 100 = 1000$ cc in 1 L. Thus, 1 cc is equal to a thousandth of a liter, or 1 *milliliter* (mL). The prefix *milli-* is read "one thousandth." The cubic centimeter and the milliliter are equivalent units of volume. However, in the nursing profession, the milliliter (mL) is preferred as a measure of liquid volume, and the cubic centimeter (cc) as a measure of dry volume.

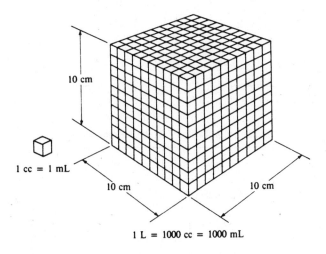

Fig. 4-3

Weight in the Metric System.   The basic unit of weight in the metric system is the *gram* (g). The gram is defined as the weight of 1 mL of distilled water at 4° Celsius. The gram is a fairly small unit of weight. In fact, it takes about 28.35 g (to the nearest hundredth) to equal 1 ounce (oz). A larger unit of weight is the *kilogram* (kg), which is 1000 g. The prefix *kilo-* means "one thousand." A kilogram is approximately equal to 2.2 pounds (lb).

Summary of Metric Units.   As you saw in the preceding discussion, various prefixes are used in the metric system to describe the relationship between units. Table 4-1 gives the meanings of the more common prefixes used in the metric system.

Table 4-1   Table of Metric Prefixes

Prefix	Meaning	Abbreviation
kilo-	thousand	k
hecto-	hundred	h
deka-	ten	da
deci-	tenth	d
centi-	hundredth	c
milli-	thousandth	m
micro-	millionth	mc or μ

Table 4-2   Metric Units of Volume

Unit	Abbreviation
liter	L
deciliter	dL
milliliter	mL
cubic centimeter	cc

Table 4-3   Metric Units of Weight

Unit	Abbreviation
kilogram	kg
gram	g
milligram	mg
microgram	mcg or μg

Table 4-4   Table of Metric Relationships

Weight	Volume
1 kg = 1000 g	1 L = 1000 mL
1 g = 1000 mg	1 dL = 100 mL
1 mg = 1000 μg	1 mL = 1 cc

The most commonly used units of weight and volume in the metric system are listed in Tables 4-2 and 4-3. Listed in Table 4-4 are the most important relationships between units in the metric system.

EXAMPLE 4.1 Explain the meaning of the following abbreviations: (*a*) 1 mL; (*b*) 1 dL; (*c*) 1 kg.

(*a*) 1 mL = 1 milliliter = one thousandth of a liter

(*b*) 1 dL = 1 deciliter = one tenth of a liter

(*c*) 1 kg = 1 kilogram = one thousand grams

Since the metric system was devised to be easily used with decimal notation, it is a common convention that measurements expressed in metric units be written with decimal numerals. For example, "one and a half grams" is written as 1.5 g, not $1\frac{1}{2}$ g; "three-fourths of a liter" is written 0.75 L, not $\frac{3}{4}$ L.

4.3 THE APOTHECARY SYSTEM

The apothecary system of measures is an older system than the metric system. The metric system has many advantages over the apothecary system and is therefore rapidly replacing the older system. Almost all medications are now measured in metric units. However, because there are some drugs which are still measured in apothecary units, you must be familiar with this system.

Weight in the Apothecary System. The only unit of weight in the apothecary system with which you need to be familiar for measuring medications is the *grain* (gr), which is approximately equal to 60 mg. One grain is approximately the weight of a drop of water.

Volume in the Apothecary System. The basic unit of volume in the apothecary system is the *minim* (m). The minim is about equal in volume to a drop of water. The various units of volume in the apothecary system are listed in Table 4-5 in order of increasing size.

The relationships between these units are given in Table 4-6.

Table 4-5   Apothecary Units of Volume

Unit	Abbreviation
minim	m
dram	dr or ʒ
ounce	oz or ʒ
pint	pt
quart	qt

Table 4-6   Table of Apothecary Relationships

m 60 = dr 1
dr 8 = oz 1
oz 16 = pt 1
pt 2 = qt 1

In the apothecary system, the abbreviation for the unit is written *before* the amount. For example, "45 minims" is written m 45; "4 drams" is written dr 4.

Another standard practice when using apothecary measures is to write parts of wholes as *fractions*, not in decimal notation. For example, "two and a half pints" is written pt $2\frac{1}{2}$, not pt 2.5; "a quarter grain" is written gr $\frac{1}{4}$.

The ounce, the pint, and the quart in the apothecary system are the same as the ordinary household ounce, pint, and quart.

EXAMPLE 4.2 Write the following quantities in abbreviated form: (*a*) 20 minims; (*b*) $\frac{1}{60}$ grain; (*c*) 12 drams; (*d*) one and a half quarts; (*e*) half an ounce; (*f*) two-thirds of a pint.

(*a*) 20 minims = m 20

(*b*) $\frac{1}{60}$ grain = gr $\frac{1}{60}$

(*c*) 12 drams = dr 12

(*d*) one and a half quarts = qt $1\frac{1}{2}$

(*e*) half an ounce = oz $\frac{1}{2}$

(*f*) two-thirds of a pint = pt $\frac{2}{3}$

4.4 ROMAN NUMERALS

Drug orders in apothecary units are still occasionally written in Roman numerals. Thus, it is necessary to know this system of numeration. Table 4-7 gives the first 30 Roman numerals and the corresponding

Table 4-7   Table of Roman Numerals from 1 to 30

1	i	11	xi	21	xxi
2	ii	12	xii	22	xxii
3	iii	13	xiii	23	xxiii
4	iv	14	xiv	24	xxiv
5	v	15	xv	25	xxv
6	vi	16	xvi	26	xxvi
7	vii	17	xvii	27	xxvii
8	viii	18	xviii	28	xxviii
9	ix	19	xix	29	xxix
10	x	20	xx	30	xxx

base ten numerals to illustrate how Roman numerals are formed. Study of this table will shown that $1 = i$, $5 = v$, and $10 = x$. Furthermore, 2 and 3 are formed by "adding ones." That is, $2 = i + i = ii$, $3 = i + i + i = iii$. However, 4 is not iiii, but rather iv. The symbol iv is interpreted as $iv = v - i = 5 - 1 = 4$. On the other hand, the symbol for 6 is vi because $vi = v + i = 5 + 1 = 6$. Similarly, $ix = 10 - 1 = 9$, and $xi = 10 + 1 = 11$. The rules can be formulated as follows:

1. If a symbol is followed by another of equal or lesser value, the values of the symbols are added.

2. If a symbol is followed by a symbol of greater value, the value of the first is subtracted from the second.

Once the Roman numerals for 1 through 9 are learned, the Roman numerals up to 39 can be formed by adding the numerals from 1 through 9 to $x = 10$, $xx = 20$, and $xxx = 30$.

EXAMPLE 4.3 Write the Roman numerals for the following base ten numerals: (*a*) 19; (*b*) 24; (*c*) 28; (*d*) 36.

(*a*) $19 = 10 + 9 = x + ix = xix$

(*b*) $24 = 20 + 4 = xx + iv = xxiv$

(*c*) $28 = 20 + 8 = xx + viii = xxviii$

(*d*) $36 = 30 + 6 = xxx + vi = xxxvi$

The Symbol s̄s̄.   In written drug orders using Roman numerals, the symbol s̄s̄ represents the fraction $\frac{1}{2}$.

EXAMPLE 4.4 Write out the meaning of each of the following in full, using base ten numerals: (*a*) pt ivs̄s̄; (*b*) gr iis̄s̄; (*c*) dr xii.

(*a*)   pt ivs̄s̄ $= 4\frac{1}{2}$ pints; (*b*) gr iis̄s̄ $= 2\frac{1}{2}$ grains; (*c*) dr xii $= 12$ drams.

4.5   THE HOUSEHOLD SYSTEM

As the name implies, the household system is the system of weights and volumes most commonly used in everyday life in the United States. Household measures are not generally used for the measurement of drugs except in home situations where accurate measurement of drugs is not available. The household units for measurement of volume which are relevant to nursing practice are listed in Table 4-8 in increasing order of size. The drop is about equal to the minim in the apothecary system. The Latin word for "drop" is *gutta*; hence the abbreviation gtt.

The relationships between the household units are listed in Table 4-9.

In the household system, as in the apothecary system, parts of wholes are written as fractions and not in decimal notation.

Table 4-8   Household Units of Volume

Unit	Abbreviation
drop	gtt
teaspoon	t or tsp
tablespoon	T or Tbs
ounce	oz
teacup	—
measuring cup	C
glass	—

Table 4-9   Table of Household Relationships

1 tsp = 60 gtt
1 Tbs = 3 t
1 oz = 2 T
1 teacup = 6 oz
1 C = 8 oz
1 glass = 8 oz

EXAMPLE 4.5 Write out the meanings of the abbreviation in full: (*a*) 30 gtt; (*b*) $1\frac{1}{2}$t; (*c*) $2\frac{1}{2}$C; (*d*) 6 oz.

(*a*)   30 gtt $= 30$ drops

(*c*) $2\frac{1}{2}$C $= 2\frac{1}{2}$ measuring cups

(*b*) $1\frac{1}{2}$t $= 1\frac{1}{2}$ teaspoons

(*d*)   6 oz $= 6$ ounces

4.6 RATIOS

A *ratio* is a comparison of two numbers by division. For example, the ratio $3:2$ (read "3 to 2") means the division, 3 divided by 2. Ratios are thus equivalent to fractions, and the ratio $3:2$ can also be written as the fraction 3/2.

EXAMPLE 4.6   The label on a bottle of ammonia reads "mix 1 part ammonia to 7 parts water." This describes the ratio $1:7$ in which ammonia and water are to be used. The same relationship can be expressed in the following two equivalent ways:

1. The amount of water is seven times the amount of ammonia.

2. The amount of ammonia is one-seventh the amount of water.

EXAMPLE 4.7   The *specific gravity* of a substance is the ratio of the mass of a unit volume of the substance to the mass of the same volume of water under the same conditions. The specific gravity of urine is usually between 1.015 and 1.025. This means that a volume of urine has between 1.015 and 1.025 times the mass of the same volume of water.

Expressing Relationships as Ratios.   The relationship between a pair of quantities can be expressed as the ratio of the two quantities. For a given relationship there are always two such ratios, one the reciprocal of the other. For example, when we say that 3 lb of bananas costs \$1.00, we are expressing a relationship between a weight (pounds) and a cost (dollars). Such a relationship can be expressed as the ratio 3 lb/\$1.00 (read "three pounds per dollar") or its reciprocal \$1.00/3 lb (read "one dollar per three pounds"). Such ratios are also called *rates* (we say, for example, that bananas sell at the rate of 3 lb per dollar).

EXAMPLE 4.8   Express each of the following relationships in ratio form in two ways: (*a*) 1 g is equal to 1000 mg; (*b*) a particular drug comes in tablets, each containing 250 mg of the drug; (*c*) the label on a vial of medication indicates that every 5 mL contains 0.1 g of the drug.

(*a*)   The two possible ratios are

$$\frac{1 \text{ g}}{1000 \text{ mg}}$$ which is read, "One gram per 1000 milligrams"

and its reciprocal

$$\frac{1000 \text{ mg}}{1 \text{ g}}$$ which is read, "1000 milligrams per gram"

(*b*)   The two possible ratios are

$$\frac{250 \text{ mg}}{1 \text{ tab}}$$ which is read, "250 milligrams per tablet"

and its reciprocal

$$\frac{1 \text{ tab}}{250 \text{ mg}}$$ which is read, "1 tablet per 250 milligrams"

(*c*)   The two possible ratios are

$$\frac{0.1 \text{ g}}{5 \text{ mL}}$$ which is read, "0.1 g per 5 mL"

and its reciprocal

$$\frac{5 \text{ mL}}{0.1 \text{ g}}$$ which is read, "5 mL per 0.1 g"

Cancelling Units in Ratios. Units which occur in ratios can be treated as though they were numerical factors. Thus, *when the same units occur in both numerator and denominator of a ratio, they can be cancelled out as common factors.*

EXAMPLE 4.9 The small intestine is about 20 feet (ft) in length, and the large intestine is about 5 ft in length. Comparing the lengths by division, the ratio is 20 ft/5 ft. The same units occur in both numerator and denominator of the ratio, and can be cancelled out as common factors. Thus the ratio of the lengths is

$$\frac{20 \text{ ft}}{5 \text{ ft}} = \frac{20}{5} = \frac{4}{1} \quad \text{or} \quad 4:1$$

4.7 DIMENSIONAL ANALYSIS

The calculations of medical dosages are problems in converting a given quantity of medication from one unit of measurement to another unit of measurement based on a known relationship between the units. For example, you may need to calculate how many milligrams are contained in 0.85 g, based on the fact that 1 g is equal to 1000 mg. Or perhaps you may need to know how many tablets of a drug are needed to give 125 mg of the drug, if there are 50 milligrams per tablet (50 mg/tab) of the drug.

Such calculations can be easily performed by a technique called *dimensional analysis*, which is routinely used in the physical sciences and engineering. In fact, as you will see, dimensional analysis is no more than a formalization of the common sense way in which one would solve such problems.

To understand the method, let us start with a familiar problem. We know that if 1 lb of apples costs 49¢, then the price of 6 lb can be calculated by multiplying the given amount 6 lb by the rate 49¢/1 lb to obtain

$$\text{Total cost} = 6 \text{ lb} \times \frac{49¢}{1 \text{ lb}} = 6 \times 49¢ = 294¢ = \$2.94$$

An apparently more complicated problem is in fact no more difficult if we use the same approach. Suppose the rate at which the apples are sold is 3 lb for \$1.39. How much would $5\frac{1}{2}$ lb cost? We could do this problem by dividing 3 into \$1.39 to find out how much 1 lb cost, then multiply this by $5\frac{1}{2}$. But we could obtain the same result by multiplying the given amount $5\frac{1}{2}$ lb by the rate $\frac{\$1.39}{3 \text{ lb}}$.

$$\text{Total cost} = 5\frac{1}{2} \text{ lb} \times \frac{\$1.39}{3 \text{ lb}} = \frac{5\frac{1}{2} \times \$1.39}{3} = \$2.55$$

This is an example of a *conversion problem*, that is, converting an amount expressed in one unit (pounds) to an equivalent amount in another unit (dollars) based on a known relationship. This can be diagrammed as follows:

$$5\frac{1}{2} \text{ lb} \rightarrow ? \text{ dollars}$$

Such a problem is solved by multiplying the given amount ($5\frac{1}{2}$ lb) by a rate (\$1.39/3 lb) obtained from the known relationship (3 lb costs \$1.39). When a rate is used in a conversion problem, it is also called a *conversion factor.*

A point to which close attention must be paid is which of the two possible ratios is the correct conversion factor to use. The rule is: *The correct conversion factor has the units of the given amount in the denominator, and the units of the answer in the numerator.* When the problem is set up correctly, all the units will cancel out between numerator and denominator except the units of the answer (in the example above, the pounds cancel out and the dollars remain).

Summary of the Method of Dimensional Analysis. In any conversion problem, there will always be three main elements:

1. The *given quantity* (what you are going to change)
2. An *unknown* answer (that to which you wish to convert the given quantity)
3. A *relationship* between the units of the given quantity and the units of the answer (which will determine the conversion factor used to solve the problem)

These three elements must always be firmly established in your mind. Then you can state the problem,

$$\text{Given quantity} \rightarrow \text{? answer}$$

and find its solution,

$$\text{Answer} = \text{given quantity} \times \text{conversion factor}$$

The examples below will illustrate the method.

EXAMPLE 4.10   If 1 kg is equal to about 2.2 lb, how many kilograms does a 140-lb person weigh? Give the answer to the nearest tenth.
   This is a conversion problem.

1. The given quantity is 140 lb.
2. The unknown is: How many kilograms?
3. The relationship is: 1 kg equals 2.2 lb.

The conversion required is: 140 lb → ? kg. The answer is

$$\text{The number of kg} = 140 \text{ lb} \times \frac{1 \text{ kg}}{2.2 \text{ lb}} = \frac{140 \times 1 \text{ kg}}{2.2} = \frac{140 \text{ kg}}{2.2} = 63.6 \text{ kg}$$

Thus, 140 lb is equal to 63.6 kg. Note that the conversion factor was set up with 2.2 lb in the denominator, so that the pounds will cancel out.

EXAMPLE 4.11   1 in is equal to about 2.54 cm. If a man's height is 180 cm, calculate his height in inches to the nearest whole.

1. The given quantity is: 180 cm
2. The unknown is: How many inches?
3. The relationship is: 1 in = 2.54 cm
4. The conversion required is: 180 cm → ? in.

The answer is

$$\text{Number of inches} = 180 \text{ cm} \times \frac{1 \text{ in}}{2.54 \text{ cm}} = \frac{180 \times 1 \text{ in}}{2.54} = \frac{180 \text{ in}}{2.54} = 71 \text{ in}$$

Thus, 180 cm = 71 in (or 5 ft 11 in).

EXAMPLE 4.12   For the following problems, refer to Table 4-6.

(*a*) How many ounces contain dr 12?

(*b*) How many drams are in oz $\frac{1}{2}$?

(c) How many ounces are contained in pt $\overline{\text{iss}}$?

(*a*) The required conversion is: dr 12 → oz ?

     The relationship to use is: oz 1 = dr 8

     Set up the calculation: $\text{dr } 12 \times \dfrac{\text{oz } 1}{\text{dr } 8}$

Perform the calculation: $= \dfrac{\cancel{12}^{\,3} \times \text{oz } 1}{\cancel{8}_{\,2}} = \text{oz} \dfrac{3}{2} = \text{oz } 1\dfrac{1}{2}$

Thus, oz $1\dfrac{1}{2}$ contains dr 12.

(b) The required conversion is: oz $\dfrac{1}{2} \rightarrow$ dr ?

The relationship to use is: oz 1 = dr 8

Set up the calculation: $\cancel{\text{oz}} \dfrac{1}{2} \times \dfrac{\text{dr } 8}{\cancel{\text{oz}} \, 1}$

Perform the calculation: $= \dfrac{1}{\cancel{2}_{\,1}} \times \dfrac{\text{dr } \cancel{8}^{\,4}}{1} = \text{dr} \dfrac{4}{1} = \text{dr } 4$

Thus, oz $\dfrac{1}{2} =$ dr 4.

(c) Since pt $\overline{\text{iss}} =$ pt $1\dfrac{1}{2}$ (see Sec. 4.4),

The required conversion is: pt $1\dfrac{1}{2} \rightarrow$ oz ?

The relationship to use is: pt 1 = oz 16

Set up the calculation: $\cancel{\text{pt}} \, 1\dfrac{1}{2} \times \dfrac{\text{oz } 16}{\cancel{\text{pt}} \, 1}$

Perform the calculation: $= 1\dfrac{1}{2} \times \dfrac{\text{oz } 16}{1} = \dfrac{3}{\cancel{2}_{\,1}} \times \dfrac{\text{oz } \cancel{16}^{\,8}}{1} = 3 \times \text{oz } 8 = \text{oz } 24$

Thus, pt $1\dfrac{1}{2} =$ oz 24.

EXAMPLE 4.13 For the following problems, refer to Table 4-9.

(a) How many tablespoons contain 6 t?

(b) How many ounces are contained in $1\dfrac{1}{2}$ T?

(c) How many ounces are contained in $1\dfrac{1}{4}$ C?

(a) The required conversion is: 6 t $\rightarrow$? T

The relationship to use is: 1 T = 3 t

Set up the calculation: $6 \cancel{t} \times \dfrac{1 \text{ T}}{3 \cancel{t}}$

Perform the calculation: $= \cancel{6}^{\,2} \times \dfrac{1 \text{ T}}{\cancel{3}_{\,1}} = 2 \times 1 \text{ T} = 2 \text{ T}$

(b) The required conversion is: $1\dfrac{1}{2}$ T $\rightarrow$? oz

The relationship to use is: 1 oz = 2 T

Set up the calculation: $1\dfrac{1}{2} \cancel{\text{T}} \times \dfrac{1 \text{ oz}}{2 \cancel{\text{T}}}$

Perform the calculation: $= 1\dfrac{1}{2} \times \dfrac{1 \text{ oz}}{2} = \dfrac{3}{2} \times \dfrac{1 \text{ oz}}{2} = \dfrac{3}{4} \text{ oz}$

(c)   The required conversion is: $1\frac{1}{4}$ C $\rightarrow$? oz

The relationship to use is: 1 C = 8 oz

Set up the calculation: $1\frac{1}{4}$ ¢ $\times \dfrac{8 \text{ oz}}{1 \text{ ¢}}$

Perform the calculation: $= 1\frac{1}{4} \times 8 \text{ oz} = \dfrac{5}{\overset{}{\underset{1}{4}}} \times \overset{2}{8} \text{ oz} = 10 \text{ oz}$

Conversions Requiring More than One Step.   The following conversions require more than one step because there is no direct relationship between the given quantity and the unknown. A third quantity related to both must be used.

EXAMPLE 4.14   Perform the following conversions.

(a)   Find the number of ounces in $1\frac{3}{4}$ qt.

(b)   Find the number of teaspoons in $\frac{1}{2}$ oz.

(a)   The required conversion is: qt $1\frac{3}{4} \rightarrow$ oz?

There is no direct relationship between quarts and ounces listed in Table 4-6. However, there is a relationship between quarts and pints, and a relationship between pints and ounces. Thus, to solve the problem, we first convert qt $1\frac{3}{4}$ into pints, then convert the resulting answer into ounces. This is done in a single calculation.

The required conversion is: qt $1\frac{3}{4} \rightarrow$ pt? $\rightarrow$ oz?

The equivalences to use are: qt 1 = pt 2 and pt 1 = oz 16

The calculation is set up as follows: qt $1\frac{3}{4} \times \dfrac{\text{pt 2}}{\text{qt 1}} \times \dfrac{\text{oz 16}}{\text{pt 1}}$

This conversion factor changes the qt into pt	This conversion factor changes the pt into oz

Note how all the units cancel out except for ounces, the unit for the answer. The calculation is now carried out:

$$1\frac{3}{4} \times \frac{2}{1} \times \frac{\text{oz } 16}{1} = \frac{7}{\overset{}{\underset{1}{4}}} \times \frac{2}{1} \times \frac{\text{oz } \overset{4}{16}}{1} = 14 \times \text{oz } 4 = \text{oz } 56$$

(b)   The required conversion is: $\frac{1}{2}$ oz $\rightarrow$? t

This requires two steps: $\frac{1}{2}$ oz $\rightarrow$? T $\rightarrow$? t

The equivalences to use are: 1 oz = 2 T and 1 T = 3 t

Set up the calculation: $\frac{1}{2}$ oz $\times \dfrac{2 \text{ T}}{1 \text{ oz}} \times \dfrac{3 \text{ t}}{1 \text{ T}}$

Perform the calculation: $= \dfrac{1}{\overset{}{\underset{1}{2}}} \times \dfrac{\overset{1}{2}}{1} \times \dfrac{3 \text{ t}}{1} = 3 \text{ t}$

EXAMPLE 4.15   Given that 1 in equals 2.54 cm, how many feet are there in 100 cm? (Give answer to the nearest hundredth.)

The required conversion is: $100 \text{ cm} \rightarrow ? \text{ ft}$

This requires two steps: $100 \text{ cm} \rightarrow ? \text{ in} \rightarrow ? \text{ ft}$

The equivalences to use are: $1 \text{ in} = 2.54 \text{ cm and } 1 \text{ ft} = 12 \text{ in}$

Set up the calculation: $100 \text{ cm} \times \dfrac{1 \text{ in}}{2.54 \text{ cm}} \times \dfrac{1 \text{ ft}}{12 \text{ in}}$

Perform the calculation: $= \dfrac{100 \text{ ft}}{2.54 \times 12} = \dfrac{100 \text{ ft}}{30.48} = 3.28 \text{ ft}$

4.8   METRIC CONVERSIONS

The method of dimensional analysis will now be applied to conversions between units in the metric system. The relationships used in these conversions are those listed in Table 4-4.

EXAMPLE 4.16   Convert the following measurements in milligrams to their equivalents in grams: (a) 750 mg; (b) 36 mg; (c) 4 mg.

(a)   The required conversion is: $750 \text{ mg} \rightarrow ? \text{ g}$

The relationship to use is: $1 \text{ g} = 1000 \text{ mg}$

Set up the calculation: $750 \text{ mg} \times \dfrac{1 \text{ g}}{1000 \text{ mg}}$

Perform the calculation: $= \dfrac{750 \text{ g}}{1000} = 0.75 \text{ g}$

Shortcut: The above calculations show that, to convert from milligrams to grams, we need only divide by 1000. In decimal notation this can be done by simply moving the decimal point 3 places to the left (see Sec. 3.7):

$$750 \text{ mg} = 750. \text{ g} = .75 \text{ g}$$

(b)   By the shortcut: 36 mg = 036. g = 0.036 g

(c)   By the shortcut: 4 mg = 004. g = 0.004 g

EXAMPLE 4.17   Convert the following measurements in grams to their equivalents in milligrams: (a) 0.35 g; (b) 1.2 g; (c) 0.06 g.

(a)   The required conversion is: $0.35 \text{ g} \rightarrow ? \text{ mg}$

The relationship to use is: $1 \text{ g} = 1000 \text{ mg}$

Set up the calculation: $0.35 \text{ g} \times \dfrac{1000 \text{ mg}}{1 \text{ g}}$

Perform the calculation: $= 0.35 \times 1000 \text{ mg} = 350 \text{ mg}$

Shortcut: The above calculations show that, to convert from grams to milligrams, we need only multiply by 1000. In decimal notation, this can be done by simply moving the decimal point 3 places to the right (see Sec. 3.7):

$$0.35 \text{ g} = 0.350 \text{ mg} = 350 \text{ mg}$$

(b)   By the shortcut: 1.2 g = 1.200 mg = 1200 mg

(c)   By the shortcut: 0.06 g = 0.060 mg = 60 mg

EXAMPLE 4.18 Convert the following measurements in liters to their equivalents in milliliters: (*a*) 3.5 L; (*b*) 0.27 L; (*c*) 0.0635 L.

(*a*) The required conversion is: $\qquad$ 3.5 L → ? mL

The relationship to use is: $\qquad$ 1 L = 1000 mL

Set up the calculation: $\qquad$ $3.5\,\cancel{L} \times \dfrac{1000\ \text{mL}}{1\,\cancel{L}}$

Perform the calculation: $\qquad$ $= 3.5 \times 1000\ \text{mL} = 3500\ \text{mL}$

Shortcut: This conversion is similar to a conversion from grams to milligrams and can be done the same way. Move the decimal point 3 places to the right:

$$3.5\ \text{L} = 3.500\ \text{mL} = 3500\ \text{mL}$$

(*b*) By the shortcut: 0.27 L = 0.270 mL = 270 mL
(*c*) By the shortcut: 0.0635 L = 0.063,5 mL = 63.5 mL

EXAMPLE 4.19 Perform the following conversions: (*a*) 26.4 g = ? kg; (*b*) 0.5 mg = ? μg; (*c*) 42 cm = ? m; (*d*) 13.5 mL = ? cc.

(*a*) The required conversion is: $\qquad$ 26.4 g → ? kg

The relationship to use is: $\qquad$ 1 kg = 1000 g

Set up the calculation: $\qquad$ $26.4\,\cancel{g} \times \dfrac{1\ \text{kg}}{1000\,\cancel{g}}$

Perform the calculation: $\qquad$ $= \dfrac{26.4}{1000}\ \text{kg} = 0.0264\ \text{kg}$

By the shortcut: 26.4 g = 026.4 kg = 0.0264 kg

(*b*) The required conversion is: $\qquad$ 0.5 mg → ? μg

The relationship to use is: $\qquad$ 1 mg = 1000 μg

Set up the calculation: $\qquad$ $0.5\,\cancel{\text{mg}} \times \dfrac{1000\ \mu\text{g}}{1\,\cancel{\text{mg}}}$

Perform the calculation: $\qquad$ $= 0.5 \times 1000\ \mu\text{g} = 500\ \mu\text{g}$

By the shortcut: 0.5 mg = 0.500 μg = 500 μg

(*c*) The required conversion is: $\qquad$ 42 cm → ? m

The relationship between meters and centimeters is not listed in Table 4-4, but the prefix *centi-* indicates that a centimeter is a hundredth of a meter. Thus,

The equivalence to use is: $\qquad$ 1 m = 100 cm

Set up the calculation: $\qquad$ $42\,\cancel{\text{cm}} \times \dfrac{1\ \text{m}}{100\,\cancel{\text{cm}}}$

Perform the calculation: $\qquad$ $= \dfrac{42}{100}\ \text{m} = 0.42\ \text{m}$

By the shortcut: 42 cm = 42 m = 0.42 m

(*d*) Since 1 cc = 1 mL, then 13.5 mL = 13.5 cc.

4.9 CONVERSIONS BETWEEN SYSTEMS

The tables below list the more important commonly accepted relationships between units of measurement in different systems. These relationships are *not exact*, but are rounded within an acceptable margin of error, as established by the United States Pharmacopeia, from more exact relationships. (The established acceptable margin of error is defined to be 10 percent of true value.)

Weight Relationships.   The exact relationship between the grain (in the apothecary system) and the gram (in the metric system) is

$$1 \text{ gram} = 15.432 \text{ grains}$$

This is approximately by the relationships in Table 4-10.

Table 4-10   Metric–Apothecary Weight Relationships

1 g = gr 15
60 mg = gr 1

Volume Relationships.   The exact relationship between the minim (in the apothecary system) and the milliliter (in the metric system) is

$$1 \text{ milliliter} = 16.23 \text{ minims}$$

The more commonly used metric–apothecary volume relationships are listed in Table 4-11. These relationships are illustrated in Fig. 4-4.

Table 4-11   Metric–Apothecary Volume Relationships

1 mL = m 15 or 16
4 mL = dr 1
30 mL = oz 1
500 mL = pt 1
1000 mL = qt 1

Table 4-12   Metric–Household Volume Relationships

5 mL = 1 t
15 mL = 1 T
30 mL = 1 oz

Given in Table 4-12 are the more commonly accepted relationships between metric and household units.

EXAMPLE 4.20   How many grains are contained in 0.2 g?

The required conversion is: $0.2 \text{ g} \rightarrow \text{gr} ?$

The relationship to use is: $1 \text{ g} = \text{gr} 15$

Set up the calculation: $0.2 \text{ g} \times \dfrac{\text{gr } 15}{1 \text{ g}}$

Perform the calculation: $= 0.2 \times \text{gr } 15 = \text{gr } 3$

That is, 0.2 g = gr 3.

EXAMPLE 4.21   Convert gr $\dfrac{1}{300}$ to milligrams.

The required conversion is: $\text{gr } \dfrac{1}{300} \rightarrow ? \text{ mg}$

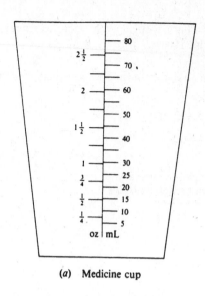

(a) Medicine cup

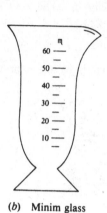

(b) Minim glass

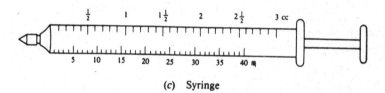

(c) Syringe

Fig. 4-4

The relationship to use is:

$$gr\ 1 = 60\ mg$$

Set up the calculation:

$$gr\ \frac{1}{300} \times \frac{60\ mg}{gr\ 1}$$

Perform the calculation:

$$= \frac{1}{300} \times 60\ mg = \frac{1}{5}\ mg = 0.2\ mg$$

That is, $gr\ \dfrac{1}{300} = 0.2$ mg.

EXAMPLE 4.22   How many milliliters are in qt $1\dfrac{1}{2}$?

The required conversion is:

$$qt\ 1\frac{1}{2} \rightarrow ?\ mL$$

The relationship to use is:

$$qt\ 1 = 1000\ mL$$

Set up the calculation:

$$qt\ 1\frac{1}{2} \times \frac{1000\ mL}{qt\ 1}$$

Perform the calculation:

$$= 1\frac{1}{2} \times 1000\ mL = 1500\ mL$$

That is, $qt\ 1\dfrac{1}{2} = 1500$ mL.

EXAMPLE 4.23   How many ounces are there in 300 mL?

The required conversion is:

$$300\ mL \rightarrow oz?$$

The relationship to use is: $\qquad$ oz 1 = 30 mL

Set up the calculation: $\qquad 300 \text{ mL} \times \dfrac{\text{oz } 1}{30 \text{ mL}}$

Perform the calculation: $\qquad = \overset{10}{300} \times \dfrac{\text{oz } 1}{\underset{1}{30}} = \text{oz } 10$

That is, 300 mL = oz 10.

EXAMPLE 4.24　How many milliliters are contained in ♏ xii?　♏ xii means ♏ 12 (see Sec. 4.4).

The required conversion is: $\qquad$ ♏ 12 → ? mL

The relationship to use is: $\qquad$ 1 mL = ♏ 15

Set up the calculation: $\qquad$ ♏ 12 $\times \dfrac{1 \text{ mL}}{♏ 15}$

Perform the calculation: $\qquad = \dfrac{\overset{4}{12} \text{ mL}}{\underset{5}{15}} = \dfrac{4}{5} \text{ mL} = 0.8 \text{ mL}$

That is, ♏ xii = 0.8 mL.

This conversion may also be performed using the relationship 1 mL = ♏ 16:

Set up the calculation: $\qquad$ ♏ 12 $\times \dfrac{1 \text{ mL}}{♏ 16}$

Perform the calculation: $\qquad = \dfrac{\overset{3}{12} \text{ mL}}{\underset{4}{16}} = \dfrac{3}{4} \text{ mL} = 0.75 \text{ mL}$

Which relationship should be used? Both approximations are within the acceptable margin of error, and either can be used according to convenience, except in situations where greater accuracy is needed. In that case, the more accurate approximation 1 mL = ♏ 16 should be used. Note that on the tuberculin syringe in Fig. 4-5, 1 cc = ♏ 16, and the syringe is graduated in *hundredths* of a cubic centimeter.

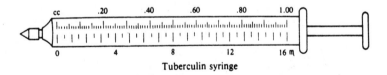

Tuberculin syringe

Fig. 4-5

EXAMPLE 4.25　How many tablespoonsful will contain 8 mL?

The required conversion is: $\qquad$ 8 mL → ? T

The relationship to use is: $\qquad$ 1 T = 15 mL

Set up the calculation: $\qquad$ 8 mL $\times \dfrac{1 \text{ T}}{15 \text{ mL}}$

Perform the calculation: $\qquad = \dfrac{8}{15} \text{ T or about } \dfrac{1}{2} \text{ T}$

EXAMPLE 4.26　How many milliliters are contained in 1 C?

The required conversion is: $\qquad$ 1 C → ? mL

This requires two steps: $\qquad$ 1 C → ? oz → ? mL

The equivalences to use are: $\qquad$ 1 C = 8 oz and 1 oz = 30 mL

Set up the calculation:

$$1 \, \cancel{C} \times \frac{8 \, \cancel{oz}}{1 \, \cancel{C}} \times \frac{30 \text{ mL}}{1 \, \cancel{oz}}$$

Perform the calculation:

$$= 8 \times 30 \text{ mL} = 240 \text{ mL}$$

EXAMPLE 4.27 Part of a patient's liquid intake consists of a beverage served in a teacup. How many milliliters of liquid intake does this represent?

A teacup contains approximately 6 oz of fluid. However, since a cup is not filled to the brim when a beverage is served in it, for the purpose of calculating the fluid intake, the capacity of a teacup is often taken to be 5 oz. Thus,

The required conversion is: $5 \text{ oz} \rightarrow ? \text{ mL}$

The relationship to use is: $1 \text{ oz} = 30 \text{ mL}$

Set up the calculation: $5 \, \cancel{oz} \times \dfrac{30 \text{ mL}}{1 \, \cancel{oz}}$

Perform the calculation: $= 5 \times 30 \text{ mL} = 150 \text{ mL}$

EXAMPLE 4.28 A patient drank orange juice from an 8-oz glass. How many milliliters of fluid intake does this represent?

The required conversion is: $8 \text{ oz} \rightarrow ? \text{ mL}$

The equivalence to use is: $1 \text{ oz} = 30 \text{ mL}$

Set up the calculation: $8 \, \cancel{oz} \times \dfrac{30 \text{ mL}}{1 \, \cancel{oz}}$

Perform the calculation: $= 8 \times 30 \text{ mL} = 240 \text{ mL}$

Thus, one full glass = 240 mL. However, since a glass is not usually filled to the brim, the more convenient figure 200 mL is often used for the purpose of calculating liquid intake.

Solved Problems

4.1 Write out the meaning of each of the following abbreviations in full, and indicate whether the unit is metric, apothecary, or household.

(a) 3.5 mL	(e) ℔ 24	(i) 250 mg	(m) $\frac{1}{3}$ C
(b) 120 mm	(f) 2 T	(j) dr 4	(n) 50 μg
(c) gr $\frac{1}{6}$	(g) 0.5 g	(k) 40 kg	(o) 24 dL
(d) oz $\frac{3}{4}$	(h) 15 gtt	(l) $\frac{1}{2}$ t	(p) pt $2\frac{1}{2}$

Solution

(a) 3.5 mL = 3.5 milliliters = 3.5 thousandths of a liter (metric)

(b) 120 mm = 120 millimeters = 120 thousandths of a meter (metric)

(c) gr $\frac{1}{6} = \frac{1}{6}$ grain (apothecary)

(d) oz $\frac{3}{4} = \frac{3}{4}$ ounce (apothecary or household)

(e) ℩ 24 = 24 minims (apothecary)

(f) 2 T = 2 tablespoons (household)

(g) 0.5 g = 0.5 grams (metric)

(h) 15 gtt = 15 drops (household)

(i) 250 mg = 250 milligrams = 250 thousandths of a gram (metric)

(j) dr 4 = 4 drams (apothecary)

(k) 40 kg = 40 kilograms = 40 thousand grams (metric)

(l) $\frac{1}{2}$ t = $\frac{1}{2}$ teaspoon (household)

(m) $\frac{1}{3}$ C = $\frac{1}{3}$ measuring cup (household)

(n) 50 μg = 50 micrograms = 50 millionths of a gram (metric)

(o) 24 dL = 24 deciliters = 24 tenths of a liter (metric)

(p) pt $2\frac{1}{2}$ = $2\frac{1}{2}$ pints (apothecary or household)

4.2 Change each of the following from one numeration system to the other (base ten or Roman).

(a) iii	(f) 21	(k) ix	(p) i$\overline{\text{ss}}$
(b) v	(g) $\frac{1}{2}$	(l) xix	(q) xxxiv
(c) vii	(h) ii$\overline{\text{ss}}$	(m) $5\frac{1}{2}$	(r) vi$\overline{\text{ss}}$
(d) $\overline{\text{ss}}$	(i) iv	(n) 16	(s) xxix
(e) xxx	(j) xiv	(o) xxiv	(t) iv$\overline{\text{ss}}$

Solution

(a) iii = 3

(b) v = 5

(c) vii = v + ii = 5 + 2 = 7

(d) $\overline{\text{ss}}$ = $\frac{1}{2}$

(e) xxx = 30

(f) 21 = 20 + 1 = xx + i = xxi

(g) $\frac{1}{2}$ = $\overline{\text{ss}}$

(h) ii$\overline{\text{ss}}$ = ii + $\overline{\text{ss}}$ = 2 + $\frac{1}{2}$ = $2\frac{1}{2}$

(i) iv = v − i = 5 − 1 = 4

(j) xiv = x + iv = 10 + 4 = 14

(k) ix = x − i = 10 − 1 = 9

(l) xix = x + ix = 10 + 9 = 19

(m) $5\frac{1}{2}$ = 5 + $\frac{1}{2}$ = v + $\overline{\text{ss}}$ = v$\overline{\text{ss}}$

(n) 16 = 10 + 6 = x + vi = xvi

(o) xxiv = xx + iv = 20 + 4 = 24

(p) $\overline{\text{iss}} = \text{i} + \overline{\text{ss}} = 1 + \dfrac{1}{2} = 1\dfrac{1}{2}$

(q) xxxiv = xxx + iv = 30 + 4 = 34

(r) $\overline{\text{viss}} = \text{vi} + \overline{\text{ss}} = 6 + \dfrac{1}{2} = 6\dfrac{1}{2}$

(s) xxix = xx + ix = 20 + 9 = 29

(t) $\overline{\text{ivss}} = \text{iv} + \overline{\text{ss}} = 4 + \dfrac{1}{2} = 4\dfrac{1}{2}$

4.3 Solve the following problems using dimensional analysis.

(a) dr 32 = oz?   (e) pt 2 = oz?   (i) $\dfrac{1}{4}$ C = ? oz

(b) 2 C = ? oz   (f) oz $\dfrac{1}{4}$ = dr?   (j) $1\dfrac{1}{2}$ t = ? T

(c) 1 T = ? oz   (g) $\dfrac{1}{4}$ oz = ? T   (k) qt $\dfrac{1}{2}$ = oz?

(d) dr 1 = oz?   (h) oz $1\dfrac{1}{2}$ = dr?   (l) dr 48 = pt?

(m) Using the relationship 1 kg = 2.2 lb, find the weight in kilograms of a person who weighs 115 lb (give the answer to the nearest tenth).

(n) Using 1 kg = 2.2 lb, find how many pounds a person weighs if she weighs 56 kg (give the answer to the nearest tenth).

(o) If 1 g of carbohydrates yields approximately 4 calories (cal), find the number of dietary calories provided by 40 g of carbohydrates (give the answer to the nearest one).

(p) Using the relationship 1 in = 2.54 cm, find the height of a person in centimeters if she is 63 in tall (give the answer to the nearest one).

(q) Using 1 in = 2.54 cm, find the height of a person in inches if he is 170 cm tall (give the answer to the nearest one).

(r) If 1 lb = 16 oz, find the number of pounds contained in 56 oz.

(s) Using the relationship 1 in = 2.54 cm, find the height of a 6-ft person in centimeters (give the answer to the nearest tenth).

(t) An adult heart weighs about 11 oz. Given that 1 lb = 16 oz and that 1 kg = 2.2 lb, find the weight of the heart in kilograms (give the answer to the nearest hundredth).

Solution

(a) The required conversion is: dr 32 → oz?

The relationship to use is: oz 1 = dr 8

Set up the calculation: $\cancel{\text{dr}}\ 32 \times \dfrac{\text{oz } 1}{\cancel{\text{dr}}\ 8}$

Perform the calculation: $= \dfrac{\overset{4}{\cancel{32}} \times \text{oz } 1}{\underset{1}{\cancel{8}}} = \text{oz } 4$

(b) The required conversion is: 2 C → ? oz

The relationship to use is: 1 C = 8 oz

Set up the calculation: $2\cancel{\text{C}} \times \dfrac{8\ \text{oz}}{1\ \cancel{\text{C}}}$

Perform the calculation: $= 2 \times 8\ \text{oz} = 16\ \text{oz}$

(c) The required conversion is:　　$1\,T \rightarrow ?\,oz$

The relationship to use is:　　$1\,oz = 2\,T$

Set up the calculation:　　$1\,\cancel{T} \times \dfrac{1\,oz}{2\,\cancel{T}}$

Perform the calculation:　　$= \dfrac{1}{2}\,T$

(d) The required conversion is:　　$dr\,1 \rightarrow oz\,?$

The relationship to use is:　　$oz\,1 = dr\,8$

Set up the calculation:　　$\cancel{dr}\,1 \times \dfrac{oz\,1}{\cancel{dr}\,8}$

Perform the calculation:　　$= oz\,\dfrac{1}{8}$

(e) The required conversion is:　　$pt\,2 \rightarrow oz\,?$

The relationship to use is:　　$pt\,1 = oz\,16$

Set up the calculation:　　$\cancel{pt}\,2 \times \dfrac{oz\,16}{\cancel{pt}\,1}$

Perform the calculation:　　$= 2 \times oz\,16 = oz\,32$

(f) The required conversion is:　　$oz\,\dfrac{1}{4} \rightarrow dr\,?$

The relationship to use is:　　$oz\,1 = dr\,8$

Set up the calculation:　　$\cancel{oz}\,\dfrac{1}{4} \times \dfrac{dr\,8}{\cancel{oz}\,1}$

Perform the calculation:　　$= \dfrac{1}{\underset{1}{\cancel{4}}} \times dr\,\overset{2}{\cancel{8}} = dr\,2$

(g) The required conversion is:　　$\dfrac{1}{4}\,oz \rightarrow ?\,T$

The equivalence to use is:　　$1\,oz = 2\,T$

Set up the calculation:　　$\dfrac{1}{4}\,\cancel{oz} \times \dfrac{2\,T}{1\,\cancel{oz}}$

Perform the calculation:　　$= \dfrac{1}{\underset{2}{\cancel{4}}} \times \overset{1}{\cancel{2}}\,T = \dfrac{1}{2}\,T$

(h) The required conversion is:　　$oz\,1\dfrac{1}{2} \rightarrow dr\,?$

The equivalence to use is:　　$oz\,1 = dr\,8$

Set up the calculation:　　$\cancel{oz}\,1\dfrac{1}{2} \times \dfrac{dr\,8}{\cancel{oz}\,1}$

Perform the calculation:　　$= 1\dfrac{1}{2} \times dr\,8 = \dfrac{3}{\underset{1}{\cancel{2}}} \times dr\,\overset{4}{\cancel{8}} = dr\,12$

(i) The required conversion is:　　$\dfrac{1}{4}\,C \rightarrow ?\,oz$

The relationship to use is:　　$1\,C = 8\,oz$

Set up the calculation:　　$\dfrac{1}{4}\,\cancel{C} \times \dfrac{8\,oz}{1\,\cancel{C}}$

Perform the calculation:　　$= \dfrac{1}{\underset{1}{\cancel{4}}} \times \overset{2}{\cancel{8}}\,oz = 2\,oz$

(j) The required conversion is:　　$1\dfrac{1}{2}\,t \rightarrow ?\,T$

The relationship to use is:　　$1\,T = 3\,t$

Set up the calculation:　　$1\dfrac{1}{2}\,\cancel{t} \times \dfrac{1\,T}{3\,\cancel{t}}$

Perform the calculation: $= 1\dfrac{1}{2} \times \dfrac{1}{3}\dfrac{T}{} = \dfrac{\overset{1}{\cancel{3}}}{2} \times \dfrac{1}{\underset{1}{\cancel{3}}}\,T = \dfrac{1}{2}\,T$

(k) The required conversion is: qt $\dfrac{1}{2} \to$ oz ?

This requires two steps: qt $\dfrac{1}{2} \to$ pt ? $\to$ oz ?

The relationships to use are: qt 1 = pt 2 and pt 1 = oz 16

Set up the calculation: $\cancel{qt}\ \dfrac{1}{2} \times \dfrac{pt\ 2}{\cancel{qt}\ 1} \times \dfrac{oz\ 16}{\cancel{pt}\ 1}$

$$\text{This converts} \atop \text{qt to pt} \qquad\qquad {\text{This converts} \atop \text{pt to oz}}$$

Perform the calculation: $= \dfrac{1}{\underset{1}{\cancel{2}}} \times \dfrac{\overset{1}{\cancel{2}}}{1} \times \dfrac{oz\ 16}{1} = oz\ 16$

(l) The required conversion is: dr 48 $\to$ pt ?

This requires two steps: dr 48 $\to$ oz ? $\to$ pt ?

The relationships to use are: oz 1 = dr 8 and pt 1 = oz 16

Set up the calculation: $\cancel{dr}\ 48 \times \dfrac{\cancel{oz}\ 1}{\cancel{dr}\ 8} \times \dfrac{pt\ 1}{\cancel{oz}\ 16}$

$$\text{This converts} \atop \text{dr to oz} \qquad\qquad {\text{This converts} \atop \text{oz to pt}}$$

Perform the calculation: $= \overset{3}{\cancel{48}} \times \dfrac{1}{8} \times \dfrac{pt\ 1}{\underset{1}{\cancel{16}}} = pt\ \dfrac{3}{8}$

(m) The required conversion is: 115 lb $\to$? kg

The relationship to use is: 1 kg = 2.2 lb

Set up the calculation: $115\ \cancel{lb} \times \dfrac{1\ kg}{2.2\ \cancel{lb}}$

Perform the calculation: $= \dfrac{115\ kg}{2.2} = 52.3\ kg$

(n) The required conversion is: 56 kg $\to$? lb

The relationship to use is: 1 kg = 2.2 lb

Set up the calculation: $56\ \cancel{kg} \times \dfrac{2.2\ lb}{1\ \cancel{kg}}$

Perform the calculation: $= 56 \times 2.2\ lb = 123.2\ lb$

(o) The required conversion is: 40 g $\to$? cal

The relationship to use is: 1 g = 4 cal

Set up the calculation: $40\ \cancel{g} \times \dfrac{4\ cal}{1\ \cancel{g}}$

Perform the calculation: $= 40 \times 4\ cal = 160\ cal$

(p) The required conversion is: 63 in $\to$? cm

The relationship to use is: 1 in = 2.54 cm

Set up the calculation: $63\ \cancel{in} \times \dfrac{2.54\ cm}{1\ \cancel{in}}$

Perform the calculation: $= 63 \times 2.54\ cm = 160\ cm$

(q) The required conversion is: 170 cm → ? in

The relationship to use is: 1 in = 2.54 cm

Set up the calculation: $170 \text{ cm} \times \dfrac{1 \text{ in}}{2.54 \text{ cm}}$

Perform the calculation: $= \dfrac{170 \text{ in}}{2.54} = 67 \text{ in}$

(r) The required conversion is: 56 oz → ? lb

The relationship to use is: 1 lb = 16 oz

Set up the calculation: $56 \text{ oz} \times \dfrac{1 \text{ lb}}{16 \text{ oz}}$

Perform the calculation: $= \dfrac{\overset{7}{56} \text{ lb}}{\underset{2}{16}} = \dfrac{7}{2} \text{ lb} = 3\dfrac{1}{2} \text{ lb}$

(s) The required conversion is: 6 ft → ? cm

This requires two steps: 6 ft → ? in → ? cm

The relationships to use are: 1 ft = 12 in and 1 in = 2.54 cm

Set up the calculation: $6 \text{ ft} \times \dfrac{12 \text{ in}}{1 \text{ ft}} \times \dfrac{2.54 \text{ cm}}{1 \text{ in}}$

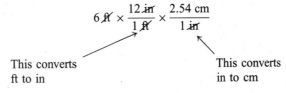

This converts   This converts
ft to in   in to cm

Perform the calculation: $= 6 \times 12 \times 2.54 \text{ cm} = 182.9 \text{ cm}$

(t) The required conversion is: 11 oz → ? kg

This requires two steps: 11 oz → ? lb → ? kg

The relationships to use are: 1 lb = 16 oz and 1 kg = 2.2 lb

Set up the calculation: $11 \text{ oz} \times \dfrac{1 \text{ lb}}{16 \text{ oz}} \times \dfrac{1 \text{ kg}}{2.2 \text{ lb}}$

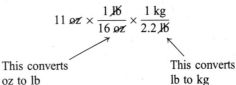

This converts   This converts
oz to lb   lb to kg

Perform the calculation: $= \dfrac{11 \text{ kg}}{16 \times 2.2} = \dfrac{11 \text{ kg}}{35.2} = 0.31 \text{ kg}$

4.4 Perform the following metric conversions (use Table 4-4).

(a) 4 g = ? mg   (k) 25 cc = ? L

(b) 2 L = ? mL   (l) 200 μg = ? mg

(c) 3.5 g = ? mg   (m) 48 μg = ? mg

(d) 0.2 kg = ? g   (n) 1.2 mL = ? L

(e) 0.03 mg = ? μg   (o) 4.3 mL = ? cc

(f) 0.002 L = ? mL   (p) 0.5 mg = ? g

(g) 2100 mL = ? L   (q) 0.3 cc = ? L

(h) 240 mg = ? g   (r) 2.40 m = ? cm

(i) 25 cc = ? mL   (s) 360 cm = ? m

(j) 360 g = ? kg   (t) 560 mm = ? cm

Solution

(a) $4 \text{ g} \times \dfrac{1000 \text{ mg}}{1 \text{ g}} = 4 \times 1000 \text{ mg} = 4000 \text{ mg}$

(b) $2 \text{ L} \times \dfrac{1000 \text{ mL}}{1 \text{ L}} = 2 \times 1000 \text{ mL} = 2000 \text{ mL}$

(c) $3.5 \text{ g} \times \dfrac{1000 \text{ mg}}{1 \text{ g}} = 3.5 \times 1000 \text{ mg} = 3500 \text{ mg}$

(d) $0.2 \text{ kg} \times \dfrac{1000 \text{ g}}{1 \text{ kg}} = 0.2 \times 1000 \text{ g} = 200 \text{ g}$

(e) $0.03 \text{ mg} \times \dfrac{1000 \text{ μg}}{1 \text{ mg}} = 0.03 \times 1000 \text{ μg} = 30 \text{ μg}$

(f) $0.002 \text{ L} \times \dfrac{1000 \text{ mL}}{1 \text{ L}} = 0.002 \times 1000 \text{ mL} = 2 \text{ mL}$

(g) $2100 \text{ mL} \times \dfrac{1 \text{ L}}{1000 \text{ mL}} = \dfrac{2100 \text{ L}}{1000} = 2.1 \text{ L}$

(h) $240 \text{ mg} \times \dfrac{1 \text{ g}}{1000 \text{ mg}} = \dfrac{240 \text{ g}}{1000} = 0.24 \text{ g}$

(i) Since cc and mL are the same, 25 cc = 25 mL

(j) $360 \text{ g} \times \dfrac{1 \text{ kg}}{1000 \text{ g}} = \dfrac{360 \text{ kg}}{1000} = 0.36 \text{ kg}$

(k) $25 \text{ cc} \times \dfrac{1 \text{ L}}{1000 \text{ cc}} = \dfrac{25 \text{ L}}{1000} = 0.025 \text{ L}$

    (1 L = 1000 cc since 1 cc = 1 mL)

(l) $200 \text{ μg} \times \dfrac{1 \text{ mg}}{1000 \text{ μg}} = \dfrac{200 \text{ mg}}{1000} = 0.2 \text{ mg}$

(m) $48 \text{ μg} \times \dfrac{1 \text{ mg}}{1000 \text{ μg}} = \dfrac{48 \text{ mg}}{1000} = 0.048 \text{ mg}$

(n) $1.2 \text{ mL} \times \dfrac{1 \text{ L}}{1000 \text{ mL}} = \dfrac{1.2 \text{ L}}{1000} = 0.0012 \text{ L}$

(o) Since mL and cc are the same, 4.3 mL = 4.3 cc

(p) $0.5 \text{ mg} \times \dfrac{1 \text{ g}}{1000 \text{ mg}} = \dfrac{0.5 \text{ g}}{1000} = 0.0005 \text{ g}$

(q) $0.3 \text{ cc} \times \dfrac{1 \text{ L}}{1000 \text{ cc}} = \dfrac{0.3 \text{ L}}{1000} = 0.0003 \text{ L}$

(r) $2.40 \text{ m} \times \dfrac{100 \text{ cm}}{1 \text{ m}} = 2.40 \times 100 \text{ cm} = 240 \text{ cm}$

    (1 m = 100 cm)

(s) $360 \text{ cm} \times \dfrac{1 \text{ m}}{100 \text{ cm}} = \dfrac{360 \text{ m}}{100} = 3.6 \text{ m}$

    (1 m = 100 cm)

(t) $560 \text{ mm} \times \dfrac{1 \text{ cm}}{10 \text{ mm}} = \dfrac{560 \text{ cm}}{10} = 56 \text{ cm}$

    (1 cm = 10 mm)

4.5   Perform the following conversions (use the relationships given in Tables 4-10, 4-11, and 4-12).

(a) 120 mg = gr ?   (m) oz iii$\overline{ss}$ = ? mL

(b) 300 mL = oz ?   (n) gr $\frac{1}{4}$ = ? mg

(c) 2 T = ? mL   (o) 1.5 mL = m ?

(d) dr vi = ? mL   (p) 0.2 g = gr ?

(e) gr $\frac{1}{10}$ = ? mg   (q) 1250 mL = qt ?

(f) 2 mL = m ?   (r) gr $\frac{3}{4}$ = ? g

(g) gr xxx = ? g   (s) 0.4 mg = gr ?

(h) 3 t = ? mL   (t) 10 mL = dr ?

(i) pt i$\overline{ss}$ = ? mL   (u) 0.3 mL = m ?

(j) 10 mL = ? t   (v) m xx = ? mL

(k) oz 3 = ? mL   (w) pt iii = ? L

(l) gr $\frac{1}{600}$ = ? mg   (x) gr $\frac{1}{300}$ = ? μg

Solution

(a) $120\ \text{mg} \times \dfrac{\text{gr } 1}{60\ \text{mg}} = \dfrac{120 \times \text{gr } 1}{60} = \text{gr } 2$

(b) $300\ \text{mL} \times \dfrac{\text{oz } 1}{30\ \text{mL}} = \dfrac{300 \times \text{oz } 1}{30} = \text{oz } 10$

(c) $2\ T \times \dfrac{15\ \text{mL}}{1\ T} = 2 \times 15\ \text{mL} = 30\ \text{mL}$

(d) $\text{dr } 6 \times \dfrac{4\ \text{mL}}{\text{dr } 1} = 6 \times 4\ \text{mL} = 24\ \text{mL}$

(e) $\text{gr } \dfrac{1}{10} \times \dfrac{60\ \text{mg}}{\text{gr } 1} = \dfrac{60\ \text{mg}}{10} = 6\ \text{mg}$

(f) $2\ \text{mL} \times \dfrac{\text{m } 15\ \text{or } 16}{1\ \text{mL}} = 2 \times \text{m } 15\ \text{or } 16 = \text{m } 30\ \text{or } 32$

(g) $\text{gr } 30 \times \dfrac{1\ \text{g}}{\text{gr } 15} = \dfrac{30\ \text{g}}{15} = 2\ \text{g}$

(h) $3\ t \times \dfrac{5\ \text{mL}}{1\ t} = 3 \times 5\ \text{mL} = 15\ \text{mL}$

(i) $\text{pt } 1\dfrac{1}{2} \times \dfrac{500\ \text{mL}}{\text{pt } 1} = \dfrac{3}{2} \times 500\ \text{mL} = 750\ \text{mL}$

(j) $10\ \text{mL} \times \dfrac{1\ t}{5\ \text{mL}} = \dfrac{10\ t}{5} = 2\ t$

(k) $\text{oz } 3 \times \dfrac{30\ \text{mL}}{\text{oz } 1} = 3 \times 30\ \text{mL} = 90\ \text{mL}$

(l) $\text{gr } \dfrac{1}{600} \times \dfrac{60\ \text{mg}}{\text{gr } 1} = \dfrac{60\ \text{mg}}{600} = \dfrac{1}{10}\ \text{mg} = 0.1\ \text{mg}$

(m) $\text{oz } 3\frac{1}{2} \times \dfrac{30 \text{ mL}}{\text{oz } 1} = \dfrac{7}{2} \times \overset{15}{30} \text{ mL} = 105 \text{ mL}$

(n) $\text{gr } \dfrac{1}{4} \times \dfrac{60 \text{ mg}}{\text{gr } 1} = \dfrac{60 \text{ mg}}{4} = 15 \text{ mg}$

(o) $1.5 \text{ mL} \times \dfrac{\text{m } 16}{1 \text{ mL}} = 1\frac{1}{2} \times \text{m } 16 = \dfrac{3}{2} \times \text{m } \overset{8}{16} = \text{m } 24$

(p) $0.2 \text{ g} \times \dfrac{\text{gr } 15}{1 \text{ g}} = 0.2 \times \text{gr } 15 = \text{gr } 3$

(q) $1250 \text{ mL} \times \dfrac{\text{qt } 1}{1000 \text{ mL}} = \text{qt } \dfrac{\overset{5}{1250}}{\underset{4}{1000}} = \text{qt} \dfrac{5}{4} = \text{qt } 1\frac{1}{4}$

(r) $\text{gr } \dfrac{3}{4} \times \dfrac{1 \text{ g}}{\text{gr } 15} = \dfrac{\overset{1}{3}}{4} \times \dfrac{1 \text{ g}}{\underset{5}{15}} = \dfrac{1}{20} \text{ g} = 0.05 \text{ g}$

(s) $0.4 \text{ mg} \times \dfrac{\text{gr } 1}{60 \text{ mg}} = \dfrac{\overset{1}{4}}{10} \times \text{gr } \dfrac{1}{\underset{15}{60}} = \text{gr } \dfrac{1}{150}$

(t) $10 \text{ mL} \times \dfrac{\text{dr } 1}{4 \text{ mL}} = \dfrac{\overset{5}{10} \times \text{dr } 1}{\underset{2}{4}} = \text{dr } \dfrac{5}{2} = \text{dr } 2\frac{1}{2}$

(u) $0.3 \text{ mL} \times \dfrac{\text{m } 15}{1 \text{ mL}} = 0.3 \times \text{m } 15 = \text{m } 4.5 \rightarrow \text{m } 5 \text{ (to the nearest unit)}$

(v) $\text{m } 20 \times \dfrac{1 \text{ mL}}{\text{m } 15} = \dfrac{20 \text{ mL}}{15} = 1.33 \text{ mL} \rightarrow 1.3 \text{ mL} \text{ (to the nearest tenth)}$

(w) $\text{pt } 3 \times \dfrac{500 \text{ mL}}{\text{pt } 1} \times \dfrac{1 \text{ L}}{1000 \text{ mL}} = \dfrac{3 \times 500}{1000} \text{ L} = \dfrac{1500}{1000} \text{ L} = 1.5 \text{ L}$

(x) $\text{gr } \dfrac{1}{300} \times \dfrac{60 \text{ mg}}{\text{gr } 1} \times \dfrac{1000 \text{ μg}}{1 \text{ mg}} = \dfrac{60{,}000 \text{ μg}}{300} = 200 \text{ μg}$

Supplementary Problems

4.6 Write out the meaning of each of the following abbreviations in full, and indicate whether the unit is metric, apothecary, or household.

(a) m 32

(b) 70 mm

(c) 5 mL

(d) gr $\dfrac{1}{4}$

(e) oz $1\frac{1}{2}$

(f) dr 2

(g) 1 T

(h) 0.25 g

(i) 30 mg

(j) 6 oz

(k) 3 t

(l) qt 2

(m) dr $2\frac{1}{2}$

(n) $\dfrac{1}{4}$ C

(o) 300 μg

(p) 3 dL

4.7   Change each of the following from one numeration system to the other (base ten or Roman).

(a) v   (f) 34   (k) 19   (p) xi

(b) iv   (g) $2\frac{1}{2}$ (l) $7\frac{1}{2}$ (q) 36

(c) viii   (h) xvii   (m) 29   (r) $4\frac{1}{2}$

(d) i$\overline{ss}$ (i) v$\overline{ss}$ (n) iii$\overline{ss}$ (s) 39

(e) xxi   (j) ix   (o) $1\frac{1}{2}$ (t) ii$\overline{ss}$

4.8   Using dimensional analysis, solve the following problems.

(a) oz 2 = dr ?   (e) dr 2 = oz ?   (i) 6 oz = ? C

(b) 2 T = ? oz   (f) pt $\frac{1}{2}$ = oz ?   (j) 2 t = ? oz

(c) qt 2 = pt ?   (g) $\frac{1}{2}$ C = ? oz   (k) oz 16 = qt ?

(d) $\frac{1}{2}$ T = ? t   (h) oz $\frac{3}{4}$ = dr ?   (l) pt $\frac{1}{2}$ = dr ?

(m) Find the weight of a child in kilograms if he weighs 86 lb, given that 1 kg = 2.2 lb (give the answer to the nearest tenth).

(n) A baby weighs 8 kg. Find her weight in pounds (to the nearest tenth).

(o) A gram of fat yields approximately 9 cal. Find the number of dietary calories provided by 60 g of fat (to the nearest one).

(p) A person is 58 in tall. Find the height in centimeters, given that 1 in = 2.54 cm (answer to the nearest one).

(q) For a child who is 96 cm tall, find the height in inches (to the nearest one).

(r) At the end of 3 months a fetus is about 7.5 cm in length. How many inches is this?

(s) The brain of an adult weighs about 1300 g. About how many pounds is this?

(t) An intravenous solution is being administered at the rate of 2.5 mL/min. How many hours will it take to give 1500 mL?

4.9   Perform the following metric conversions (use Table 4-4).

(a) 3 L = ? mL   (k) 40 g = ? kg

(b) 1.65 kg = ? g   (l) 320 cc = ? mL

(c) 6 mL = ? cc   (m) 750 µg = ? mg

(d) 2.275 g = ? mg   (n) 50 mL = ? L

(e) 0.3 L = ? mL   (o) 6.5 mg = ? g

(f) 0.070 mg = ? µg   (p) 0.2 mL = ? L

(g) 0.009 g = ? mg   (q) 3.2 m = ? cm

(h) 3160 mg = ? g   (r) 0.25 m = ? mm

(i) 410 mL = ? L   (s) 450 cm = ? m

(j) 300 mg = ? g   (t) 65 mm = ? cm

4.10 Perform the following conversions (use the relationships of Sec. 4.9).

(a) oz 2 = ? mL (m) gr $\frac{1}{150}$ = ? mg

(b) 2 t = ? mL (n) 750 mL = pt ?

(c) 180 mg = gr ? (o) oz $\overline{ss}$ = ? mL

(d) pt ii = ? mL (p) 0.5 g = gr ?

(e) dr 2 = ? mL (q) dr i$\overline{ss}$ = ? mL

(f) 2 g = gr ? (r) 10 mL = ? T

(g) 30 mg = gr ? (s) 0.2 mL = ᵯ ?

(h) 60 mL = oz ? (t) gr iii = ? g

(i) 15 mL = dr ? (u) 0.75 mL = ᵯ ?

(j) gr $\frac{1}{6}$ = ? mg (v) pt $\overline{ss}$ = ? mL

(k) $\frac{1}{2}$ T = ? mL (w) gr $\frac{1}{600}$ = ? μg

(l) 0.5 mL = ᵯ ? (x) 0.25 L = qt ?

Answers to Supplementary Problems

4.6
(a) 32 minims (apothecary) (i) 30 milligrams (metric)

(b) 70 millimeters (metric) (j) 6 ounces (household)

(c) 5 milliliters (metric) (k) 3 teaspoons (household)

(d) $\frac{1}{4}$ grain (apothecary) (l) 2 quarts (apothecary)

(e) 1$\frac{1}{2}$ ounces (apothecary) (m) 2$\frac{1}{2}$ drams (apothecary)

(f) 2 drams (apothecary) (n) $\frac{1}{4}$ measuring cup (household)

(g) 1 tablespoon (household) (o) 300 micrograms (metric)

(h) 0.25 gram (metric) (p) 3 deciliters (metric)

4.7
(a)	5	(f)	xxxiv	(k)	xix	(p)	11
(b)	4	(g)	ii$\overline{ss}$	(l)	vii$\overline{ss}$	(q)	xxxvi
(c)	8	(h)	17	(m)	xxix	(r)	iv$\overline{ss}$
(d)	1$\frac{1}{2}$	(i)	5$\frac{1}{2}$	(n)	3$\frac{1}{2}$	(s)	xxxix
(e)	21	(j)	9	(o)	i$\overline{ss}$	(t)	2$\frac{1}{2}$

4.8
(a)	dr 16	(f)	oz 8	(k)	qt $\frac{1}{2}$	(p)	147 cm
(b)	oz 1	(g)	4 oz	(l)	dr 64	(q)	38 in
(c)	pt 4	(h)	dr 6	(m)	39.1 kg	(r)	3 in
(d)	1$\frac{1}{2}$ t	(i)	$\frac{3}{4}$ C	(n)	17.6 lb	(s)	2.9 lb
(e)	oz $\frac{1}{4}$	(j)	$\frac{1}{3}$ oz	(o)	540 cal	(t)	10 h

4.9   (*a*) 3000 mL   (*f*) 70 μg   (*k*) 0.04 kg   (*p*) 0.0002 L
        (*b*) 1650 g   (*g*) 9 mg   (*l*) 320 mL   (*q*) 320 cm
        (*c*) 6 cc   (*h*) 3.16 g   (*m*) 0.75 mg   (*r*) 250 mm
        (*d*) 2275 mg   (*i*) 0.41 L   (*n*) 0.05 L   (*s*) 4.5 m
        (*e*) 300 mL   (*j*) 0.3 g   (*o*) 0.0065 g   (*t*) 6.5 cm

4.10 (*a*) 60 mL   (*g*) gr $\frac{1}{2}$ (*m*) 0.4 mg   (*s*) m 3

        (*b*) 10 mL   (*h*) oz 2   (*n*) pt $1\frac{1}{2}$ (*t*) 0.2 g

        (*c*) gr 3   (*i*) dr $3\frac{3}{4}$ (*o*) 15 mL   (*u*) m 12

        (*d*) 1000 mL   (*j*) 10 mg   (*p*) gr $7\frac{1}{2}$ (*v*) 250 mL

        (*e*) 8 mL   (*k*) 7.5 mL   (*q*) 6 mL   (*w*) 100 μg

        (*f*) gr 30   (*l*) m 8   (*r*) $\frac{2}{3}$ T   (*x*) qt $\frac{1}{4}$

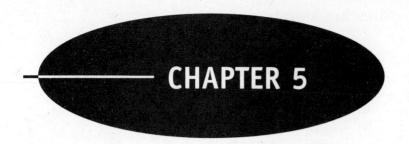

CHAPTER 5

Oral Medication

5.1 CONVERTING MEDICAL DOSAGES

In this chapter you will learn how to convert a medical dosage from a doctor's order to a form in which it can be administered orally. Oral medication is given in solid or liquid form. When the available form is solid, the units of measurement will be tablets (tab) or capsules (cap). Thus, the problem will be to convert the doctor's order to the appropriate number of tablets or capsules:

$$\text{Doctor's order} \rightarrow ? \text{ tab or cap}$$

When the available form is liquid, the administered drug will be measured in units of volume, for example, milliliters. Thus, the problem will be to convert the doctor's order to the appropriate number of milliliters:

$$\text{Doctor's order} \rightarrow ? \text{ mL}$$

5.2 ORAL MEDICATION IN SOLID FORM

Typical solid forms of medication are tablets and capsules (see Fig. 5-1). Capsules are never broken into smaller parts but are dispensed whole. Whenever possible, tablets are also given whole. In situations where tablets of the required size are not available, it may be necessary to break a tablet in half. A tablet is suitable for breaking if it is *scored*, that is, etched with a line which facilitates breaking it into halves (see Fig. 5-1). Since even a scored tablet is difficult to break in half, breaking should be avoided whenever possible.

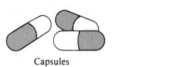

Capsules

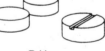

Tablets

Fig. 5-1

When the medication to be administered is in solid form, the relationship to use for the conversion (doctor's order→tab or cap) is the *strength* of the tablets or capsules available, that is, the amount of drug per tablet or capsule. Tablets or capsules of a particular drug may be manufactured in different strengths. For example, vitamin C (ascorbic acid) comes in 250-mg and 500-mg tablets. The relationship to use to convert the doctor's order will then be either 250 mg per tablet or 500 mg per tablet, depending on which strength is used.

EXAMPLE 5.1   The doctor has ordered 20 mg of Prozac for a patient. The label for the tablets on hand is shown in Fig. 5-2. How many tablets should be given?

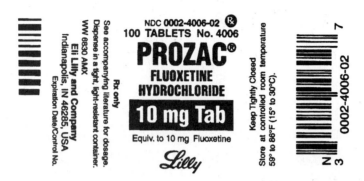

Fig. 5-2

The required conversion is: 20 mg → ? tab

The relationship to use is: 1 tab = 10 mg

Set up the calculation: $20 \text{ mg} \times \dfrac{1 \text{ tab}}{10 \text{ mg}}$

Perform the calculation: $\dfrac{20}{10} \text{ tab} = 2 \text{ tab}$

For a problem like this, you should also develop the ability to reason as suggested by Fig. 5-3.

1 tab		1 tab		2 tabs
10 mg	+	10 mg	=	20 mg

Fig. 5-3

EXAMPLE 5.2   The order is for 15 mg of codeine. The available tablets are scored and each contains 30 mg. How many tablets should you give?

The required conversion is: 15 mg → ? tab

The relationship to use is: 1 tab = 30 mg

Set up the calculation: $15 \text{ mg} \times \dfrac{1 \text{ tab}}{30 \text{ mg}}$

Perform the calculation: $\dfrac{\overset{1}{15}}{\underset{2}{30}} \text{ tab} = \dfrac{1}{2} \text{ tab}$

Thus, to give 15 mg of codeine using tablets containing 30 mg each, give half a tablet.

Again, you should develop the ability to see that the answer makes sense by reasoning as shown in Fig. 5-4.

EXAMPLE 5.3   The order is for 5 mg of Zyprexa. The labels for the tablets on hand are shown in Fig. 5-5. How many tablets of each dosage should be given?

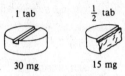

Fig. 5-4

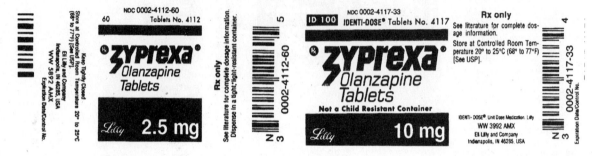

Fig. 5-5

The required conversion is: 5 mg → ? tab

For the 2.5-mg tablets: $5 \text{ mg} \times \dfrac{1 \text{ tab}}{2.5 \text{ mg}} = \dfrac{5}{2.5} \text{ tab} = 2 \text{ tab}$

For the 10-mg tablets: $5 \text{ mg} \times \dfrac{1 \text{ tab}}{10 \text{ mg}} = \dfrac{5}{10} \text{ tab} = \dfrac{1}{2} \text{ tab}$

The best choice is the 2.5-mg tablets, since you will not be required to break tablets.

EXAMPLE 5.4   The order is for Gantrisin 1500 mg PO. The bottle of tablets is labeled "Gantrisin 0.5 g." How many tablets should you administer?

The required conversion is: 1500 mg → ? tab

This requires two steps because the
order is given in milligrams
but the strength of the
tablets is given in grams: 1500 mg → ? g → ? tab

The relationships to use are: 1 g = 1000 mg and 1 tab = 0.5 g

Set up the calculation: $1500 \text{ mg} \times \dfrac{1 \text{ g}}{1000 \text{ mg}} \times \dfrac{1 \text{ tab}}{0.5 \text{ g}}$

Perform the calculation: $\dfrac{1500}{1000 \times 0.5} \text{ tab} = \dfrac{\overset{3}{\cancel{1500}}}{\underset{1}{\cancel{500}}} \text{ tab} = 3 \text{ tab}$

Thus, you would give 3 tablets of 0.5 g each to administer 1500 mg.

EXAMPLE 5.5   The order is for 200 mg tid of Difulcan. The labels for the tablets on hand are shown in Fig. 5-6. How many tablets of each dosage should be given?

The required conversion is: 200 mg → ? tab

For the 50-mg tablets: $200 \text{ mg} \times \dfrac{1 \text{ tab}}{50 \text{ mg}} = \dfrac{200}{50} \text{ tab} = 4 \text{ tab}$

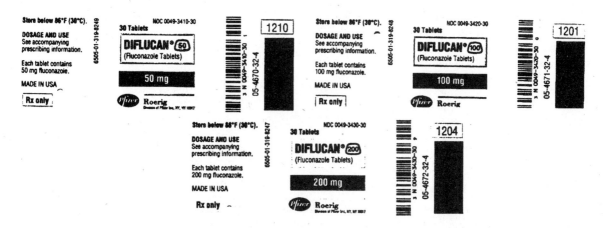

Fig. 5-6

For the 100-mg tablets:

$$200 \; \text{mg} \times \frac{1 \; \text{tab}}{100 \; \text{mg}} = \frac{200}{100} \; \text{tab} = 2 \; \text{tab}$$

For the 200-mg tablets:

$$200 \; \text{mg} \times \frac{1 \; \text{tab}}{200 \; \text{mg}} = \frac{200}{200} \; \text{tab} = 1 \; \text{tab}$$

EXAMPLE 5.6   The doctor orders 150 mg of a medication. On hand are two bottles, one containing tablets of 100 mg each and the other containing tablets of 75 mg each. Which tablets should you give, and how many?

The problem is to give the exact amount of medication ordered using the smallest number of whole tablets. Calculate the answer for both strengths.

1.   For the 100-mg tablets:

$$\overset{3}{150} \; \text{mg} \times \frac{1 \; \text{tab}}{\underset{2}{100} \; \text{mg}} = \frac{3}{2} \; \text{tab} = 1\frac{1}{2} \text{tab}$$

2.   For the 75-mg tablets:

$$\overset{2}{150} \; \text{mg} \times \frac{1 \; \text{tab}}{\underset{1}{75} \; \text{mg}} = \frac{2}{1} \; \text{tab} = 2 \; \text{tab}$$

Since it is best to avoid breaking tablets, you should give two 75-mg tablets containing a total of 2×75 mg = 150 mg.

Drugs Measured by Units.   Some drugs are measured according to their active strength by standards of measurement known as units (U). Some examples are penicillin, insulin, vitamins, and heparin. The meaning of the term "unit" differs according to the type of drug to which it is applied. For example, a unit of penicillin and a unit of insulin have different meanings. The definitions of these terms are beyond the scope of this book. It is sufficient to say that these units are used in drug conversion problems in the same way that units of weight are used.

EXAMPLE 5.7   Penicillin G potassium 1.6 million U is to be administered in 4 equal doses. The tablets on hand each contain 400,000 U. How many tablets should be given per dose?

The required conversion is: 1,600,000 U → ? tab

The relationship to use is: 1 tab = 400,000 U

Set up the calculation:

$$1{,}600{,}000 \; \text{U} \times \frac{1 \; \text{tab}}{400{,}000 \; \text{U}}$$

The order is to be administered
in 4 equal doses. Therefore,
divide the dosage by 4. This
can be done by multiplying the

calculation by $\frac{1}{4}$:

$$\frac{1}{4} \times 1,600,000 \, \cancel{U} \times \frac{1 \text{ tab}}{400,000 \, \cancel{U}}$$

$$= \frac{1,600,000}{4 \times 400,000} \text{ tab} = 1 \text{ tab}$$

5.3   ORAL MEDICATION IN LIQUID FORM

Typical liquid medications for oral administration are solutions and suspensions, which consist of an active ingredient contained in a liquid vehicle. The amount of active ingredient (the drug) contained in a certain volume of the liquid is the *concentration* of the medication. The concentration is the relationship used to perform the required conversion, doctor's order→ ? mL. For example, tetracycline is available as a syrup, in which 5 mL of the syrup contains 125 mg of the drug. The relationship used to perform the conversion is: 5 mL syrup = 125 mg drug.

EXAMPLE 5.8   The doctor orders tetracycline 250 mg PO. The bottle of tetracycline syrup indicates that the concentration is 125 mg per 5 mL. How many milliliters would you give?

The problem is to find the volume of syrup which contains 250 mg of tetracycline.

The required conversion is: 250 mg → ? mL

The relationship to use is: 5 mL = 125 mg

Set up the calculation: $250 \, \cancel{mg} \times \dfrac{5 \text{ mL}}{125 \, \cancel{mg}}$

Perform the calculation: $\dfrac{\overset{2}{\cancel{250}} \times 5 \text{ mL}}{\underset{1}{\cancel{125}}} = 10 \text{ mL}$

Thus, 250 mg of tetracycline is contained in 10 mL of the syrup.

You should also recognize that: 250 mg = 125 mg + 125 mg. Therefore, 5 mL + 5 mL = 10 mL will contain 250 mg.

Drugs Measured in Milliequivalents.   An *equivalent* (Eq) is a measure of the number of ionic charges contained in a certain amount of an electrolytic compound. Therefore, an equivalent measures the active strength, or chemical combining power, of a compound. A *milliequivalent* (mEq) is one-thousandth of an equivalent. Dosages of certain drugs are measured in milliequivalents. One such drug is potassium chloride, which is available in a concentration of 40 mEq in 30 mL. The concentration, whatever it may be in a given problem, is used as the relationship to perform the dosage conversion.

EXAMPLE 5.9   The patient is to receive potassium chloride 20 mEq. You have on hand a bottle labeled "potassium chloride (KCl) 40 mEq per 30 mL." How many milliliters will you administer to the patient?

The required conversion is: 20 mEq → ? mL

The relationship to use is: 30 mL = 40 mEq

Set up the calculation: $20 \, \cancel{mEq} \times \dfrac{30 \text{ mL}}{40 \, \cancel{mEq}}$

Perform the calculation: $\dfrac{\overset{1}{\cancel{20}} \times 30 \text{ mL}}{\underset{2}{\cancel{40}}} = \dfrac{\overset{15}{\cancel{30}} \text{ mL}}{\underset{1}{\cancel{2}}} = 15 \text{ mL}$

Thus, to administer 20 mEq, you would give 15 mL of the solution.

EXAMPLE 5.10   You are to administer 0.2 g of a drug PO. On hand is a bottle labeled "125 mg per 5 mL." How many milliliters of the medication should you give?

The required conversion is:	$0.2\ \text{g} \rightarrow ?\ \text{mL}$

The order is in grams, but the concentration relates milligrams to milliliters; therefore convert the grams to milligrams, then convert the milligrams to milliliters.

This requires two steps:	$0.2\ \text{g} \rightarrow ?\ \text{mg} \rightarrow ?\ \text{mL}$
The relationships to use are:	$1\ \text{g} = 1000\ \text{mg}$ and $125\ \text{mg} = 5\ \text{mL}$
Set up the calculation:	$0.2\ \cancel{\text{g}} \times \dfrac{1000\ \cancel{\text{mg}}}{1\ \cancel{\text{g}}} \times \dfrac{5\ \text{mL}}{125\ \cancel{\text{mg}}}$
Perform the calculation:	$\dfrac{0.2 \times \overset{8}{\cancel{1000}} \times 5\ \text{mL}}{\underset{1}{\cancel{125}}} = 0.2 \times 8 \times 5\ \text{mL} = 8\ \text{mL}$

Thus, you would administer 8 mL of the solution, which will contain 0.2 g of the drug.

EXAMPLE 5.11   The order is for 25 mg of Thorazine syrup. The label for the bottle on hand is shown in Fig. 5-7. How many milliliters of Thorazine should be given?

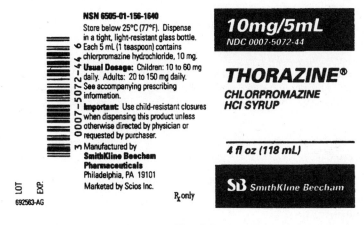

Fig. 5-7

The required conversion is:	$25\ \text{mg} \rightarrow ?\ \text{mL}$
The relationship to use is:	$10\ \text{mg} = 5\ \text{mL}$
Set up the calculation:	$25\ \cancel{\text{mg}} \times \dfrac{5\ \text{mL}}{10\ \cancel{\text{mg}}}$
Perform the calculation:	$\dfrac{25 \times 5\ \text{mL}}{10} = \dfrac{125\ \text{mL}}{10} = 12.5\ \text{mL}$

EXAMPLE 5.12   The order is for 2 g of a drug to be given PO in 4 equally divided doses. The drug label reads, "200 mg per 2 mL." How many milliliters should be given per dose?

The required conversion is:	$2\ \text{g} \rightarrow ?\ \text{mL}$
This requires two steps:	$2\ \text{g} \rightarrow ?\ \text{mg} \rightarrow ?\ \text{mL}$

The relationships to use are:

$$1 \text{ g} = 1000 \text{ mg and } 200 \text{ mg} = 2 \text{ mL}$$

Set up the calculation:

$$2 \text{ g} \times \frac{1000 \text{ mg}}{1 \text{ g}} \times \frac{2 \text{ mL}}{200 \text{ mg}}$$

The order is to be administered in 4 equal doses, so at this point the dosage will be divided by 4. Do this by multiplying the calculation by $\frac{1}{4}$:

$$\frac{1}{4} \times 2 \cancel{g} \times \frac{1000 \cancel{mg}}{1 \cancel{g}} \times \frac{2 \text{ mL}}{200 \cancel{mg}}$$

$$= \frac{2 \times \overset{5}{\cancel{1000}} \times 2 \text{ mL}}{4 \times \underset{1}{\cancel{200}}} = \frac{\overset{5}{\cancel{20}} \text{ mL}}{\underset{1}{\cancel{4}}} = 5 \text{ mL}$$

The order is administered in 4 equal doses of 5 mL per dose.

5.4   RECONSTITUTING POWDERS OR CRYSTALS TO LIQUID FORM

Some medications which are administered in liquid form are packaged as dry powder or crystals of the drug. This is because the drug is not stable and tends to deteriorate when in liquid form. Such drugs must be reconstituted to liquid form before administration by adding water to the container according to the directions on the package. For example, amoxicillin is packaged as a dry powder in variously sized bottles, with directions for reconstituting the powder to liquid form. The relationship to use for the conversion is the concentration stated on the package.

EXAMPLE 5.13   The order is for amoxicillin 750 mg PO. You have on hand a 150-mL bottle of dry powder. The directions read, "Add 105 mL of water and shake well to obtain 150 mL of suspension containing 250 mg per 5 mL." (*a*) How many milliliters will contain 750 mg? (*b*) Divided into 3 equal doses, how many milliliters will there be per dose?

(*a*)   Calculate the total order.

The required conversion is:

$$750 \text{ mg} \rightarrow \text{ ? mL}$$

The relationship to use is:

$$5 \text{ mL} = 250 \text{ mg}$$

Set up the calculation:

$$750 \cancel{mg} \times \frac{5 \text{ mL}}{250 \cancel{mg}}$$

Perform the calculation:

$$\frac{\overset{3}{\cancel{750}} \times 5 \text{ mL}}{\underset{1}{\cancel{250}}} = 15 \text{ mL}$$

Thus, 15 mL contains 750 mg.

(*b*)   Divided into 3 equal doses, each dose is $\dfrac{15 \text{ mL}}{3} = 5 \text{ mL}$ per dose.

Solved Problems

5.1   The doctor orders Tylenol 650 mg. If 325-mg tablets are available, how many tablets would you give?

Solution

The required conversion is:	650 mg → ? tab
The relationship to use is:	1 tab = 325 mg
Set up the calculation:	$650 \, \text{mg} \times \dfrac{1 \, \text{tab}}{325 \, \text{mg}}$
Perform the calculation:	$\dfrac{\overset{2}{650}}{\underset{1}{325}} \, \text{tab} = 2 \, \text{tab}$

5.2 The physician orders 200 mg of a drug. The bottle containing the drug is labeled "125 mg per 5 mL." How many milliliters should you give?

Solution

The required conversion is:	200 mg → ? mL
The relationship to use is:	125 mg = 5 mL
Set up the calculation:	$200 \, \text{mg} \times \dfrac{5 \, \text{mL}}{125 \, \text{mg}}$
Perform the calculation:	$\dfrac{200 \times \overset{1}{\cancel{5}} \, \text{mL}}{\underset{25}{\cancel{125}}} = \dfrac{\overset{8}{200}}{\underset{1}{25}} \, \text{mL} = 8 \, \text{mL}$

5.3 Vitamin A 100,000 U PO daily is ordered. The capsules on hand contain 25,000 U each. How many capsules should you administer?

Solution

The required conversion is:	100,000 U → ? cap
The relationship to use is:	1 cap = 25,000 U
Set up the calculation:	$100,000 \, \text{U} \times \dfrac{1 \, \text{cap}}{25,000 \, \text{U}}$
Perform the calculation:	$\dfrac{\overset{4}{100,000}}{\underset{1}{25,000}} \, \text{cap} = 4 \, \text{cap}$

5.4 Potassium gluconate 25 mEq is to be administered. The bottle of elixir is labeled "20 mEq per 15 mL." How many milliliters will contain the order?

Solution

The required conversion is:	25 mEq → ? mL
The relationship to use is:	20 mEq = 15 mL
Set up the calculation:	$25 \, \text{mEq} \times \dfrac{15 \, \text{mL}}{20 \, \text{mEq}}$
Perform the calculation:	$\dfrac{\overset{5}{25} \times 15 \, \text{mL}}{\underset{4}{20}} = \dfrac{75 \, \text{mL}}{4}$

$$= 18.8 \, \text{mL (nearest tenth)}$$

5.5 The order is for Zithromax PO 500 mg on day 1, then 250 mg qd on days 2–5 for a total dose of 1.5 g. The label of the bottle on hand is shown in Fig. 5-8.

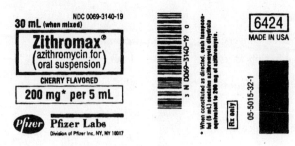

Fig. 5-8

(a)   How many milliliters should be administered on day 1?

(b)   How many milliliters should be administered on days 2–5?

(c)   Would the 30-mL size be large enough for the full course?

Solution

(a)   The required conversion is: 500 mg → mL

The relationship to use is: 5 mL = 200 mg

Set up the calculation: $500 \text{ mg} \times \dfrac{5 \text{ mL}}{200 \text{ mg}}$

Perform the calculation: $\dfrac{500 \times 5 \text{ mL}}{200} = \dfrac{2500 \text{ mL}}{200} = 12.5 \text{ mL}$

(b)   The required conversion is: 250 mg → mL

The relationship to use is: 5 mL = 200 mg

Set up the calculation: $250 \text{ mg} \times \dfrac{5 \text{ mL}}{200 \text{ mg}}$

Perform the calculation: $\dfrac{250 \times 5 \text{ mL}}{200} = \dfrac{1250 \text{ mL}}{200} = 6.25 \text{ mL}$

(c)   The 30-mL bottle would not contain enough drug for the full course of the ordered therapy, since 12.5 mL + 4 × 6.25 mL = 37.5 mL exceeds 30 mL.

5.6   You are to give Prostaphlin (oxacillin sodium) 2 g daily using 500-mg capsules. How many capsules should you give each day?

Solution

The required conversion is: 2 g → ? cap

This requires two steps: 2 g → ? mg → ? cap

The relationships to use are: 1 g = 1000 mg and 1 cap = 500 mg

Set up the calculation: $2 \text{ g} \times \dfrac{1000 \text{ mg}}{1 \text{ g}} \times \dfrac{1 \text{ cap}}{500 \text{ mg}}$

Perform the calculation: $2 \times \dfrac{1000}{500} \text{ cap} = 4 \text{ cap}$

5.7   The order is for Zoloft 50 mg qd. The label of the tablets on hand is shown in Fig. 5-9. How many tablets should you give daily?

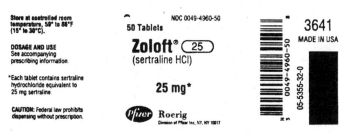

Store at controlled room
temperature, 59° to 86°F
(15° to 30°C).

DOSAGE AND USE
See accompanying
prescribing information.

*Each tablet contains sertraline
hydrochloride equivalent to
25 mg sertraline.

CAUTION: Federal law prohibits
dispensing without prescription.

NDC 0049-4960-50

50 Tablets

Zoloft® ⬭25⬭
(sertraline HCl)

25 mg*

Pfizer **Roerig**
Division of Pfizer Inc, NY, NY 10017

3641
MADE IN USA

Fig. 5-9

Solution

The required conversion is: 50 mg → ? tab

The relationship to use is: 1 tab = 25 mg

Set up the calculation: $50 \text{ mg} \times \dfrac{1 \text{ tab}}{25 \text{ mg}}$

Perform the calculation: $\dfrac{50 \text{ tab}}{25} = 2 \text{ tab}$

5.8   The order calls for 1 g of amoxicillin PO tid. The label reads "amoxicillin 250 mg/5 mL." How many milliliters should be given for each dose?

Solution

The required conversion is: 1 g → ? mL

This requires two steps: 1 g → 1000 mg → ? mL

Set up the calculation: $1 \text{ g} \times \dfrac{1000 \text{ mg}}{1 \text{ g}} \times \dfrac{5 \text{ mL}}{250 \text{ mg}}$

Perform the calculation: $\dfrac{1000 \times 5 \text{ mL}}{250} = 20 \text{ mL}$

5.9   Terramycin syrup contains oxytetracycline HCl 125 mg per 5 mL. You are to give 1 g in 4 equal doses. How many milliliters should be given per dose?

Solution

The required conversion is: 1 g → ? mL

This requires two steps: 1 g → ? mg → ? mL

The relationships to use are: 1 g = 1000 mg and 125 mg = 5 mL

Set up the calculation: $\dfrac{1}{4} \times 1 \text{ g} \times \dfrac{1000 \text{ mg}}{1 \text{ g}} \times \dfrac{5 \text{ mL}}{125 \text{ mg}}$

Perform the calculation: $\dfrac{\overset{8}{1000} \times 5 \text{ mL}}{4 \times \underset{1}{125}} = \dfrac{\overset{2}{8} \times 5 \text{ mL}}{\underset{1}{4}} = 10 \text{ mL}$

5.10   A bottle contains penicillin V potassium powder for reconstitution. The directions read, "Add 60 mL of water to package to obtain 100 mL of solution containing 200,000 U per 5 mL." How many milliliters are needed to administer 300,000 U of the drug?

Solution

The required conversion is:	$300,000 \text{ U} \rightarrow ? \text{ mL}$
The relationship to use is:	$200,000 \text{ U} = 5 \text{ mL}$
Set up the calculation:	$300,000 \text{ U} \times \dfrac{5 \text{ mL}}{200,000 \text{ U}}$
Perform the calculation:	$\dfrac{\overset{3}{\cancel{300,000}} \times 5 \text{ mL}}{\underset{2}{\cancel{200,000}}} = \dfrac{15}{2} \text{ mL} = 7.5 \text{ mL}$

5.11 The physician orders 1 g of an antibiotic to be given PO. The drug is in powdered form. The directions for reconstitution read, "Add 65 mL of sterile water to obtain 100 mL of suspension containing 300 mg per 5 mL." How many milliliters will contain the order?

Solution

The required conversion is:	$1 \text{ g} \rightarrow ? \text{ mL}$
This requires two steps:	$1 \text{ g} \rightarrow ? \text{ mg} \rightarrow ? \text{ mL}$
The relationships to use are:	$1 \text{ g} = 1000 \text{ mg}$ and $300 \text{ mg} = 5 \text{ mL}$
Set up the calculation:	$1 \text{ g} \times \dfrac{1000 \text{ mg}}{1 \text{ g}} \times \dfrac{5 \text{ mL}}{300 \text{ mg}}$
Perform the calculation:	$\dfrac{\overset{10}{\cancel{1000}} \times 5 \text{ mL}}{\underset{3}{\cancel{300}}} = \dfrac{50 \text{ mL}}{3}$
	$= 16.3 \text{ mL} \qquad \text{(nearest tenth)}$

5.12 The order is for Lorabid PO 400 mg q12h for 14 days. The labels for the capsules on hand is shown in Fig. 5-10.

(*a*) How many capsules are to be given per dose?

(*b*) How many total capsules will be needed for the 14 days of therapy?

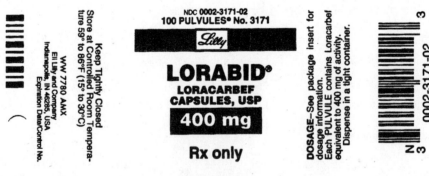

Fig. 5-10

Solution

(*a*) The required conversion is:	$400 \text{ mg} \rightarrow ? \text{ cap}$
The relationship to use is:	$1 \text{ cap} = 400 \text{ mg}$

Set up the calculation: $400 \text{ mg} \times \dfrac{1 \text{ cap}}{400 \text{ mg}}$

Perform the calculation: $\dfrac{400 \text{ cap}}{400} = 1 \text{ cap}$

(b) Two capsules are to be taken per day for 14 days, that is, 2 cap → 1 day.

The required conversion is: 14 days → ? cap

The relationship to use is: 1 day = 2 cap

Set up the calculation: $14 \text{ days} \times \dfrac{2 \text{ cap}}{1 \text{ day}}$

Perform the calculation: $\dfrac{14 \times 2 \text{ cap}}{1} = 28 \text{ cap}$

Supplementary Problems

5.13 The physician orders 150 mg of a medication to be given PO. The tablets on hand contain 75 mg each. How many tablets do you administer?

5.14 You are to give cortisone acetate 75 mg PO. The tablets each contain 25 mg. How many tablets should you administer?

5.15 The order is for Chlor-Trimeton 3 mg. The bottle of syrup is labeled "2 mg per 5 mL." How many milliliters should be given?

5.16 The doctor's order is for Dilaudid 6 mg. The tablets on hand contain 2 mg each of the drug. How many tablets should you give?

5.17 Tablets of penicillin G potassium containing 400,000 U each are available. How many tablets are needed to give 800,000 U?

5.18 Cimetidine 400 mg PO is ordered. The available medication is labeled, "cimetidine 300 mg per 5 mL." How many milliliters should be administered? Give answer to nearest tenth.

5.19 Coumadin (warfarin sodium) 15 mg is ordered. The only tablets available are scored tablets containing 10 mg each. How would you administer the medication?

5.20 Phenergan tablets containing 12.5 mg each are available. You are to give 25 mg PO. How many tablets should you administer?

5.21 You are to administer 325 mg of a drug from a bottle which is labeled "50 mg/mL." How many milliliters should you administer?

5.22 The order is for 0.25 mg of Lanoxin pediatric elixir. The label for the bottle on hand is shown in Fig. 5-11. How many teaspoons should be given?

5.23 You are to give 15 mEq of potassium gluconate from a bottle containing 20 mEq per 15 mL. How many milliliters are needed? Give answer to nearest tenth.

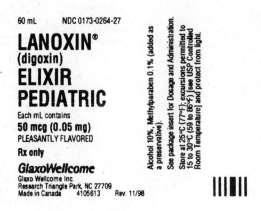

Fig. 5-11

5.24   The order is for 0.25 mg of atropine sulfate. The bottle of elixir contains 0.039 mg/mL of the drug. How many milliliters should you give? Give answer to nearest tenth.

5.25   The doctor's order is for 50 mg of Amoxil tid. The label for the Amoxil on hand is shown in Fig. 5-12. When 12 mL of water is added, the Amoxil is reconstituted to 15 mL of 50 mg/mL. The order is for 50 mg tid. (*a*) How many milliliters is each dose? (*b*) How many total milliliters will the patient receive each day? (*c*) How many total doses does the bottle contain?

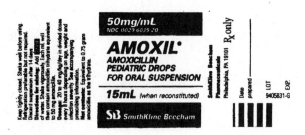

Fig. 5-12

5.26   The doctor orders 55 mg of Choledyl. Choledyl pediatric syrup contains 50 mg per 5 mL of the drug. How many milliliters should the child receive?

5.27   Ordinase (tolbutamide) 1.5 g is to be administered using 500-mg tablets. How many tablets should you give?

5.28   Thiosulfil (sulfamethizole) 1000 mg is to be given from tablets containing 0.5 g each of the drug. How many tablets should you administer?

5.29   You are to administer Gantrisin (sulfisoxazole) 2 g. The tablets contain 500 mg each. How many tablets should you give?

5.30   A bottle of digoxin elixir is labeled "digoxin 50 μg/mL." How many milliliters contain 0.3 mg?

5.31   You are to give Talwin 0.05 g PO. On hand are 50-mg tablets. How many tablets are required?

5.32   The label on a bottle of medication indicates a concentration of 125 mg/mL. You are directed to administer 0.8 g. How many milliliters will you give?

5.33   The doctor orders 0.04 g of Lasix (furosemide) PO. On hand are 40-mg tablets. How many do you give?

5.34   On hand are aminophylline capsules containing 250 mg each of the drug. How many capsules are needed to give 0.5 g?

5.35   The doctor orders 125 μg of Synthroid. On hand are 0.125-mg uncoated tablets. How many do you give?

5.36   The order is for 25 mg of Vioxx. The label for the tablets on hand is shown in Fig. 5-13. How many Vioxx tablets should you administer?

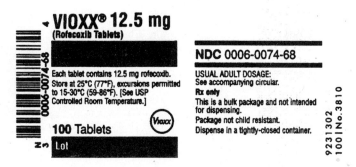

Fig. 5-13

5.37   You have tablets containing 15 mg of codeine on hand. How many tablets do you need to administer 30 mg of codeine?

5.38   If one scored tablet contains 250 mg of a drug, how many tablets will be needed to give 0.5 g of the drug?

5.39   The physician's assistant orders 0.5 g rectal of chloral hydrate. Suppositories of 500 mg are available. How many should be administered?

5.40   A medication is available 20 mg per 5 mL. The doctor orders 120 mg, to be divided into 4 equal doses. How many cc's should be given per dose?

5.41   You are to administer 100 mg of phenobarbital. The phenobarbital is available as 100-mg tablets and as an oral elixir 20 mg/5 mL. (*a*) How many tablets would be needed? (*b*) How many milliliters of oral elixir would be needed?

5.42   The nurse practitioner orders 90 mg of a drug. The concentration stated on the label is 30 mg per 5 mL. How many milliliters should be administered?

5.43   The directions for ampicillin for oral suspension read, "Add 66 mL of distilled water to the powder to obtain 100 mL of suspension containing 250 mg per 5 mL." How many milliliters per dose will you give if you are to give 900 mg divided into three equal doses?

5.44   The directions for Coly-Mycin for oral suspension read, "Reconstitute with 37 mL of water to obtain 60 mL containing 25 mg per 5 mL." The order is for 115 mg divided into 3 equal doses. How many milliliters per dose will you administer? Give answers to nearest tenth.

5.45   The order is for 8 mg of Cardura. The labels for the bottles on hand are shown in Fig. 5-14. How should you administer the order?

5.46   If the order in Problem 5.45 is for 4 mg of Cardura, how should you administer the order?

5.47   If the order in Problem 5.45 is for 6 mg of Cardura, how should you administer the order?

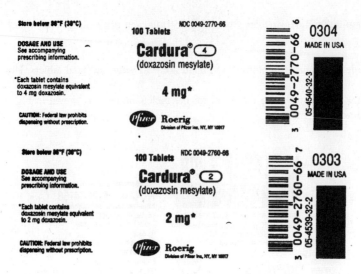

Fig. 5-14

Answers to Supplementary Problems

5.13	2 tablets	**5.25**	(*a*) 1 mL; (*b*) 3 mL; (*c*) 15 doses	**5.37**	2 tablets	
5.14	3 tablets	**5.26**	5.5 mL	**5.38**	2 tablets	
5.15	7.5 mL	**5.27**	3 tablets	**5.39**	1 suppository	
5.16	3 tablets	**5.28**	2 tablets	**5.40**	7.5 cc per dose	
5.17	2 tablets	**5.29**	4 tablets	**5.41**	(*a*) 1 tablet; (*b*) 25 mL	
5.18	6.7 mL	**5.30**	6 mL	**5.42**	15 mL	
5.19	$1\frac{1}{2}$ tablets	**5.31**	1 tablet	**5.43**	6 mL	
5.20	2 tablets	**5.32**	6.4 mL	**5.44**	7.7 mL	
5.21	6.5 mL	**5.33**	1 tablet	**5.45**	Give two 4-mg Cardura tablets	
5.22	1 teaspoon	**5.34**	2 capsules	**5.46**	Give one 4-mg Cardura tablet	
5.23	11.3 mL	**5.35**	1 tablet	**5.47**	Give one 2-mg Cardura tablet and one 4-mg Cardura tablet	
5.24	6.4 mL	**5.36**	2 tablets			

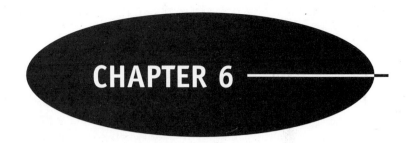

Parenteral Drug Administration

6.1 DRUGS ADMINISTERED BY INJECTION

Parenterally administered drugs are those that are administered by any route other than the alimentary canal. They include drugs administered by several methods, including *subcutaneous* (SC), *intravenous* (IV), and *intramuscular* (IM) methods. Drugs that are administered subcutaneously or intramuscularly are *injected* by syringe. Drugs that are administered intravenously may be injected into a vein but are usually *infused* over some period of time.

When a drug is to be injected parenterally, the active agent is contained in an injectable liquid vehicle. The amount of drug to be administered will be measured in milligrams. Therefore, the dosage conversion problem is to convert the doctor's order to the appropriate number of milliliters:

$$\text{Doctor's order} \rightarrow \text{? mL}$$

EXAMPLE 6.1 The physician orders 8 mg of a drug. A 1-mL ampule contains 10 mg of the drug. How many milliliters do you administer?

The calculation required here is the same as for oral liquid medication (Sec. 5.2).

The required conversion is:	$8 \text{ mg} \rightarrow \text{? mL}$
The relationship to use is:	$10 \text{ mg} = 1 \text{ mL}$
Set up the calculation:	$8 \text{ mg} \times \dfrac{1 \text{ mL}}{10 \text{ mg}}$
Perform the calculation:	$\dfrac{8 \text{ mL}}{10} = 0.8 \text{ mL}$

You would draw 0.8 mL of solution out of the ampule into the syringe and inject this amount into the patient.

EXAMPLE 6.2 The physician has ordered 50 mg IM of Thorazine. Fig. 6-1 shows the label for the Thorazine on hand. How many milliliters do you administer?

The required conversion is:	$50 \text{ mg} \rightarrow \text{? mL}$
The relationship to use is:	$25 \text{ mg} = 1 \text{ mL}$

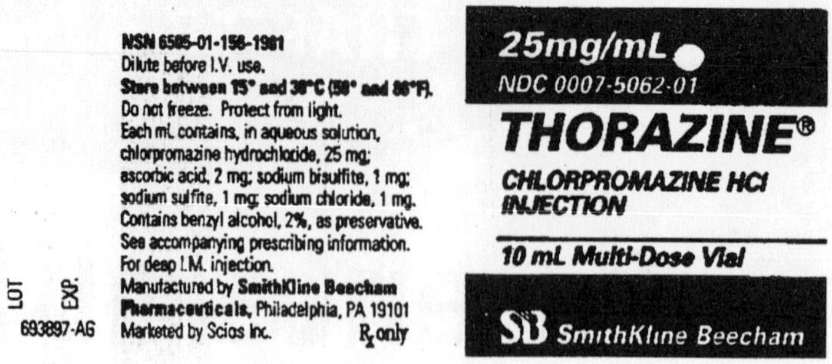

NSN 6505-01-156-1981
Dilute before I.V. use.
Store between 15° and 30°C (59° and 86°F).
Do not freeze. Protect from light.
Each mL contains, in aqueous solution,
chlorpromazine hydrochloride, 25 mg;
ascorbic acid, 2 mg; sodium bisulfite, 1 mg;
sodium sulfite, 1 mg; sodium chloride, 1 mg.
Contains benzyl alcohol, 2%, as preservative.
See accompanying prescribing information.
For deep I.M. injection.
Manufactured by **SmithKline Beecham**
Pharmaceuticals, Philadelphia, PA 19101
693897-AG   Marketed by Scios Inc.   R only

LOT   EXP.

25mg/mL ●
NDC 0007-5062-01
THORAZINE®
CHLORPROMAZINE HCl
INJECTION

10 mL Multi-Dose Vial

SB SmithKline Beecham

Fig. 6-1

Set up the calculation:

$$50 \text{ mg} \times \frac{1 \text{ mL}}{25 \text{ mg}}$$

Perform the calculation:

$$\frac{50 \text{ mL}}{25} = 2 \text{ mL}$$

Thus, you would withdraw 2 mL from the vial and inject this amount.

EXAMPLE 6.3 A 1-mL vial containing 1 mg/mL of scopolamine hydrobromide is available, and the order is for 400 μg SC. How many milliliters should you administer?

The required conversion is: $400 \ \mu g \rightarrow ? \text{ mL}$

This requires two steps: $400 \ \mu g \rightarrow ? \text{ mg} \rightarrow ? \text{ mL}$

The relationships to use are: $1000 \ \mu g = 1 \text{ mg}$ and $1 \text{ mg} = 1 \text{ mL}$

Set up the calculation:

$$400 \ \mu g \times \frac{1 \text{ mg}}{1000 \ \mu g} \times \frac{1 \text{ mL}}{1 \text{ mg}}$$

Perform the calculation:

$$\frac{400}{1000} \text{ mL} = 0.4 \text{ mL}$$

Thus, you would administer 0.4 mL from the vial.

EXAMPLE 6.4 The order is 1 mg IV of Lanoxin. Fig. 6-2 shows the label of the Lanoxin on hand. There are 10 ampuls in the box from which this label was taken. How many milliliters do you administer?

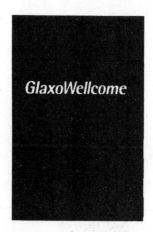

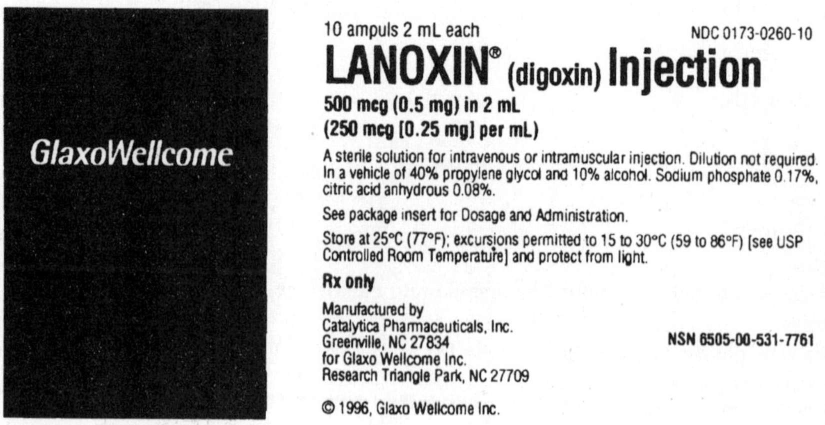

GlaxoWellcome

10 ampuls 2 mL each   NDC 0173-0260-10
LANOXIN® (digoxin) Injection
500 mcg (0.5 mg) in 2 mL
(250 mcg [0.25 mg] per mL)

A sterile solution for intravenous or intramuscular injection. Dilution not required.
In a vehicle of 40% propylene glycol and 10% alcohol. Sodium phosphate 0.17%,
citric acid anhydrous 0.08%.

See package insert for Dosage and Administration.

Store at 25°C (77°F); excursions permitted to 15 to 30°C (59 to 86°F) [see USP
Controlled Room Temperature] and protect from light.

Rx only

Manufactured by
Catalytica Pharmaceuticals, Inc.
Greenville, NC 27834   NSN 6505-00-531-7761
for Glaxo Wellcome Inc.
Research Triangle Park, NC 27709

© 1996, Glaxo Wellcome Inc.

Fig. 6-2

The required conversion is:	$1 \text{ mg} \rightarrow ? \text{ mL}$
The relationship to use is:	$0.5 \text{ mg} = 2 \text{ mL}$
Set up the calculation:	$1 \text{ mg} \times \dfrac{2 \text{ mL}}{0.5 \text{ mg}}$
Perform the calculation:	$\dfrac{2 \text{ mL}}{0.5} = 4 \text{ mL}$

Since each ampul contains 2 mL, you would need to administer 2 ampuls IV.

EXAMPLE 6.5   A drug is supplied 4 mg/mL in a multiple-dose vial. The order is for 8 mg injected IM. How many milliliters should you give?

The required conversion is:	$8 \text{ mg} \rightarrow ? \text{ mL}$
The relationship to use is:	$4 \text{ mg} = 1 \text{ mL}$
Set up the calculation:	$8 \text{ mg} \times \dfrac{1 \text{ mL}}{4 \text{ mg}}$
Perform the calculation:	$\dfrac{8 \text{ mL}}{4} = 2 \text{ mL}$

Thus, 2 mL of the drug injected IM will supply 8 mg.

6.2   INJECTABLES IN POWDER OR CRYSTAL FORM

A parenterally injected medication may be supplied in powder or crystal form. In order to administer the medication by injection, the drug must first be reconstituted to liquid form according to directions. The resulting concentration is the relationship that is used to convert the doctor's order to the appropriate number of milliliters for administration. See Fig. 6-3.

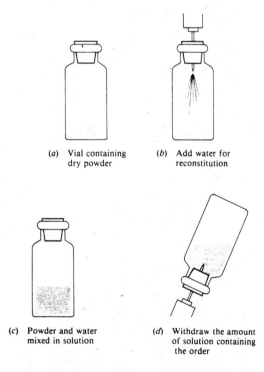

(a) Vial containing   (b) Add water for
     dry powder   reconstitution

(c) Powder and water   (d) Withdraw the amount
     mixed in solution   of solution containing
                                 the order

Fig. 6-3   Steps in preparing powders for injection

EXAMPLE 6.6 The order is for 200 mg of drug to be administered IM. The directions on a vial containing 1 g of powder indicate that adding 7.2 mL of sterile water for injection will yield a concentration of 125 mg/mL. How many milliliters must you withdraw to obtain 200 mg of the drug?

The order for 200 mg must be converted to milliliters. The concentration is given to be 125 mg/mL.

The required conversion is: $200 \text{ mg} \rightarrow ? \text{ mL}$

The relationship to use is: $125 \text{ mg} = 1 \text{ mL}$

Set up the calculation: $200 \text{ mg} \times \dfrac{1 \text{ mL}}{125 \text{ mg}}$

Perform the calculation: $\dfrac{\overset{8}{200} \text{ mL}}{\underset{5}{125}} = \dfrac{8 \text{ mL}}{5} = 1.6 \text{ mL}$

Thus, after you have reconstituted the powder according to directions, you will withdraw 1.6 mL of the liquid to be injected IM.

6.3   INTRAVENOUS INFUSION

When a solution is *infused intravenously*, it is delivered over an extended period of time, which may be, for example, as brief as 15 min or as long as 24 h or more. The solution is delivered by means of an *intravenous delivery system* (Fig. 6-4), which consists of (1) an *IV bag or bottle* to contain the solution, (2) an *IV line or tubing* through which the solution flows, (3) an *IV needle* at the injection site, and (4) a *means of controlling the flow*. The IV solution is either gravity-fed or electromechanically pumped. In a gravity-fed system, the flow is controlled by manipulating a variable switch which constricts the tubing to slow the flow. In a pumped system, the flow is controlled by setting the pump to deliver the solution at the desired rate.

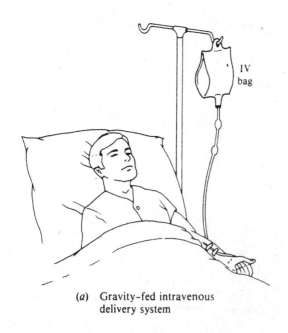

(*a*) Gravity-fed intravenous
delivery system

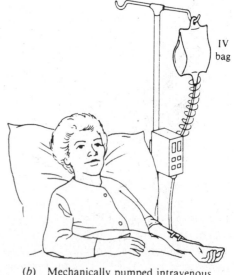

(*b*) Mechanically pumped intravenous
delivery system

Fig. 6-4

The *rate of delivery* or *flow rate* is the ratio of the total amount of solution delivered to the time in which this amount is delivered:

$$\text{Flow rate} = \frac{\text{amount of solution delivered}}{\text{time in which it is delivered}}$$

The flow rate may be expressed in various units, for example, in mL/h or in gtt/min. A flow rate expressed in gtt/min is called a *drop rate*.

In this section you will learn how to convert a flow rate from one unit to another. For example, it may be ordered by the doctor that 1200 mL of 5% dextrose in water (D_5W) be given intravenously over a period of 8 h. It is important to observe that the doctor's order is a flow rate, i.e., an amount to be administered over a period of time, and *not* just an amount to be administered. The flow rate is $\dfrac{1200 \text{ mL}}{8 \text{ h}}$. To carry out the order, you may need to convert this to a drop rate:

$$\frac{1200 \text{ mL}}{8 \text{ h}} \rightarrow ? \frac{\text{gtt}}{\text{min}}$$

This conversion requires two steps:

$$\frac{1200 \text{ mL}}{8 \text{ h}} \rightarrow ? \frac{\text{mL}}{\text{min}} \rightarrow ? \frac{\text{gtt}}{\text{min}}$$

The first conversion changes hours to minutes, and the second changes milliliters to drops. Examples 6.7 and 6.8 will deal with each step separately.

EXAMPLE 6.7 A 1200-mL solution of D_5W is to be infused over a period of 8 h. What is the flow rate in milliliters per minute?

The required conversion is:

$$\frac{1200 \text{ mL}}{8 \text{ h}} \rightarrow ? \frac{\text{mL}}{\text{min}}$$

This conversion requires only that hours be changed into minutes. Thus, the relationship to use is:

$$1 \text{ h} = 60 \text{ min}$$

Set up the calculation:

$$\frac{1200 \text{ mL}}{8 \text{ \cancel{h}}} \times \frac{1 \text{ \cancel{h}}}{60 \text{ min}}$$

Note that the hours have cancelled out, and the units that remain are what we wanted, $\dfrac{\text{mL}}{\text{min}}$. Perform the calculation:

$$\frac{\overset{20}{\cancel{1200}} \text{ mL}}{8 \times \underset{1}{\cancel{60}} \text{ min}} = \frac{20 \text{ mL}}{8 \text{ min}} = 2.5 \text{ mL/min}$$

Thus, to deliver 1200 mL in 8 h, the flow rate must be 2.5 mL/min.

Example 6.8 will show how to convert a rate in mL/min to a rate in gtt/min. To perform this conversion, a relationship must be known between milliliters and drops. This relationship depends on the IV tubing used, and is given by the manufacturer's specifications for the tubing. The number of drops contained in 1 mL is called the *drop factor*. The most common drop factors are 10 gtt/mL, 15 gtt/mL, 20 gtt/mL, and 60 gtt/mL. A delivery system with a drop factor of 60 is called a *microdrop delivery system*, and the drops it delivers are called microdrops.

EXAMPLE 6.8 An IV solution is flowing at the rate of 2.5 mL/min. Calculate the drop rate for the following drop factors: (*a*) 10 gtt/mL; (*b*) 15 gtt/mL.

The required conversion is:

$$\frac{2.5 \text{ mL}}{1 \text{ min}} \rightarrow ? \frac{\text{gtt}}{\text{min}}$$

This conversion will require only that milliliters be changed into drops. The answer will depend on the drop factor.

(a) Drop factor = 10

The relationship to use is: 1 mL = 10 gtt

Set up the calculation: $\dfrac{2.5 \text{ mL}}{1 \text{ min}} \times \dfrac{10 \text{ gtt}}{1 \text{ mL}}$

Perform the calculation: $\dfrac{2.5 \times 10 \text{ gtt}}{1 \text{ min}} = 25 \text{ gtt/min}$

(b) Drop factor = 15

The relationship to use is: 1 mL = 15 gtt

Set up the calculation: $\dfrac{2.5 \text{ mL}}{1 \text{ min}} \times \dfrac{15 \text{ gtt}}{1 \text{ mL}}$

Perform the calculation: $\dfrac{2.5 \times 15 \text{ gtt}}{1 \text{ min}} = 37.5 \text{ gtt/min}$

An answer in drops should always be rounded to the nearest whole number, since it is impossible to measure a fraction of a drop. Thus, the answer is 38 gtt/min.

Note that for the same flow rate, a drop factor of 10 gave a drop rate of 25 gtt/min, while a drop factor of 15 gave a drop rate of 38 gtt/min.

EXAMPLE 6.9   Five hundred milliliters of an 0.45% normal saline solution is to be infused IV over a 4-h period. The drop factor is 20. Calculate the flow rate in gtt/min.

The required conversion is: $\dfrac{500 \text{ mL}}{4 \text{ h}} \rightarrow ? \dfrac{\text{mL}}{\text{min}} \rightarrow ? \dfrac{\text{gtt}}{\text{min}}$

The relationships to use are: 1 h = 60 min and 1 mL = 20 gtt

Set up the calculation: $\dfrac{500 \text{ mL}}{4 \text{ h}} \times \dfrac{1 \text{ h}}{60 \text{ min}} \times \dfrac{20 \text{ gtt}}{1 \text{ mL}}$

Perform the calculation: $\dfrac{500 \times \overset{1}{20} \text{ gtt}}{4 \times \underset{3}{60} \text{ min}} = \dfrac{\overset{125}{500} \text{ gtt}}{\underset{1}{4} \times 3 \text{ min}} = \dfrac{125 \text{ gtt}}{3 \text{ min}} = 42 \text{ gtt/min}$

Thus, to infuse 500 mL of solution in 4 h, with a drop factor of 20, you would set the drop rate at 42 gtt/min.

A drug may be administered diluted in an IV solution in two ways: (1) the drug may be added to the solution in the IV bag itself, or (2) the drug may be added to the solution by means of a controlled volume infusion attached to the main line. This is called an IV *piggyback* (IVPB, see Fig. 6-5).

EXAMPLE 6.10   One gram of Mefoxin (cefoxin sodium) in 100 mL of D_5W is to be administered in half an hour IVPB. If the drop factor is 10 drops per milliliter, calculate the drop rate.

The problem is to convert the flow rate $\dfrac{100 \text{ mL}}{1/2 \text{ h}}$ to gtt/min.

The required conversion is: $\dfrac{100 \text{ mL}}{1/2 \text{ h}} \rightarrow ? \dfrac{\text{mL}}{\text{min}} \rightarrow ? \dfrac{\text{gtt}}{\text{min}}$

The relationships to use are: 1 h = 60 min and 1 mL = 10 gtt

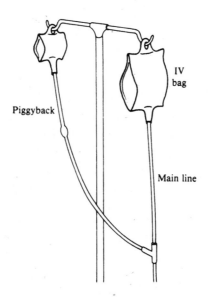

Fig. 6-5

Set up the calculation:
$$\frac{100\ \cancel{mL}}{1/2\ \cancel{h}} \times \frac{1\ \cancel{h}}{60\ min} \times \frac{10\ gtt}{1\ \cancel{mL}}$$

Perform the calculation:
$$\frac{100}{1} \times \frac{2}{1} \times \frac{1}{\underset{6}{\cancel{60}}} \times \frac{\overset{1}{\cancel{10}}\ gtt}{1\ min}$$

$$= \frac{100 \times \overset{1}{\cancel{2}}}{\underset{3}{\cancel{6}}}\ \frac{gtt}{min} = 33.3\ gtt/min$$

Round the answer to 33 gtt/min to deliver 100 mL in half an hour.

EXAMPLE 6.11   An IV solution is flowing at the rate of 30 gtt/min. What is the equivalent rate in mL/h if the drop factor is 60 gtt/mL?
    The problem is to convert the drop rate of 30 gtt/min to a flow rate of mL/h.

The required conversion is:
$$\frac{30\ gtt}{1\ min} \rightarrow ?\ \frac{mL}{min} \rightarrow ?\ \frac{mL}{h}$$

The relationships to use are: 60 gtt = 1 mL and 60 min = 1 h

Set up the calculation:
$$\frac{30\ \cancel{gtt}}{1\ \cancel{min}} \times \frac{1\ mL}{60\ \cancel{gtt}} \times \frac{60\ \cancel{min}}{1\ h}$$

Perform the calculation:
$$\frac{30 \times \overset{1}{\cancel{60}}\ mL}{\underset{1}{\cancel{60}}\ h} = 30\ mL/h$$

Thus, a drop rate of 30 gtt/min will deliver 30 mL/h with a drop factor of 60, i.e., with a microdrop delivery system.

    Example 6.11 illustrates the following fact: *With a drop factor of 60, the flow rate in ML/h is equal to the drop rate in gtt/min.*

EXAMPLE 6.12   One thousand milliliters of an IV solution is to be infused over a period of 8 h. A check of the time tape after 4 h showed that only 350 mL of the solution has been infused. Recalculate a new drop rate that will finish the infusion in 4 h. The drop factor is 10 gtt/mL.
    The amount remaining in the bottle is 1000 mL − 350 mL = 650 mL. Therefore, 650 mL must be infused in 4 h. The problem then is to convert 650 mL/4 h to gtt/min.

The required conversion is:

$$\frac{650 \text{ mL}}{4 \text{ h}} \rightarrow ? \frac{\text{mL}}{\text{min}} \rightarrow ? \frac{\text{gtt}}{\text{min}}$$

The relationships to use are:

$$1 \text{ h} = 60 \text{ min} \text{ and } 1 \text{ mL} = 10 \text{ gtt}$$

Set up the calculation:

$$\frac{650 \text{ mL}}{4 \text{ h}} \times \frac{1 \text{ h}}{60 \text{ min}} \times \frac{10 \text{ gtt}}{1 \text{ mL}}$$

Perform the calculation:

$$\frac{650 \times \overset{1}{\cancel{10}} \text{ gtt}}{4 \times \underset{6}{\cancel{60}} \text{ min}} = \frac{650 \text{ gtt}}{24 \text{ min}} = 27 \text{ gtt/min}$$

You must reset the drop rate to 27 gtt/min to deliver the 650 mL in 4 h.

EXAMPLE 6.13   You have set the drop rate to infuse 1000 mL of 0.9% saline solution in 8 h. The drop factor is 15. You return an hour later to check the IV and find that 125 mL has been delivered. Is the solution flowing at the correct rate?

You must determine whether a flow rate of 1000 mL/8 h is equal to a flow rate of 125 mL/h. Yes, the flow rates are equal, because:

$$\frac{\overset{125}{\cancel{1000}} \text{ mL}}{\underset{1}{\cancel{8}} \text{ h}} = \frac{125 \text{ mL}}{1 \text{ h}}$$

EXAMPLE 6.14   You check the patient's IV and find that there is 200 mL of fluid remaining in the bag. If you are to hang a new bag by the time there are 50 mL remaining, how soon should you return? The drop factor is 15 and the drop rate is 25 gtt/min.

The problem is to find how long it will take to deliver 200 mL − 50 mL = 150 mL. Thus, you must convert 150 mL into its equivalent in minutes.

The required conversion is:

$$150 \text{ mL} \rightarrow ? \text{ gtt} \rightarrow ? \text{ min}$$

The relationships to use are:

$$1 \text{ mL} = 15 \text{ gtt} \text{ and } 25 \text{ gtt} = 1 \text{ min}$$

Set up the calculation:

$$150 \text{ mL} \times \frac{15 \text{ gtt}}{1 \text{ mL}} \times \frac{1 \text{ min}}{25 \text{ gtt}}$$

Perform the calculation:

$$\frac{\overset{6}{\cancel{150}} \times 15}{\underset{1}{\cancel{25}}} \text{ min} = 90 \text{ min}$$

Thus, you should return in 90 min.

6.4   INSULIN ADMINISTRATION

Insulin is measured according to therapeutic activity in USP units (U). The drug is available in U-100 strength. This means the drug is available in the strength that contains 100 U/mL. The drug may be administered in three different size syringes: 3/10, 1/2, and 1 cc. The three sizes of syringes accommodate those small to large dosages.

U-100 Insulin.   U-100 insulin is administered with syringes specially calibrated to be used with U-100 insulin. There are three types of U-100 insulin syringes. One is marked in insulin units up to 100 U, one is marked up to 50 U, and the third is marked up to 30 U (see Fig. 6-6). It will be easier to read the smallest of the three when less than 30 units are given.

EXAMPLE 6.15   You are to give 60 units of U-100 using a U-100 syringe. Simply locate 60 units on the U-100 syringe and fill the syringe to that point. The other two syringes are not suitable for administering 60 units.

EXAMPLE 6.16   You are to give 25 U of U-100 insulin using a 3/10-, a 1/2-, and a 1-cc syringe. Any one of the three sizes of syringes can be used to administer the 25 units of U-100 insulin. Just go to the 25 U mark on the appropriate syringe.

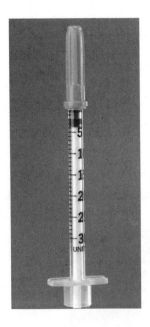 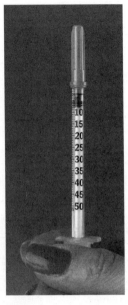 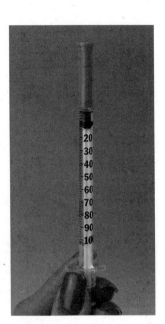

Fig. 6-6

When an Insulin Syringe Is Not Available.   Sometimes an insulin syringe of the required type may not be available. A tuberculin syringe must then be used, and the order must be converted to the appropriate volume in milliliters using the strength of the insulin being administered as the conversion factor.

EXAMPLE 6.17   The order is for 75 units of U-100 insulin. How would you administer this order using a tuberculin syringe?
    Since you are using a tuberculin syringe, the order must be converted into milliliters.

The required conversion is: $75\ U \rightarrow ?\ mL$

The label "U-100" means that 100 units
of insulin is contained in 1 mL of solution.
Thus, the relationship to use is: $100\ U = 1\ mL$

Set up the calculation: $75\ \cancel{U} \times \dfrac{1\ mL}{100\ \cancel{U}}$

Perform the calculation: $\dfrac{75}{100}\ mL = 0.75\ mL$

Thus, 0.75 mL of U-100 solution contains 75 U of insulin.

Solved Problems

DRUGS ADMINISTERED BY INJECTION

6.1   Phenergan (promethazine hydrochloride) 40 mg IM is to be given for sedation. The syringe contains 50 mg/mL. How many milliliters will you give?

Solution

The required conversion is:	$40 \text{ mg} \rightarrow ? \text{ mL}$
The relationship to use is:	$50 \text{ mg} = 1 \text{ mL}$
Set up the calculation:	$40 \text{ mg} \times \dfrac{1 \text{ mL}}{50 \text{ mg}}$
Perform the calculation:	$\dfrac{40}{50} \text{ mL} = 0.8 \text{ mL}$

6.2 The order is 1 mg IV of Stelazine. Figure 6-7 shows the label for the Stelazine on hand.

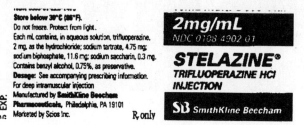

Fig. 6-7

Solution

The required conversion is:	$1 \text{ mg} \rightarrow ? \text{ mL}$
The relationship to use is:	$2 \text{ mg} = 1 \text{ mL}$
Set up the calculation:	$1 \text{ mg} \times \dfrac{1 \text{ mL}}{2 \text{ mg}}$
Perform the calculation:	$\dfrac{1}{2} \text{ mL or } 0.5 \text{ mL}$

6.3 Penicillin G procaine 1,000,000 U IM is ordered. You have a disposable 2-mL syringe containing 1,200,000 U. How many milliliters should be administered?

Solution

The required conversion is:	$1,000,000 \text{ U} \rightarrow ? \text{ mL}$
The relationship to use is:	$1,200,000 \text{ U} = 2 \text{ mL}$
Set up the calculation:	$1,000,000 \text{ U} \times \dfrac{2 \text{ mL}}{1,200,000 \text{ U}}$
Perform the calculation:	$\dfrac{\overset{5}{1,000,000} \times 2 \text{ mL}}{\underset{6}{1,200,000}} = \dfrac{10 \text{ mL}}{6}$
	$= 1.7 \text{ mL}$ (nearest tenth)

6.4 Benadryl 0.04 g is ordered IM. The drug is available 10 mg/mL. How many milliliters should you give?

Solution

The required conversion is: $0.04\ \text{g} \to ?\ \text{mg} \to ?\ \text{mL}$

The relationships to use are: $1\ \text{g} = 1000\ \text{mg}$ and $10\ \text{mg} = 1\ \text{mL}$

Set up the calculation: $0.04\ \text{g} \times \dfrac{1000\ \cancel{\text{mg}}}{1\ \text{g}} \times \dfrac{1\ \cancel{\text{mL}}}{10\ \cancel{\text{mg}}}$

Perform the calculation: $\dfrac{0.04 \times \overset{100}{\cancel{1000}}\ \text{mL}}{\underset{1}{\cancel{10}}} = 4\ \text{mL}$

6.5   The physician ordered 0.35 mg of a drug. A 1-mL ampul on hand contains 400 µg. How many milliliters will contain the order of 0.35 mg?

Solution

The required conversion is: $0.35\ \text{mg} \to ?\ \mu\text{g} \to ?\ \text{mL}$

The relationships to use are: $1\ \text{mg} = 1000\ \mu\text{g}$ and $400\ \mu\text{g} = 1\ \text{mL}$

Set up the calculation: $0.35\ \cancel{\text{mg}} \times \dfrac{1000\ \cancel{\mu\text{g}}}{1\ \cancel{\text{mg}}} \times \dfrac{1\ \text{mL}}{400\ \cancel{\mu\text{g}}}$

Perform the calculation: $\dfrac{0.35 \times \overset{5}{\cancel{1000}}}{\underset{2}{\cancel{400}}}\ \text{mL} = \dfrac{1.75}{2}\ \text{mL}$

                                            $= 0.9\ \text{mL}$ (nearest tenth)

6.6   A dosette vial of morphine sulfate containing 10 mg/mL is on hand. You are to give 20 mg IM. How many milliliters should you give?

Solution

The required conversion is: $20\ \text{mg} \to ?\ \text{mL}$

The relationship to use is: $10\ \text{mg} = 1\ \text{mL}$

Set up the calculation: $20\ \cancel{\text{mg}} \times \dfrac{1\ \text{mL}}{10\ \cancel{\text{mg}}}$

Perform the calculation: $2\ \text{mL}$

6.7   The label on a vial containing a drug states that the concentration is 0.4 mg/mL. You are to give 0.3 mg. How many milliliters should you give?

Solution

The required conversion is: $0.3\ \text{mg} \to ?\ \text{mL}$

The relationship to use is: $0.4\ \text{mg} = 1\ \text{mL}$

Set up the calculation: $0.3\ \cancel{\text{mg}} \times \dfrac{1\ \text{mL}}{0.4\ \cancel{\text{mg}}}$

Perform the calculation: $0.8\ \text{mL}$ (nearest tenth)

6.8 You have available Thorazine 25 mg/mL in a 10-mL vial. The order is for 50 mg of the drug IM. How much should you give?

Solution

The required conversion is:	50 mg → ? mL
The relationship to use is:	25 mg = 1 mL
Set up the calculation:	$50 \text{ mg} \times \dfrac{1 \text{ mL}}{25 \text{ mg}}$
Perform the calculation:	2 mL

6.9 Ten milligrams of Compazine is to be given IM from a 10-mL multidose vial containing 5 mg/mL. How many milliliters should you give?

Solution

The required conversion is:	10 mg → ? mL
The relationship to use is:	5 mg = 1 mL
Set up the calculation:	$10 \text{ mg} \times \dfrac{1 \text{ mL}}{5 \text{ mg}}$
Perform the calculation:	2 mL

6.10 You are to administer 1.2 million units of Bicillin L-A IM as a single dose. You have on hand for injection a 4-mL disposable syringe containing 2,400,000 units. How many milliliters must you administer to give the correct dose?

Solution

The required conversion is:	1.2 million units → ? mL
The relationship to use is:	2,400,000 units = 4 mL
Set up the calculation:	$1,200,000 \text{ units} \times \dfrac{4 \text{ mL}}{2,400,000 \text{ units}}$ (Recall that 1.2 million units is the same as 1,200,000 units.)
Perform the calculation:	2 mL; you use half the disposable syringe

INTRAVENOUS INFUSION PROBLEMS

6.11 Normal saline 750 mL is to be infused IV over a period of 12 h. Calculate the flow rate in drops per minute if the drop factor is 15 gtt/mL.

Solution

The required conversion is:	$\dfrac{750 \text{ mL}}{12 \text{ h}} \rightarrow ? \dfrac{\text{mL}}{\text{min}} \rightarrow ? \dfrac{\text{gtt}}{\text{min}}$
The relationships to use are:	1 h = 60 min and 1 mL = 15 gtt

Set up the calculation:

$$\frac{750 \; \cancel{mL}}{12 \; \cancel{h}} \times \frac{1 \; \cancel{h}}{60 \; min} \times \frac{15 \; gtt}{1 \; \cancel{mL}}$$

Perform the calculation:

$$\frac{750 \times \overset{1}{\cancel{15}} \; gtt}{12 \times \underset{4}{\cancel{60}} \; min} = \frac{750 \; gtt}{48 \; min} = 16 \; gtt/min \qquad \text{(nearest whole)}$$

6.12 The IV is set to deliver 75 microdrops per minute. What is the rate of flow in milliliters per hour?

Solution

The required conversion is:

$$\frac{75 \; gtt}{1 \; min} \to ? \; \frac{mL}{min} \to ? \; \frac{mL}{h}$$

The relationships to use are: $60 \; gtt = 1 \; mL$ and $60 \; min = 1 \; h$

Set up the calculation:

$$\frac{75 \; \cancel{gtt}}{1 \; \cancel{min}} \times \frac{1 \; mL}{60 \; \cancel{gtt}} \times \frac{60 \; \cancel{min}}{1 \; h}$$

Perform the calculation:

$$\frac{75 \times \overset{1}{\cancel{60}}}{\underset{1}{\cancel{60}}} \; mL/h = 75 \; mL/h$$

6.13 Garamycin 250 mg is to be infused IV in 100-mL piggyback over 30 min. Calculate the drop rate if the drop factor is 10.

Solution

The required conversion is:

$$\frac{100 \; mL}{30 \; min} \to ? \; \frac{gtt}{min}$$

The relationship to use is: $1 \; mL = 10 \; gtt$

Set up the calculation:

$$\frac{100 \; \cancel{mL}}{30 \; min} \times \frac{10 \; gtt}{1 \; \cancel{mL}}$$

Perform the calculation:

$$\frac{100 \times 10}{30} \; gtt/min = 33 \; gtt/min \qquad \text{(nearest whole)}$$

6.14 One liter of sodium lactate is to be infused IV in 8 h. (*a*) Calculate the flow rate in milliliters per minute. (*b*) Calculate the flow rate in drops per minute for a drop factor of 15.

Solution

(*a*)   The required conversion is:

$$\frac{1 \; L}{8 \; h} \to ? \; \frac{mL}{h} \to ? \; \frac{mL}{min}$$

The relationships to use are: $1 \; L = 1000 \; mL$ and $1 \; h = 60 \; min$

Set up the calculation:

$$\frac{1 \; \cancel{L}}{8 \; \cancel{h}} \times \frac{1000 \; mL}{1 \; \cancel{L}} \times \frac{1 \; \cancel{h}}{60 \; min}$$

Perform the calculation:

$$\frac{1000}{8 \times 60} \; mL/min = 2.1 \; mL/min \quad \text{(nearest tenth)}$$

(*b*)   Convert the answer from part (*a*) to a drop rate for a drop factor of 15.

The required conversion is:

$$\frac{2.1 \; mL}{1 \; min} \to ? \; \frac{gtt}{min}$$

The relationship to use is: $1 \; mL = 15 \; gtt$

Set up the calculation:

$$\frac{2.1\ \text{mL}}{1\ \text{min}} \times \frac{15\ \text{gtt}}{1\ \text{mL}}$$

Perform the calculation:

$$2.1 \times 15\ \text{gtt/min} = 32\ \text{gtt/min} \qquad \text{(nearest whole)}$$

6.15 Pitocin (oxytocin) is ordered to induce labor. You are to prepare the IV infusion by adding the contents of a 10-U ampule to 1000 mL of D_5 Ringer's lactate. This is to be infused at the rate of 1 milliunit per minute. What should the drop rate be if the drop factor is 60? One *milliunit* (mU) is a thousandth of a USP unit.

Solution

The required conversion is:

$$\frac{1\ \text{mU}}{\text{min}} \to ?\ \frac{\text{U}}{\text{min}} \to ?\ \frac{\text{mL}}{\text{min}} \to ?\ \frac{\text{gtt}}{\text{min}}$$

The relationships to use are:

$$1000\ \text{mU} = 1\ \text{U},\ 10\ \text{U} = 1000\ \text{mL, and } 1\ \text{mL} = 60\ \text{gtt}$$

Set up the calculation:

$$\frac{1\ \text{mU}}{1\ \text{min}} \times \frac{1\ \text{U}}{1000\ \text{mU}} \times \frac{1000\ \text{mL}}{10\ \text{U}} \times \frac{60\ \text{gtt}}{1\ \text{mL}}$$

Perform the calculation:

$$\frac{1000 \times 60}{1000 \times 10}\ \text{gtt/min} = 6\ \text{gtt/min}$$

6.16 Potassium chloride 30 mEq is to be given in 1 L of IV fluid. Available are ampules containing 20 mEq in 10 mL and 40 mEq in 20 mL. (*a*) Which size ampules should you use, and how many milliliters of the drug should you add to the IV bag? (*b*) If the flow rate is 125 mL/h, how many milliequivalents per hour are being infused?

Solution

(*a*) First, determine the number of milliliters to be added to the IV bag. Use the vial containing 40 mEq because you need more than 20 mEq.

The required conversion is: 30 mEq → ? mL

The relationship to use is: 40 mEq = 20 mL

Set up the calculation:

$$30\ \text{mEq} \times \frac{20\ \text{mL}}{40\ \text{mEq}}$$

Perform the calculation:

$$\frac{30 \times 20\ \text{mL}}{40} = 15\ \text{mL}$$

(*b*) Now, calculate the rate of delivery.

The required conversion is:

$$\frac{125\ \text{mL}}{1\ \text{h}} \to ?\ \frac{\text{L}}{\text{h}} \to ?\ \frac{\text{mEq}}{\text{h}}$$

The relationships to use are: 1000 mL = 1 L and 1 L = 30 mEq

Set up the calculation:

$$\frac{125\ \text{mL}}{1\ \text{h}} \times \frac{1\ \text{L}}{1000\ \text{mL}} \times \frac{30\ \text{mEq}}{1\ \text{L}}$$

Perform the calculation:

$$\frac{125 \times 30}{1000}\ \text{mEq/h} = 3.75\ \text{mEq/h}$$

6.17 You have set up the IV apparatus to infuse 2 L of D_5W in 24 h. You return 15 min later to check the rate of delivery and see that about 27 mL has been infused. Is the rate of delivery correct?

Solution

Find the amount in milliliters that should have been infused in 15 min.

The required conversion is: 　　　　$15 \text{ min} \rightarrow ? \text{ h} \rightarrow ? \text{ L} \rightarrow ? \text{ mL}$

The relationships to use are: 　　　$60 \text{ min} = 1 \text{ h}, 24 \text{ h} = 2 \text{ L, and } 1 \text{ L} = 1000 \text{ mL}$

Set up the calculation: 　　　　　$15 \text{ min} \times \dfrac{1 \text{ h}}{60 \text{ min}} \times \dfrac{2 \text{ L}}{24 \text{ h}} \times \dfrac{1000 \text{ mL}}{1 \text{ L}}$

Perform the calculation: 　　　　　$\dfrac{15 \times 2 \times 1000 \text{ mL}}{60 \times 24} = 21 \text{ mL}$ 　(nearest whole)

About 21 mL should have been infused in 15 min. The IV is flowing too quickly.

6.18 The IV was set to infuse 600 mL of a 5% glucose solution in 8 h. A check of the IV showed that 120 mL had been infused in 2 h. Recalculate the drop rate to finish the infusion in 6 h. The drop factor is 20.

Solution

The amount to be infused is 600 mL − 120 mL = 480 mL. Thus,

The required conversion is: 　　　　$\dfrac{480 \text{ mL}}{6 \text{ h}} \rightarrow ? \dfrac{\text{mL}}{\text{min}} \rightarrow ? \dfrac{\text{gtt}}{\text{min}}$

The relationships to use are: 　　　$1 \text{ h} = 60 \text{ min and } 1 \text{ mL} = 20 \text{ gtt}$

Set up the calculation: 　　　　　$\dfrac{480 \text{ mL}}{6 \text{ h}} \times \dfrac{1 \text{ h}}{60 \text{ min}} \times \dfrac{20 \text{ gtt}}{1 \text{ mL}}$

Perform the calculation: 　　　　　$\dfrac{480 \times 20}{6 \times 60} \text{ gtt/min} = 27 \text{ gtt/min}$ 　　(nearest whole)

6.19 You check the patient's IV and observe that there is 110 mL of solution remaining in the bottle. The drop rate is 20 gtt/min and the drop factor is 15 gtt/mL. If you are to hang a new bottle by the time there is 50 mL remaining, how much later should you return?

Solution

Calculate the remaining amount to be given: 110 mL − 50 mL = 60 mL. How long will it take to deliver this amount?

The required conversion is: 　　　　$60 \text{ mL} \rightarrow ? \text{ gtt} \rightarrow ? \text{ min}$

The relationships to use are: 　　　$1 \text{ mL} = 15 \text{ gtt and } 20 \text{ gtt} = 1 \text{ min}$

Set up the calculation: 　　　　　$60 \text{ mL} \times \dfrac{15 \text{ gtt}}{1 \text{ mL}} \times \dfrac{1 \text{ min}}{20 \text{ gtt}}$

Perform the calculation: 　　　　　$\dfrac{60 \times 15}{20} \text{ min} = 45 \text{ min}$

INSULIN INJECTION PROBLEMS

6.20 The order is for insulin 45 U. How would you administer this order using a U-100 insulin syringe?

Solution

From a vial of U-100 insulin, draw the solution up to the 45-U mark.

6.21   The order is for 60 U of regular insulin. You have on hand a vial of U-100 insulin. How would you administer the order using a tuberculin syringe?

Solution

The label "U-100" means that the concentration of insulin is 100 U/mL. Therefore,

The required conversion is: $60 \text{ U} \rightarrow \text{? mL}$

The relationship to use is: $100 \text{ U} = 1 \text{ mL}$

Set up the calculation: $60 \cancel{U} \times \dfrac{1 \text{ mL}}{100 \cancel{U}}$

Perform the calculation: $\dfrac{60 \text{ mL}}{100} = 0.6 \text{ mL}$

6.22   Which of the three insulin syringes (3/10 cc, 1/2 cc, and 1 cc) are usable to administer the following orders for regular insulin? (*a*) 75 units;   (*b*) 40 units;   (*c*) 20 units.

Solution

(*a*)   Only the 1-cc insulin syringe can be used to administer 75 units.

(*b*)   The 1/2-cc or the 1-cc insulin syringe can be used to administer 40 units.

(*c*)   The 3/10-cc, 1/2-cc, or 1-cc insulin syringe can be used to administer 20 units.

Supplementary Problems

DRUGS ADMINISTERED BY INJECTION

6.23   The physician orders 0.4 mg of a drug. The label on the vial states that the concentration is 0.5 mg per 2 mL. How many milliliters should be administered?

6.24   The doctor orders Garamycin (gentamycin sulfate) 70 mg. A 2-mL vial contains 40 mg/mL. How many milliliters should be administered? Give answer to nearest tenth.

6.25   A drug is ordered, 7500 U to be administered SC. A prefilled disposable syringe containing 10,000 U in 1 mL is on hand. How many milliliters should be administered?

6.26   Atropine sulfate 0.4 mg IM is to be given preoperatively. You have a prefilled disposable syringe containing 0.5 mg per 5 mL. How many milliliters will you administer?

6.27   You are to give vitamin B_{12} (cyanocobalamin) 60 μg SC using a prefilled disposable syringe containing 100 μg/mL. How many milliliters should you administer?

6.28   Meperidine hydrochloride 75 mg is to be given IM from a vial containing 50 mg/mL. How many milliliters should be administered?

6.29   The doctor orders 250 μg of a drug. The vial states that 1 mL of the drug contains 100 μg. How many milliliters should be given?

6.30   The order is for 400 mg of a drug to be given IM. A disposable syringe contains 500 mg per 2 mL. How many milliliters should be administered?

6.31   A vial contains a drug in powder form for reconstitution. Adding 10 mL of sterile water for injection will yield a concentration of 600,000 U/mL. How many milliliters will you withdraw from the vial to administer 400,000 U? Give answer to the nearest hundredth.

6.32   Penicillin G procaine 3,000,000 U is contained in 10 mL of solution. How many milliliters of solution must you withdraw from the vial to administer 600,000 U?

6.33   The directions for a vial of Polycillin-N (ampicillin sodium) containing 500 mg of dry powder state that the addition of 1.8 mL of sterile water for injection will yield 2 mL of solution. How many milliliters should be administered to give 250 mg of the drug?

6.34   A vial contains 1,000,000 U of penicillin G potassium in dry powder form. The directions say to add 3.6 mL of diluent to obtain a concentration of 250,000 U/mL. How many milliliters of solution are needed to administer 200,000 U?

6.35   Nembutal (pentobarbital sodium injection) 70 mg IM is ordered. The pharmacy has sent a 2-mL ampule containing 100 mg. How many milliliters are needed to administer the order?

6.36   Kefzol (cefazolin sodium) 300 mg IM q8h is ordered. You have on hand a 500-mg vial to which you have added 2 mL of 0.9% sodium chloride for injection, and mixed according to directions. The reconstituted solution contains 225 mg/mL. How many milliliters will you administer? Give answer to the nearest hundredth.

6.37   Talwin 20 mg SC q3h prn is ordered. Disposable prefilled syringes containing 30 mg in 1 mL were sent from the pharmacy. How many milliliters do you give? Give answer to the nearest hundredth.

6.38   A bolus of 20 mg of Reopro is ordered. Reopro is supplied in a vial containing 10 mg per 5 mL. How many milliliters of Reopro is needed in the bolus?

6.39   You have prepared penicillin G sodium from dry powder by adding 3 mL of a diluent to a vial containing 5,000,000 U. This provides a concentration of 1,000,000 U/mL. You are to administer 1,500,000 U. How many milliliters will contain this amount?

6.40   You are to give Lasix (furosemide) 40 mg IM. Lasix is available 10 mg/mL in 2-mL ampules, 4-mL ampules, and 10-mL ampules. Which size ampule will you select and how many milliliters will you administer?

6.41   You are to give 60 mg of a drug. The label on the vial states that each milliliter contains 10 mg. How many milliliters will contain 60 mg?

6.42   How many milligrams of Compazine will there be in 1 teaspoon? How many in 1 tablespoon? The label for the Compazine to be used is shown in Fig. 6-8.

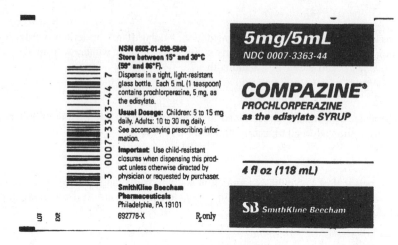

Fig. 6-8

6.43   The label on a vial of Kantrex (kanamycin sulfate) states that 1 g of the drug is contained in 3 mL of solution. How many milliliters would you administer if the order is for 700 mg?

6.44 · Fifty milligrams of haloperidol decanoate IM every 4 weeks is to be administered. The drug is available in 5-mL vials containing 100 mg/mL. How many milliliters should be administered?

6.45   The order is for 0.25 mg of medication. The label on the vial states that each milliliter contains 50 μg of the medication. How many milliliters will you administer to the patient?

6.46   Fifteen milligrams of Phenobarbital is to be administered to the patient before surgery. The pharmacy has provided a Tubex syringe containing 30 mg in 1 mL. How many milliliters should you give?

6.47   You are to give 10 mg of a drug which is available in a vial containing 15 mg/mL. How many milliliters should the patient receive? Give the answer to the nearest hundredth.

6.48   Scopolamine 0.4 mg is to be administered SC. If a 1-mL dosette vial contains 400 μg, how many milliliters should be given?

6.49   A drug is supplied in ampules containing 0.4 mg/mL. You are directed to give 400 μg. How many milliliters will contain this amount?

6.50   A drug is available 50 mg/mL. The order is for 45 mg. How many milliliters will contain the order?

6.51   Seven and one-half milligrams of morphine sulfate is to be given IV from a vial containing 10 mg/mL. How many milliliters will contain the amount ordered?

INTRAVENOUS INFUSION PROBLEMS

6.52   Calculate the drop rate of an IV if 1000 mL of a 5% glucose solution is to be administered over a period of 8 h and the drop factor is 20 gtt/mL.

6.53   Gentamycin sulfate is diluted in 200 mL of sterile isotonic saline and infused over 2 h. The drop factor is 15 gtt/mL. Calculate the flow rate in drops per minute (gtt/min).

6.54   Penicillin 600,000 U is to be given IV in 100 mL by piggyback over a period of 1 h. The drop factor is 15 gtt/mL. Calculate the flow rate in drops per minute.

6.55   Calculate the rate of infusion for an IV in microdrops per minute if the order is for 300 mL of 0.45% normal saline to be delivered over a period of 4 h.

6.56   MVI (multivitamin infusion) is added to 1000 mL of D_5W for intravenous infusion. The solution is infused at the rate of 1000 mL in 8 h. What is the rate in drops per minute for a drop factor of 15?

6.57   You are to administer 500 mg of ampicillin in 50 mL by IVPB over a period of 15 min. The drop factor is 10 gtt/mL. Calculate the rate of flow in drops per minute.

6.58   The order is for 300 mL of D_5 normal saline to be administered IV over a 6-h period. Calculate the drop rate in drops per minute for a drop factor of 15.

6.59   Xylocaine (lidocaine HCl) 250 mg is contained in 250 mL of D_5W for IV administration. Calculate the drop rate to give a flow rate of 1 mg/min. The drop factor is 20.

6.60   The drop factor for the IV line is 15. The order is to infuse the IV solution at the rate of 100 mL/h. What should the drop rate be?

6.61   The drop rate for an IV line is set at 30 gtt/min. Calculate the rate of infusion of the solution in milliliters per hour. The drop factor is 15.

6.62   Sodium lactate is being infused by microdrip (drop factor 60) at the rate of 175 gtt/min. To how many milliliters per hour is this equivalent?

6.63 Pitocin is ordered IV for a postpartum patient. You are to add 20 U to 1000 mL of D_5 Ringer's injection. You have on hand a 10-mL vial containing 10 U/mL. (*a*) How many milliliters of the medication do you add to the solution? (*b*) If the medication is to be administered at the rate of 20 mU/mm and the drop factor is 15, what should the drop rate be?

6.64 You have set up an IV to deliver 150 mL of D_5 normal saline over 10 h via a microdrip delivery system. You return in 1 h to check the flow rate and observe that 15 mL has been given. Is the IV flowing at the correct rate?

6.65 Normal saline 750 mL is to be infused over 4 h. The drop factor is 10. A check of the IV shows that 150 mL has been delivered in 1 h. Recalculate the drop rate to finish the infusion in 3 h.

6.66 You have set up the IV to deliver 1500 mL of normal saline over an 8-h period. You return after 15 min to check the rate of infusion and see that about 47 mL has been given. Is the IV flowing at the correct rate?

6.67 You check the patient's IV and see that there is 100 mL of fluid remaining. The flow rate is 15 gtt/min and the drop factor is 15. If you are to hang a new bottle by the time there is 50 mL remaining, how much time do you have?

INSULIN INJECTION PROBLEMS

6.68 Using a tuberculin syringe, give 65 U of insulin from a vial of Humulin N U-100 insulin. How many milliliters should you give?

6.69 Give 25 U of Regular Humulin R, U-100. (*a*) Using a 3/10-cc insulin syringe, how many milliliters do you put in the syringe? (*b*) Using a 1/2-cc insulin syringe, how many milliliters do you put in the syringe? (*c*) Using a 1-cc insulin syringe, how many milliliters do you put in the syringe?

6.70 You are to give 70 U of Regular Humulin R, U-100 insulin. How many millimeters will you give using a tuberculin syringe?

6.71 If you are to administer 60 units of Humulin N, U-100, would you use a 3/10-cc insulin syringe, a 1/2-cc insulin syringe, or a 1-cc insulin syringe?

Answers to Supplementary Problems

6.23	1.6 mL	**6.28**	1.5 mL	**6.33**	1 mL	**6.38**	10 mL
6.24	1.8 mL	**6.29**	2.5 mL	**6.34**	0.8 mL	**6.39**	1.5 mL
6.25	0.75 mL	**6.30**	1.6 mL	**6.35**	1.4 mL	**6.40**	4 mL
6.26	4 mL	**6.31**	0.67 mL	**6.36**	1.33 mL	**6.41**	6 mL
6.27	0.6 mL	**6.32**	2 mL	**6.37**	0.67 mL	**6.42**	5 mg; 15 mg

6.43	2.1 mL	**6.51**	0.75	**6.59**	20 gtt/min	**6.67**	50 min
6.44	0.5 mL	**6.52**	42 gtt/min	**6.60**	25 gtt/min	**6.68**	0.65 mL
6.45	5 mL	**6.53**	25 gtt/min	**6.61**	120 mL/h	**6.69**	(*a*) 0.25 mL (*b*) 0.25 mL (*c*) 0.25 mL
6.46	0.5 mL	**6.54**	25 gtt/min	**6.62**	175 mL/h	**6.70**	0.7 mL
6.47	0.67 mL	**6.55**	75 gtt/min	**6.63**	(*a*) 2 mL (*b*) 15 gtt/min	**6.71**	1-cc insulin syringe
6.48	1 mL	**6.56**	31 gtt/min	**6.64**	yes		
6.49	1 mL	**6.57**	33 gtt/minL	**6.65**	33 gtt/min		
6.50	0.9 mL	**6.58**	13 gtt/min	**6.66**	yes		

CHAPTER 7

Pediatric Dosages

7.1 DOSAGES BASED ON BODY WEIGHT

For many medications the amount to be administered is proportional to the weight of the recipient. That is, a patient receives a certain amount of a drug *per unit of body weight*. For example, a doctor may prescribe for a patient a certain number of milligrams of a medication per kilogram of body weight, or a certain number of micrograms per pound of body weight, and so on. The nurse, therefore, must calculate the total amount of the drug to be administered based on the weight of the patient.

Converting Body Weight between Pounds and Kilograms. To convert from pounds to kilograms and vice versa, the relationship to use is

$$1 \text{ kg} = 2.2 \text{ lb}$$

EXAMPLE 7.1 Convert the following weights from pounds to kilograms or vice versa: (*a*) 42 lb; (*b*) 38 kg; (*c*) 5 lb 9 oz.

Each of the conversions will use the relationship 1 kg = 2.2 lb.

(*a*) The required conversion is: $\qquad$ 42 lb → ? kg

Set up the calculation: $\qquad$ $42 \text{ lb} \times \dfrac{1 \text{ kg}}{2.2 \text{ lb}}$

Perform the calculation: $\qquad$ $\dfrac{42 \text{ kg}}{2.2} = 19.1 \text{ kg}$

Thus, 42 lb is equal to 19.1 kg.

(*b*) The required conversion is: $\qquad$ 38 kg → ? lb

Set up the calculation: $\qquad$ $38 \text{ kg} \times \dfrac{2.2 \text{ lb}}{1 \text{ kg}}$

Perform the calculation: $\qquad$ $38 \times 2.2 \text{ lb} = 83.6 \text{ lb}$

Thus, 38 kg is equal to 83.6 lb.

162

(c)   For this problem, 9 oz must first be converted into pounds using the relationship 16 oz = 1 lb. Thus,

The required conversion is: $9\,oz \rightarrow ?\,lb$

Set up the calculation: $9\,\cancel{oz} \times \dfrac{1\,lb}{16\,\cancel{oz}}$

Set up the calculation: $\dfrac{9}{16}\,lb = 0.6\,lb$ (nearest tenth)

Thus, 5 lb 9 oz = 5.6 lb. Now convert this into kilograms.

Set up the calculation: $5.6\,\cancel{lb} \times \dfrac{1\,kg}{2.2\,\cancel{lb}}$

Perform the calculation: $\dfrac{5.6}{2.2}\,kg = 2.5\,kg$ (nearest tenth)

Therefore, 5 lb 9 oz is equal to 2.5 kg.

Calculating Dosage from Body Weight.   If the patient's weight in kilograms is known and the dosage rate is given as an amount of drug per kilogram, the dosage is calculated directly from the patient's body weight:

$$Patient's\ weight \rightarrow dosage$$

EXAMPLE 7.2   A patient is to receive medication at the rate of 0.25 mg per kilogram of body weight. How many milligrams will you administer if the patient weighs 75 kg?
   The idea is to convert the weight (75 kg) of the patient directly into the appropriate amount of medication based on the relationship 1 kg (body weight) = 0.25 mg (medication).

The required conversion is: $75\,kg \rightarrow ?\,mg$

The relationship to use is: $1\,kg = 0.25\,mg$

Set up the calculation: $75\,\cancel{kg} \times \dfrac{0.25\,mg}{1\,\cancel{kg}}$

Perform the calculation: $75 \times 0.25\,mg = 18.75\,mg$

Thus, the total dosage for a 75-kg patient is 18.75 mg.

   When the weight of the patient is known in pounds but the dosage rate is given as amount of drug per kilogram, the patient's weight must first be converted from pounds to kilograms. The result is then converted into the proper dosage:

$$Patient's\ weight\ (lb) \rightarrow patient's\ weight\ (kg) \rightarrow dosage$$

EXAMPLE 7.3   The patient weighs 176 lb. The dosage rate ordered for a drug is 10 mg per kilogram of body weight. How many milligrams should you administer to the patient?
   To convert the patient's weight into the proper amount of medication, the weight in pounds must first be converted into kilograms since the dosage rate relates the weight in kilograms to the medication in milligrams.

The required conversion is: $176\,lb \rightarrow ?\,kg \rightarrow ?\,mg$

The relationships to use are: $2.2\,lb = 1\,kg$ and $1\,kg = 10\,mg$

Set up the calculation: $176\,\cancel{lb} \times \dfrac{1\,\cancel{kg}}{2.2\,\cancel{lb}} \times \dfrac{10\,mg}{1\,\cancel{kg}}$

Perform the calculation: $\dfrac{176 \times 10 \text{ mg}}{2.2} = 800 \text{ mg}$

A 176-lb patient will therefore receive 800 mg of the medication.

EXAMPLE 7.4 A patient weighs 110 lb. The order is for 0.25 mg of a drug per kilogram of body weight. If the drug label indicates the concentration to be 5 mg/mL, how many milliliters should you administer?

The weight of the patient in pounds must be converted into kilograms. Then this must be converted into the proper amount of medication in milligrams, which in turn must be converted into the dose in milliliters.

The required conversion is: $110 \text{ lb} \rightarrow ? \text{ kg} \rightarrow ? \text{ mg} \rightarrow ? \text{ mL}$

The relationships to use are: $2.2 \text{ lb} = 1 \text{ kg}, \; 1 \text{ kg} = 0.25 \text{ mg}, \text{ and } 5 \text{ mg} = 1 \text{ mL}$

Set up the calculation: $110 \text{ lb} \times \dfrac{1 \text{ kg}}{2.2 \text{ lb}} \times \dfrac{0.25 \text{ mg}}{1 \text{ kg}} \times \dfrac{1 \text{ mL}}{5 \text{ mg}}$

Perform the calculation: $\dfrac{110 \times 0.25}{2.2 \times 5} \text{ mL} = 2.5 \text{ mL}$

Administer 2.5 mL to a 110-lb patient.

EXAMPLE 7.5 Achromycin (tetracycline hydrochloride) is to be administered 10 mg per pound in 4 equal doses to a patient weighing 30 kg. Oral suspension is available 125 mg per 5 mL. How many milliliters should you give per dose?

First calculate the total amount to be administered, then divide this into 4 equal doses.

The required conversion is: $30 \text{ kg} \rightarrow ? \text{ lb} \rightarrow ? \text{ mg} \rightarrow ? \text{ mL}$

The relationships to use are: $1 \text{ kg} = 2.2 \text{ lb}, \; 1 \text{ lb} = 10 \text{ mg}, \text{ and } 125 \text{ mg} = 5 \text{ mL}$

Set up the calculation: $30 \text{ kg} \times \dfrac{2.2 \text{ lb}}{1 \text{ kg}} \times \dfrac{10 \text{ mg}}{1 \text{ lb}} \times \dfrac{5 \text{ mL}}{125 \text{ mg}}$

Divide into 4 equal doses: $\dfrac{1}{4} \times 30 \text{ kg} \times \dfrac{2.2 \text{ lb}}{1 \text{ kg}} \times \dfrac{10 \text{ mg}}{1 \text{ lb}} \times \dfrac{5 \text{ mL}}{125 \text{ mg}}$

Perform the calculation: $\dfrac{30 \times 2.2 \times 10 \times 5 \text{ mL}}{4 \times 125} = 6.6 \text{ mL/dose}$

EXAMPLE 7.6 Penicillin G sodium is supplied in vials containing 5 million U of crystalline penicillin, to which the addition of 18 mL of diluent will provide a concentration of 250,000 U/mL. You are to administer 50,000 U per kilogram of body weight daily to a child weighing 80 lb, divided into doses q4h, given in 30-mL IVPB. (*a*) How many units will be administered each day? (*b*) How many units will be given per dose? (*c*) How many milliliters will one dose contain?

(*a*) To calculate the total amount to be administered, convert the child's weight, 80 lb, to the proper amount of medication in units.

The required conversion is: $80 \text{ lb} \rightarrow ? \text{ kg} \rightarrow ? \text{ U}$

The relationships to use are: $2.2 \text{ lb} = 1 \text{ kg} \text{ and } 1 \text{ kg} = 50,000 \text{ U}$

Set up the calculation: $80 \text{ lb} \times \dfrac{1 \text{ kg}}{2.2 \text{ lb}} \times \dfrac{50,000 \text{ U}}{1 \text{ kg}}$

Perform the calculation: $\dfrac{80 \times 50,000 \text{ U}}{2.2} = 1,818,181 \text{ U}$

The total amount to be administered is 1,800,000 U (rounded to the nearest hundred thousand) over a 24-h period.

(b) To divide this into doses q4h, divide 1,800,000 U into 6 equal doses (24 h ÷ 4 h = 6 doses): 1,800,00 U ÷ 6 doses = 300,000 U per dose.

(c) We must find the number of milliliters containing 300,000 U.

The required conversion is:	$300{,}000\,U \to ?\,mL$
The relationship to use is:	$250{,}000\,U = 1\,mL$
Set up the calculation:	$300{,}000\,\cancel{U} \times \dfrac{1\,mL}{250{,}000\,\cancel{U}}$
Perform the calculation:	$\dfrac{300{,}000}{250{,}000}\,mL = 1.2\,mL$

Each dose will be contained in 1.2 mL, which will be further diluted in 30 mL to be administered IVPB.

EXAMPLE 7.7 A patient weighing 110 lb is to receive Dextran 40, 1 g per kilogram of body weight, intravenously over a 24-h period. The IV solution contains 10 g per 100 mL. (a) How many milliliters of the solution should be infused over 24 h? (b) Calculate the correct drop rate for a microdrop delivery system.

(a) First, calculate the number of milliliters that will contain the dosage.

The required conversion is:	$110\,lb \to ?\,mL$
This requires three steps:	$110\,lb \to ?\,kg \to ?\,g \to ?\,mL$
The relationships to use are:	$1\,kg = 2.2\,lb$, $1\,kg = 1\,g$, and $100\,mL = 10\,g$
Set up the calculation:	$110\,\cancel{lb} \times \dfrac{1\,\cancel{kg}}{2.2\,\cancel{lb}} \times \dfrac{1\,\cancel{g}}{1\,\cancel{kg}} \times \dfrac{100\,mL}{10\,\cancel{g}}$
Perform the calculation:	$\dfrac{110 \times 100}{2.2 \times 10}\,mL = 500\,mL$

500 mL of solution is to be infused over 24 h.

(b) Next convert the rate of delivery 500 mL/24 h to a drop rate for a drop factor of 60.

The required conversion is:	$\dfrac{500\,mL}{24\,h} \to ?\,\dfrac{gtt}{min}$
The relationships to use are:	$1\,h = 60\,min$ and $1\,mL = 60\,gtt$

You may use the fact that for a microdrop delivery system, the flow rate in milliliters per hour is equal to the drop rate in drops per minute, or you may set up the problem as below.

Set up the calculation:	$\dfrac{500\,\cancel{mL}}{24\,\cancel{h}} \times \dfrac{1\,\cancel{h}}{60\,min} \times \dfrac{60\,gtt}{1\,\cancel{mL}}$
Perform the calculation:	$\dfrac{500 \times \cancel{60}^{\,1}\,gtt}{24 \times \cancel{60}_{\,1}\,min} = 21\,gtt/min$

The drop rate is 21 gtt/min.

7.2 DOSAGES BASED ON BODY SURFACE AREA

The dosages of some drugs are calculated proportionally to the body surface area of the recipient. Body surface area is calculated in square meters (m^2). A square meter is an area equivalent to that of a square that is 1 m on each side; it is therefore approximately equal to 1 square yard. When the total body surface area of the patient is known in square meters, the proper amount of medication can be calculated.

EXAMPLE 7.8 A drug is to be administered 2.5 g per square meter. The total body surface area of the patient is 1.2 m². Calculate the dose the patient should receive.

The body surface area of the patient is to be converted to the proper amount of medication. Thus,

The required conversion is: $1.2\,\text{m}^2 \rightarrow ?\,\text{g}$

The relationship to use is: $1\,\text{m}^2 = 2.5\,\text{g}$

Set up the calculation: $1.2\,\cancel{\text{m}^2} \times \dfrac{2.5\,\text{g}}{1\,\cancel{\text{m}^2}}$

Perform the calculation: $1.2 \times 2.5\,\text{g} = 3\,\text{g}$

The patient should be given 3 g of the drug, based on body surface area.

Body Surface Area Charts. To give medication according to body surface area, a way to find the body surface area of a patient is needed. A chart for determining body surface area based only on the weight of the patient is given in Fig. 7-1. The weight of the patient in pounds is read on the left-hand scale, and the corresponding surface area in square meters is read on the right-hand scale.

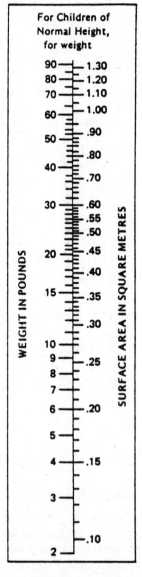

Fig. 7-1 Weight–surface area chart.

EXAMPLE 7.9 A drug is to be administered 200 mg per square meter PO. The patient weighs 85 lb. Based on the body surface area of the patient as determined from the chart of Fig. 7-1, how many milligrams should the patient receive?

The surface area of the patient should be found from the chart by locating 85 lb in the left-hand scale. The surface area found opposite the 85 lb is approximately $1.27\,m^2$. This is to be converted into the desired amount of medication.

The required conversion is: $\qquad\qquad\qquad 1.27\,m^2 \to ?\,mg$

The relationship to use is: $\qquad\qquad\qquad 1\,m^2 = 200\,mg$

Set up the calculation: $\qquad\qquad\qquad 1.27\,\cancel{m^2} \times \dfrac{200\,mg}{1\,\cancel{m^2}}$

Perform the calculation: $\qquad\qquad\qquad 1.27 \times 200\,mg = 254\,mg$

Thus, you would administer 254 mg to the patient.

The chart in Fig. 7-1 gives the surface area for a patient of "normal" weight. However, surface area varies according to both the weight *and* height of the patient. The *West nomogram* in Fig. 7-2 gives a more accurate determination of the surface area of a patient. To find the surface area of a patient, use a straightedge to join the height of the patient (in the height scale) to the weight of the patient (in the weight scale). The surface area is given by the point at which the straightedge crosses the surface area scale. For example, the straight line shown, joining 65 in to 135 lb, crosses the surface area scale at approximately $1.7\,m^2$.

EXAMPLE 7.10 A patient is 5 ft 3 in tall and weighs 100 lb. A drug is to be administered 25 mg per square meter. Based on the West nomogram, calculate the correct dosage for the patient.

Since 5 ft 3 in equals 63 in, a straightedge joining 63 in to 100 lb should cross the surface area scale at approximately $1.44\,m^2$. This is to be converted to the proper amount of medication.

The required conversion is: $\qquad\qquad\qquad 1.44\,m^2 \to ?\,mg$

The relationship to use is: $\qquad\qquad\qquad 1\,m^2 = 25\,mg$

Set up the calculation: $\qquad\qquad\qquad 1.44\,\cancel{m^2} \times \dfrac{25\,mg}{1\,\cancel{m^2}}$

Perform the calculation: $\qquad\qquad\qquad 1.44 \times 25\,mg = 36\,mg$

The correct amount to administer is 36 mg.

Surface Area Formula for Pediatric Dosages. When there is no relationship given between body surface area and amount of drug, the medication can still be administered proportionally to the body surface area using the formula:

$$\text{Child's dose} = \text{adult's dose} \times \frac{\text{child's surface area}}{1.73\ m^2}$$

This formula converts the adult's dose to the proper child's dose, based on the assumption that the body surface area of an average adult is $1.73\,m^2$.

EXAMPLE 7.11 The adult dose for pentobarbital is 30 mg PO. Calculate a safe dosage for a child weighing 50 lb, using body surface area.

Using the chart in Fig. 7-1, you find that the child's body surface area is approximately $0.87\,m^2$. Now convert the adult's dose to the proper child's dose using $0.87\,m^2$ as the child's surface area and $1.73\,m^2$ as the average adult's body surface area.

The required conversion is: $\qquad\qquad\qquad 30\,mg\ (\text{adult's}) \to ?\,mg\ (\text{child's})$

The ratio to use is: $\qquad\qquad\qquad \dfrac{0.87\ m^2}{1.73\ m^2}$

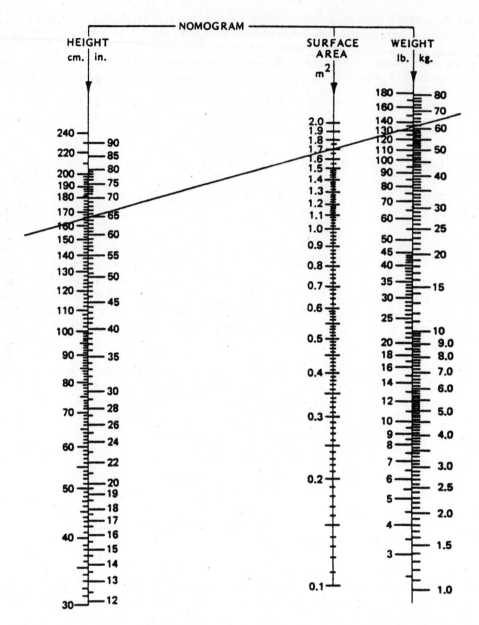

Fig. 7-2 West nomogram. (From R. E. Behrman, et al. "Nelson Textbook of Pediatrics," 16th edition, 2000. *Courtesy W. B. Saunders Co., Philadelphia.*)

Set up the calculation:

$$30 \text{ mg} \times \frac{0.87 \text{ m}^2}{1.73 \text{ m}^2}$$

Perform the calculation:

$$\frac{30 \times 0.87}{1.73} \text{ mg} = 15.1 \text{ mg} \qquad \text{(nearest tenth)}$$

Based on body surface area, 15.1 mg is a safe dose for a 50-lb child if the adult dose is 30 mg.

Another procedure for computing surface area is Mosteller's formula:

$$\text{Surface area (m}^2) = \sqrt{\frac{\text{height (cm)} \times \text{weight (kg)}}{3600}}$$

EXAMPLE 7.12   Use Mosteller's formula to compute the surface area of a patient who is 5 ft 3 in tall and who weighs 100 lb. A drug is to be administered 25 mg per square meter. Calculate the correct dosage for the patient.

First convert 63 in to centimeters and 100 lb to kilograms.

The conversion from inches to centimeters is: $63 \text{ in} \times \dfrac{2.54 \text{ cm}}{1 \text{ in}} = 160 \text{ cm}$

The conversion from pounds to kilograms is: $100 \text{ lb} \times \dfrac{1 \text{ kg}}{2.2 \text{ lb}} = 45 \text{ kg}$

The surface area using Mosteller's formula is: $\text{Surface area (m}^2) = \sqrt{\dfrac{160 \text{ (cm)} \times 45 \text{ (kg)}}{3600}} = 1.41 \text{ m}^2$

The required conversion is: $1.41 \text{ m}^2 \rightarrow ? \text{ mg}$

The relationship to use is: $1 \text{ m}^2 = 25 \text{ mg}$

Set up the calculation: $1.41 \text{ m}^2 \times \dfrac{25 \text{ mg}}{1 \text{ m}^2} = 35.25 \text{ mg}$

Solved Problems

CONVERSIONS BETWEEN POUNDS AND KILOGRAMS

7.1   Convert each of the following from pounds to kilograms or vice versa. Give answers to nearest tenth.

   (*a*)   26 kg   (*c*)   34.7 lb   (*e*)   6 lb 4 oz
   (*b*)   73 lb   (*d*)   49.5 kg   (*f*)   12 lb 10 oz

Solution

   (*a*) $26 \text{ kg} \times \dfrac{2.2 \text{ lb}}{1 \text{ kg}} = 26 \times 2.2 \text{ lb} = 57.2 \text{ lb}$

   (*b*) $73 \text{ lb} \times \dfrac{1 \text{ kg}}{2.2 \text{ lb}} = \dfrac{73}{2.2} \text{ kg} = 33.2 \text{ kg}$

   (*c*) $34.7 \text{ lb} \times \dfrac{1 \text{ kg}}{2.2 \text{ lb}} = \dfrac{34.7}{2.2} \text{ kg} = 15.8 \text{ kg}$

   (*d*) $49.5 \text{ kg} \times \dfrac{2.2 \text{ lb}}{1 \text{ kg}} = 49.5 \times 2.2 \text{ lb} = 108.9 \text{ lb}$

   (*e*)   First change oz to lb: $4 \text{ oz} \times \dfrac{1 \text{ lb}}{16 \text{ oz}} = \dfrac{4}{16} \text{ lb} = 0.25 \text{ lb}$

           So $6 \text{ lb } 4 \text{ oz} = 6.25 \text{ lb}$

           Then change lb to kg: $6.25 \text{ lb} \times \dfrac{1 \text{ kg}}{2.2 \text{ lb}} = \dfrac{6.25}{2.2} \text{ kg} = 2.8 \text{ kg}$

   (*f*)   First change oz to lb: $10 \text{ oz} \times \dfrac{1 \text{ lb}}{16 \text{ oz}} = \dfrac{10}{16} \text{ lb} = 0.6 \text{ lb}$

           So $12 \text{ lb } 10 \text{ oz} = 12.6 \text{ lb}$

Then change lb to kg: $\qquad$ $12.6\ \cancel{lb} \times \dfrac{1\ kg}{2.2\ \cancel{lb}} = \dfrac{12.6}{2.2}\ kg = 5.7\ kg$

DOSAGES BASED ON BODY WEIGHT

7.2 Lanoxin is to be administered to a child weighing 15 kg. Loading dose is 0.035 mg/kg in 3 divided doses over 24 h. The label of the available medication is shown in Fig. 7-3. How many milliliters should be given every 8 h?

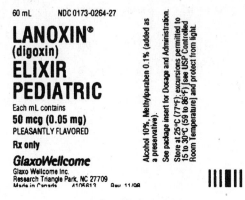

Fig. 7-3

Solution

The 24-h loading dose is

$$15\ \cancel{kg} \times \frac{0.035\ \cancel{mg}}{1\ \cancel{kg}} \times \frac{1\ mL}{0.05\ \cancel{mg}} = 10.5\ mL$$

Each 8-h dose is one-third of 10.5 mL or 3.5 mL.

7.3 You are to administer Aldactone 3.3 mg per kilogram PO daily divided into 2 doses. You have 25-mg tablets available. How would you administer the medication to a child weighing 30 kg?

Solution

$$\frac{1}{2} \times 30\ \cancel{kg} \times \frac{3.3\ mg}{1\ \cancel{kg}} = \frac{30 \times 3.3\ mg}{2} = 49.5\ mg$$

You are to give 49.5 mg, or approximately 50 mg per dose. Therefore, you will give two 25-mg tablets every 12 h.

7.4 Dilantin is prescribed at the rate of 4 mg per kilogram for a child weighing 55 lb. How many milligrams should the child receive?

Solution

$$55\ \cancel{lb} \times \frac{1\ \cancel{kg}}{2.2\ \cancel{lb}} \times \frac{4\ mg}{1\ \cancel{kg}} = \frac{55 \times 4}{2.2}\ mg = 100\ mg$$

Give 100 mg to a 55-lb child.

7.5   Thirty mg/kg/day of Ceftin oral suspension PO, in 2 divided doses for 10 days, is ordered for a 30-lb child. The label of the Ceftin available is shown in Fig. 7-4. How many milliliters should be in each daily divided dose?

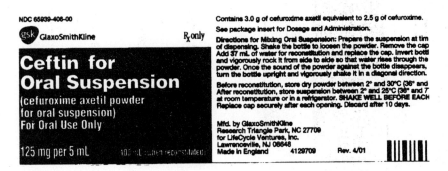

Fig. 7-4

Solution

$$30 \text{ lb} \times \frac{1 \text{ kg}}{2.2 \text{ lb}} \times \frac{30 \text{ mg}}{1 \text{ kg}} \times \frac{5 \text{ mL}}{125 \text{ mg}} = 16.4 \text{ mL}$$

The dosage is 16.4 mL per day or 8.2 mL in each of the 2 daily doses.

7.6   Unipen (nafcillin sodium) 50 mg per kilogram PO daily divided q6h is to be administered to a child weighing 40 lb. When reconstituted, the powder for oral solution yields 250 mg per 5 mL. (*a*) How many milliliters will the child receive in 24 h? (*b*) How many milliliters per dose will the child receive?

Solution

(*a*) $40 \text{ lb} \times \dfrac{1 \text{ kg}}{2.2 \text{ lb}} \times \dfrac{50 \text{ mg}}{1 \text{ kg}} \times \dfrac{5 \text{ mL}}{250 \text{ mg}} = \dfrac{40 \times 50 \times 5}{2.2 \times 250} \text{ mL} = 18.2 \text{ mL}$

The total dosage is 18.2 mL (nearest tenth).

(*b*)   To divide this into doses q6h, divide it into 4 doses (24 h ÷ 6 h = 4 doses). 18.2 mL ÷ 4 doses = 4.6 mL per dose (nearest tenth).

7.7   Abelcet is to be administered IV at a rate of 2.5 mg/kg/h to a patient weighing 70 lb.

(*a*)   What is the rate of delivery in milligrams per hour?

(*b*)   The IV solution contains 100 mg/20 mL. What is the flow rate in mL/h?

Solution

(*a*) $70 \text{ lb} \times \dfrac{1 \text{ kg}}{2.2 \text{ lb}} \times \dfrac{2.5 \text{ mg}}{1 \text{ kg}} = \dfrac{70 \times 2.5}{2.2} \text{ mg} = 80 \text{ mg}$

The rate of delivery is 80 mg/h to the nearest whole number.

(*b*) $\dfrac{80 \text{ mg}}{1 \text{ h}} \times \dfrac{20 \text{ mL}}{100 \text{ mg}} = \dfrac{80 \times 20 \text{ mL}}{100 \text{ h}} = 16 \text{ mL/h}$

The flow rate is 16 mL/h.

7.8   Dobutrex (dobutamine hydrochloride) is administered IV at the rate of 2.5 μg/min per kilogram to a patient weighing 140 lb. (*a*) What is the rate of delivery in micrograms per minute? (*b*) The IV solution contains 250 μg/mL. What is the flow rate in mL/h? (*c*) Using a microdrop, calculate the correct drop rate.

Solution

(*a*) $140 \text{ lb} \times \dfrac{1 \text{ kg}}{2.2 \text{ lb}} \times \dfrac{2.5 \text{ μg}}{1 \text{ kg}} = \dfrac{140 \times 2.5}{2.2} \text{ μg} = 159 \text{ μg}$

The rate of delivery is 159 μg/min (nearest whole).

(*b*) $\dfrac{159 \text{ μg}}{1 \text{ min}} \times \dfrac{60 \text{ min}}{1 \text{ h}} \times \dfrac{1 \text{ mL}}{250 \text{ μg}} = \dfrac{159 \times 60}{250} \dfrac{\text{mL}}{\text{h}} = 38.2 \text{ mL/h}$

The flow rate is 38.2 mL/h (nearest tenth).

(*c*) $\dfrac{38.2 \text{ mL}}{1 \text{ h}} \times \dfrac{1 \text{ h}}{60 \text{ min}} \times \dfrac{60 \text{ gtt}}{1 \text{ mL}} = \dfrac{38.2 \times 60}{60} \dfrac{\text{gtt}}{\text{min}} = 38.2 \text{ gtt/min}$

The drop rate is 38 gtt/min (to the nearest whole).

DOSAGES BASED ON BODY SURFACE AREA

7.9   Use the weight–surface area chart (Fig. 7-1) to find the body surface area corresponding to each of the following body weights: (*a*) 28 lb; (*b*) 45 lb; (*c*) 72 lb; (*d*) 85 lb.

Solution

(*a*) 0.57 m^2; (*b*) 0.81 m^2; (*c*) 1.13 m^2; (*d*) 1.27 m^2.

7.10   Use the West nomogram (Fig. 7-2) to find the body surface area corresponding to the following heights and weights: (*a*) 45 lb and 3 ft 6 in; (*b*) 45 lb and 4 ft; (*c*) 67 lb and 4 ft 2 in; (*d*) 67 lb and 4 ft 8 in.

Solution

(*a*) 0.78 m^2; (*b*) 0.83 m^2; (*c*) 1.04 m^2; (*d*) 1.08 m^2.

7.11   A drug is to be administered 250 mg/m². The patient weighs 75 lb. (*a*) Use the chart of Fig. 7-1 to find the patient's body surface area. (*b*) Calculate the proper dosage for the patient.

Solution

(*a*) 1.16 m^2

(*b*) $1.16 \text{ m}^2 \times \dfrac{250 \text{ mg}}{1 \text{ m}^2} = 290$ mg. 290 mg is an acceptable dose for this patient.

7.12   Gantrisin (sulfisoxazole) is to be given 2 g per square meter PO daily divided in doses q6h. (*a*) How many grams should be administered to a child whose body surface area is 0.8 m²? (*b*) Gantrisin syrup contains 0.5 g per 5 mL. How many milliliters should be given per dose?

Solution

(*a*) $0.8 \text{ m}^2 \times \dfrac{2 \text{ g}}{1 \text{ m}^2} = 0.8 \times 2 \text{ g} = 1.6 \text{ g}$

(b) $\dfrac{1}{4} \times 1.6 \text{ g} \times \dfrac{5 \text{ mL}}{0.5 \text{ g}} = 4 \text{ mL}$

Give 4 mL per dose.

7.13 The average adult dose of Prostaphlin (oxacillin sodium) is 3 g daily divided into doses q6h. The patient is a child 49 in tall and weighing 53 lb. (a) Use the West nomogram (Fig. 7-2) to find the body surface area of the child. (b) Convert the child's body surface area into a safe dosage for the child. (c) Prostaphlin oral solution contains 250 mg per 5 mL. How many milliliters should be given per dose?

Solution

(a) 0.91 m^2

(b) $3 \text{ g} \times \dfrac{0.91 \text{ m}^2}{1.73 \text{ m}^2} = \dfrac{3 \times 0.91}{1.73} \text{ g} = 1.6 \text{ g daily}$

$1.6 \text{ g} \div 4 = 0.4 \text{ g per dose (nearest tenth)}$

(c) $0.4 \text{ g} \times \dfrac{1000 \text{ mg}}{1 \text{ g}} \times \dfrac{5 \text{ mL}}{250 \text{ mg}} = \dfrac{0.4 \times 1000 \times 5}{250} \text{ mL} = 8 \text{ mL}$

8 mL per dose would be safe.

7.14 A child is 127 cm tall and weighs 30 kg. (a) Use the West nomogram (Fig. 7-2) to find the surface area of the child. (b) Use Mosteller's formula to find the surface area and compare it to the surface area found in part (a).

Solution

(a) Using a ruler and Fig. 7-2, the surface area is found to be 1.05 m^2.

(b) Surface area $(\text{m}^2) = \sqrt{\dfrac{127 \text{ (cm)} \times 30 \text{ (kg)}}{3600}} = 1.03 \text{ m}^2$

Supplementary Problems

CONVERSIONS BETWEEN POUNDS AND KILOGRAMS

7.15 Convert each of the following from pounds to kilograms and vice versa. Give answers to nearest tenth.

(a) 165 lb   (c) 57.4 kg   (e) 10 lb 8 oz

(b) 49 kg   (d) 148.8 lb   (f) 5 lb 3 oz

DOSAGES BASED ON BODY WEIGHT

7.16 How many milligrams of a medication should a patient weighing 82 kg receive if the dosage rate is 3 mg per kilogram of body weight?

7.17 A patient weighs 43.5 kg. The doctor orders a drug at the rate of 5 μg per kilogram of body weight. How many micrograms would you administer? Give answer to nearest whole.

7.18   Ampicillin sulbactam is to be administered 75 mg/kg IV q6h. How many grams per dose should a child weighing 30 kg receive?

7.19   Oxacillin is ordered 15 mg per kilogram PO. On hand are 250-mg and 500-mg capsules. How would you administer the medication to a child weighing 33 kg?

7.20   Chlorpromazine 0.25 mg per pound of body weight PO is prescribed for a child who weighs 40 lb. Thorazine tablets available contain 10 mg, 25 mg, and 50 mg chlorpromazine. How would you administer the order?

7.21   Ampicillin is to be given 100 mg per kilogram IV daily, divided q6h. The patient weighs 40 kg. Piggyback vials containing 500 mg, 1 g, and 2 g are available. How would you administer the medication?

7.22   The patient weighs 40 lb. Phenergan injection (promethazine hydrochloride) is prescribed 0.5 mg per pound of body weight. A 1-mL Tubex syringe contains 25 mg of promethazine. How many milliliters will you administer?

7.23   The RDA (Recommended Daily Allowance) of protein for an adult is 0.8 g per kilogram of body weight. How many grams of protein daily is recommended for an adult who weighs 150 lb? Give answer to nearest tenth.

7.24   The doctor orders 20 mg per kilogram of a drug. An infant weighs 28 lb. How many milligrams of the drug should be administered? Give answer to nearest whole.

7.25   Lasix (furosemide) is to be administered 2 mg per kilogram to an infant weighing 23 lb. How many milligrams should the infant receive? Give answer to nearest tenth.

7.26   Potassium chloride is being administered to a patient who weighs 65 lb. If the total daily dose for a child is not to exceed 3 mEq per kilogram, what should be the maximum dosage for this patient? Give answer to nearest whole.

7.27   Epinephrine 1 : 1000 is to be administered SC to a child, 0.01 mL per kilogram of body weight, q20min prn. The child weighs 62 lb. How many milliliters should you administer per dose? Give answer to nearest hundredth.

7.28   Garamycin (gentamicin sulfate) is to be infused IV, 3 mg per kilogram in divided doses q8h. How many milligrams per dose should a 110-lb patient receive?

7.29   A child weighing 48 lb is to receive phenobarbital, 6 mg per kilogram PO divided tid. (*a*) How many milligrams total will the child receive? (*b*) How many milligrams are contained in one dose? Give answer to nearest tenth.

7.30   Kantrex (kanamycin sulfate) 15 mg per kilogram divided q12h is to be infused IV to a patient weighing 73 lb. How many milligrams will the patient receive per dose? Give answer to nearest whole.

7.31 Penicillin V potassium is to be administered to a child weighing 47 lb. The dosage rate is 15 mg per kilogram. Betapen-VK oral solution on hand contains 250 mg/5 mL. How many milliliters of the oral solution should be administered to the child? Give answer to nearest tenth.

7.32 Guaifenesin is to be administered 12 mg per kilogram PO daily to a child in 6 equal doses. The bottle of Robitussin contains 100 mg guaifenesin per 5 mL. If the child weighs 56 lb, how many milliliters of Robitussin will the child receive per dose? Give answer to nearest tenth.

7.33 Dopamine hydrochloride is given IV at the rate of 2 μg/min per kilogram. The patient weighs 175 lb. (*a*) What is the rate of delivery in μg/min? Give answer to nearest whole. (*b*) The IV solution contains 400 μg/mL. What is the flow rate in mL/h? Give answer to nearest tenth.

DOSAGES BASED ON BODY SURFACE AREA

7.34 Dilantin is to be administered 250 mg per square meter of body surface area PO daily. A child has body surface area 0.6 m^2. (*a*) How many milligrams should be administered daily? (*b*) Dilantin suspension contains 125 mg per 5 mL. How many milliliters should be given?

7.35 Sulfadiazine is to be administered 4 g per square meter PO in 6 equal doses. (*a*) How many grams total should be administered to a patient whose body surface area is 0.9 m^2? (*b*) Sulfadyne tablets contain 125 mg each. How many tablets should be given per dose?

7.36 Chlorambucil is to be administered 4.5 mg per square meter per day PO to a child who weighs 50 lb and is 3 ft 6 in tall. (*a*) Use the West nomogram (Fig. 7-2) to find the child's body surface area. (*b*) Calculate the dosage for this patient. Give answer to the nearest tenth. (*c*) Chlorambucil is supplied in tablets containing 2 mg. How many tablets are needed?

7.37 A child is 36 in tall and weighs 30 lb. (*a*) Use the West nomogram to find the body surface area of this child. (*b*) Use the body surface area formula to calculate the proper dose of Demerol for this child if the average adult dose is 75 mg. Give answer to the nearest tenth.

7.38 A child weighs 95 lb and is 59 in tall. (*a*) Use the West nomogram to find the child's body surface area. (*b*) If an adult dose of epinephrine 1 : 1000 is 0.3 mL, calculate a safe dosage for the child using the body surface formula. Give answer to the nearest tenth.

7.39 An infant weighs 30 lb and is 32 in in length. Bicillin is to be administered to the infant, the adult dosage of which is 1.2 million U IM. (*a*) Use the West nomogram to find the body surface area of the infant. (*b*) Use the body surface area formula to find a safe dose for the infant. (*c*) You have an ampule containing 1.2 million U in 2 mL. How many milliliters should you give? Give answer to the nearest hundredth.

7.40 (*a*) Use the West nomogram to find the surface area for a child who is 44 in tall and weighs 50 lb. (*b*) If the adult dose of Tagamet is 300 mg, use the body surface area formula to find an acceptable dose for the child. (*c*) The bottle of Tagamet contains 300 mg per 5 mL. How many milliliters should be administered?

7.41 A child who is 4 ft 6 in tall and weighs 70 lb is to be given chloral hydrate, the adult dose of which is 250 mg PO. (*a*) Find the body surface area of the child from the West nomogram. (*b*) Use the body surface area formula to find a safe dose for the child. Give answer to nearest tenth. (*c*) Chloral hydrate syrup contains 500 mg per 5 mL. How many milliliters should you give? Give answer to the nearest tenth.

7.42   A child is 100 cm tall and weighs 40 kg. (*a*) Use the West nomogram (Fig. 7-2) to find the surface area of the child. (*b*) Use Mosteller's formula to find the surface area and compare it to the surface area found in part (*a*).

Answers to Supplementary Problems

7.15   (*a*)   75 kg   (*c*)   126.3 lb   (*e*)   4.8 kg
           (*b*)   107.8 lb   (*d*)   67.6 kg   (*f*)   2.4 kg

7.16   Give 246 mg

7.17   Give 218 μg

7.18   2.25 g

7.19   Give one 500-mg capsule

7.20   Give one 10-mg tablet

7.21   Use the 1-g vial

7.22   Give 0.8 mL

7.23   54.5 g of protein daily

7.24   Give 255 mg

7.25   Give 20.9 mg

7.26   Not more than 89 mEq/day

7.27   Give 0.28 mL per dose

7.28   Give 50 mg per dose

7.29   (*a*)   130.9 mg total   (*b*)   43.6 mg per dose

7.30   Give 249 mg per dose

7.31   Give 6.4 mL

7.32   Give 2.5 mL per dose

7.33   (*a*)   159 μg/min   (*b*)   23.9 mL/h

7.34   (*a*)   150 mg   (*b*)   Give 6 mL

7.35   (*a*)   Give 3.6 g total   (*b*)   Give 5 tablets per dose

7.36   (*a*)   0.83 m^2 (*b*)   3.7 mg daily   (*c*)   Give 2 tablets daily

7.37   (*a*)   0.59 m^2 (*b*)   Give 25.6 mg

7.38   (*a*)   1.36 m^2 (*b*)   0.24 mL is safe

7.39   (*a*)   0.57 m^2 (*b*)   400,000 U is safe   (*c*)   Give 0.67 mL

7.40   (*a*)   0.85 m^2 (*b*)   147 mg is acceptable   (*c*)   Give 2.5 mL

7.41   (*a*)   1.1 m^2 (*b*)   159 mg is safe   (*c*)   Give 1.6 mL

7.42   (*a*)   1.10 m^2 (*b*)   1.05 m^2

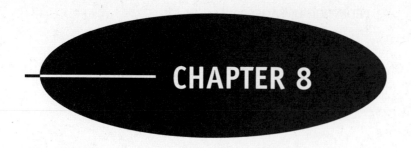

CHAPTER 8

Percentages

8.1 PERCENTAGE

The symbol "%" is called a *percent sign* and means "per hundred." A *percentage* is a number written with a percent sign after it; it represents a fraction whose numerator is the given number and whose denominator is 100. For example, the percentage 15% (read "fifteen percent") means the fraction $\dfrac{15}{100}$. Thus, when one says that a solution is 15% alcohol, this means that out of 100 parts of solution, 15 parts are alcohol.

8.2 CHANGING PERCENTAGES TO EQUIVALENT FRACTIONS

To change a percentage into an equivalent fraction, (1) remove the percent sign, then (2) write the number over 100 and simplify the resulting fraction.

EXAMPLE 8.1 Write the following percentages as equivalent simple fractions reduced to lowest terms: (a) 7%; (b) 35%; (c) $\dfrac{1}{2}$%; (d) 0.4%; (e) 125%; (f) $33\dfrac{1}{3}$%.

(a) Remove the percent sign and write the number over 100:

$$7\% = \frac{7}{100}$$

(b) Remove the percent sign and write the number over 100:

$$35\% = \frac{35}{100}$$

Reduce the fraction:

$$= \frac{7}{20}$$

(c) Remove the percent sign and write the number over 100:

$$\frac{1}{2}\% = \frac{1/2}{100}$$

Simplify the fraction:

$$= \frac{1}{2} \times \frac{1}{100} = \frac{1}{200}$$

(*d*) Remove the percent sign and write the number over 100:

$$0.4\% = \frac{0.4}{100}$$

Simplify the fraction:

$$= \frac{4/10}{100} = \frac{\overset{1}{\cancel{4}}}{10} \times \frac{1}{\underset{25}{\cancel{100}}} = \frac{1}{250}$$

(*e*) Remove the percent sign and write the number over 100:

$$125\% = \frac{125}{100}$$

Reduce and change the fraction to a mixed number:

$$= \frac{5}{4} = 1\frac{1}{4}$$

(*f*) Remove the percent sign and write the number over 100:

$$33\frac{1}{3}\% = \frac{33\frac{1}{3}}{100}$$

Simplify the fraction:

$$= 33\frac{1}{3} \times \frac{1}{100} = \frac{\overset{1}{\cancel{100}}}{3} \times \frac{1}{\underset{1}{\cancel{100}}} = \frac{1}{3}$$

8.3 CHANGING PERCENTAGES TO EQUIVALENT DECIMAL NUMERALS

The percentage 37.5% represents the fraction $\frac{37.5}{100}$. This is the same as .375 since you can divide a number by 100 by moving the decimal point two places to the left (see Sec. 3.6). This illustrates the following rule for changing a percentage to an equivalent decimal numeral: (1) Remove the percent sign, then (2) write the number in decimal form and move the decimal point two places to the left.

EXAMPLE 8.2 Write the following percentages as equivalent decimal numerals: (*a*) 24.5%; (*b*) 0.3%; (*c*) 45%; (*d*) 250%; (*e*) $\frac{1}{4}$%; (*f*) $12\frac{1}{2}$%.

(*a*) Remove the percent sign and move the decimal point two places to the left:

$$24.5\% \rightarrow 0.24.5 = 0.245$$

(*b*) Remove the percent sign and move the decimal point two places to the left:

$$0.3\% \rightarrow 0.00.3 = 0.003$$

(*c*) Remove the percent sign and move the decimal point two places to the left:

$$45\% \rightarrow 0.45. = 0.45$$

(d)   Remove the percent sign and move the decimal point two places to the left:

$$250\% \to 2{,}50. = 2.50$$

(e)   Write $\frac{1}{4}$ as the decimal 0.25:

$$\frac{1}{4}\% = 0.25\%$$

Remove the percent sign and move the decimal point two places to the left:

$$0.25\% \to 0{,}00{,}25 = 0.0025$$

(f)   Write $12\frac{1}{2}$ as the decimal 12.5:

$$12\frac{1}{2}\% = 12.5\%$$

Remove the percent sign and move the decimal point two places to the left:

$$12.5\% \to 0{,}12{.}5 = 0.125$$

It is useful to memorize the fractional and decimal equivalents of some common percentages. Some of these are listed in Tables 8-1 and 8-2.

Table 8-1   Percentage Equivalents for the Tenths

Percentage	Decimal	Fraction
10%	0.1	1/10
20%	0.2	2/10
30%	0.3	3/10
40%	0.4	4/10
50%	0.5	5/10
60%	0.6	6/10
70%	0.7	7/10
80%	0.8	8/10
90%	0.9	9/10
100%	1.0	10/10

Table 8-2   Other Common Percentages

Percentage	Decimal	Fraction
25%	0.25	1/4
$33\frac{1}{3}\%$	$0.33\frac{1}{3}$	1/3
50%	0.50	1/2
$66\frac{2}{3}\%$	$0.66\frac{2}{3}$	2/3
75%	0.75	3/4

8.4   CHANGING DECIMAL NUMERALS TO EQUIVALENT PERCENTAGES

Since changing a decimal numeral to its equivalent percentage is the reverse of changing a percentage to an equivalent decimal numeral, the opposite steps are taken. That is, to change a decimal numeral to an equivalent percentage, (1) move the decimal point two places to the *right*, then (2) attach the percent sign.

EXAMPLE 8.3   Write the following decimal numerals as equivalent percentages: (a) 0.25; (b) 0.033; (c) 1.4; (d) 6; (e) 24.3.

(a)   Move the decimal point two places to the right and add the percent sign:

$$0.25 \to 0{.}25{,}\% = 25\%$$

(b) Move the decimal point two places to the right and add the percent sign:

$$0.033 \rightarrow 0.03\,3\% = 3.3\%$$

(c) Move the decimal point two places to the right and add the percent sign:

$$1.4 \rightarrow 1.40\,\% = 140\%$$

(d) Move the decimal point two places to the right and add the percent sign:

$$6 \rightarrow 6.00\,\% = 600\%$$

(e) Move the decimal point two places to the right and add the percent sign:

$$24.3 \rightarrow 24.30\,\% = 2430\%$$

8.5 CHANGING FRACTIONS TO EQUIVALENT PERCENTAGES

To change a fraction into an equivalent percentage, (1) change the fraction into an equivalent decimal, then (2) change the decimal into the equivalent percentage.

EXAMPLE 8.4   Write the following fractions as equivalent percentages: (a) $\frac{3}{4}$; (b) $\frac{1}{500}$; (c) $2\frac{1}{2}$; (d) $\frac{2}{3}$; (e) $\frac{1}{30}$.

(a) Write $\frac{3}{4}$ as a decimal by performing the division:

$$\begin{array}{r} .75 \\ 4\overline{)3.00} \end{array}$$

Move the decimal point two places to the right and add the percent sign:

$$0.75 \rightarrow 0.75\,\% = 75\%$$

Thus, $\frac{3}{4} = 75\%$.

(b) Write $\frac{1}{500}$ as a decimal by performing the division:

$$\begin{array}{r} .002 \\ 500\overline{)1.000} \end{array}$$

Move the decimal point two places to the right and add the percent sign:

$$.002 \rightarrow .00\,2\% = 0.2\%$$

(c) Write $2\frac{1}{2}$ as a decimal:

$$2\frac{1}{2} = 2.50$$

Move the decimal point two places to the right and add the percent sign:

$$2.50 \rightarrow 2.50\,\% = 250\%$$

(d) To write $\frac{2}{3}$ as a decimal, the division is performed as in the above examples. Since this division does not end, the usual procedure is to approximate the answer by rounding to some degree of accuracy. An alternative is to write the answer with a fractional part as follows:

$$\begin{array}{r} .66 \\ 3\overline{)2.00} \\ \underline{18} \\ 20 \\ \underline{18} \\ 2 \end{array} = 0.66\frac{2}{3} \begin{array}{l} \leftarrow \text{remainder} \\ \leftarrow \text{divisor} \end{array}$$

$$\leftarrow \text{remainder}$$

Thus, $\frac{2}{3} = 0.66\frac{2}{3}$. Move the decimal point two places to the right and add the percent sign:

$$0.66\frac{2}{3} \rightarrow 0.\underset{\smile}{66}\,\frac{2}{3}\% = 66\frac{2}{3}\%$$

(e) Write $\frac{1}{30}$ as a decimal by performing the division (note the remainder):

$$\begin{array}{r} .03\frac{1}{3} \\ 30\overline{)1.00} \end{array}$$

Move the decimal point two places to the right and add the percent sign:

$$.03\frac{1}{3} \rightarrow .\underset{\smile}{03}\,\frac{1}{3}\% = 3\frac{1}{3}\%$$

8.6 PERCENTAGE OF A NUMBER

Since $35\% = \frac{35}{100}$, a phrase such as "35% of 80" means $\frac{35}{100}$ of 80, which means to multiply $\frac{35}{100}$ times 80. Performing this calculation yields the value 28. Thus,

$$28 = 35 \text{ percent of } 80$$

In the above equation, the number (80) that follows the phrase "percent of" is called the *base* (also called the *whole*), and the result (28) of the calculation is called the *part*.

Every problem in percentages consists of solving:

$$\text{Part} = \text{percentage of the base}$$

when one of the three quantities (1) percentage, (2) part, or (3) base is unknown and the other two are given.

8.7 FINDING THE PERCENTAGE GIVEN THE PART AND THE BASE

When the part and the base are given, to find the percentage use the formula:

$$\text{Percentage} = \frac{\text{part}}{\text{base}} \times 100\%$$

EXAMPLE 8.5 Find the percentage in each of the following problems:

(a) 36 is what percent of 144?

(b) What percent of 36 is 144?

(c) What percent of 300 is 2?

(d) 45 is what percent of 45?

In each of these problems, the percentage is the unknown quantity. The base is always the number that comes after the phrase "percent of," and the part is the result of finding a percentage of the base.

(*a*) Since the problem says "percent of 144," the base is 144 and the part is 36. Thus, from the formula:

$$\text{Percentage} = \frac{\overset{1}{\cancel{36}}}{\underset{4}{\cancel{144}}} \times 100\% = \frac{100}{4}\% = 25\%$$

Thus, 36 is 25% of 144.

(*b*) Since the problem says "percent of 36," the base is 36 and the part is 144. Thus, from the formula:

$$\text{Percentage} = \frac{\overset{4}{\cancel{144}}}{\underset{1}{\cancel{36}}} \times 100\% = 400\%$$

Thus, 144 is 400% of 36.

(*c*) Since the problem says "percent of 300," the base is 300 and the part is 2. Thus, from the formula:

$$\text{Percentage} = \frac{2}{\underset{3}{\cancel{300}}} \times \overset{1}{\cancel{100}}\% = \frac{2}{3}\% \text{ or } 0.66\frac{2}{3}\%$$

Thus, 2 is 0.67% of 300 (rounded to the nearest hundredth).

(*d*) Since the problem says "percent of 45," the base is 45 and the part is also 45. Thus, from the formula:

$$\text{Percentage} = \frac{\overset{1}{\cancel{45}}}{\underset{1}{\cancel{45}}} \times 100\% = 100\%$$

Thus, 45 is 100% of 45.

The following facts should be noted from the above example:

1. The percentage is less than 100% when the part is smaller than the base.
2. The percentage is greater than 100% when the part is larger than the base.
3. The percentage is equal to 100% when the part and the base are equal.

8.8   FINDING THE PART GIVEN THE PERCENTAGE AND THE BASE

When the percentage and base are known, to find the part use the formula:

$$\text{Part} = \frac{\text{percentage}}{100\%} \times \text{base}$$

EXAMPLE 8.6   Solve the following problems:

(*a*) What is 60% of 350?

(*b*) Find 125% of 40.

(*c*) 0.7% of 50 is equal to what number?

(*d*) What number is equal to $2\frac{1}{2}\%$ of 1000?

In each of these problems, the base and the percentage are known, and the part is to be found.

(*a*)   Since the problem says "% of 350," the base is 350. The percentage is 60%. From the formula:

$$\text{Part} = \frac{\overset{3}{\cancel{60\%}}}{\underset{5}{\cancel{100\%}}} \times 350 = 210$$

Thus, 210 is 60% of 350.

(*b*)   Since the problem says "% of 40," the base is 40. The percentage is 125%. From the formula:

$$\text{Part} = \frac{\overset{5}{\cancel{125\%}}}{\underset{4}{\cancel{100\%}}} \times 40 = 50$$

Thus, 50 is 125% of 40.

(*c*)   Since the problem says "% of 50," the base is 50. The percentage is 0.7%. From the formula:

$$\text{Part} = \frac{0.7\%}{100\%} \times 50 = \frac{0.7 \times 50}{100} = 0.35$$

Thus, 0.7% of 50 is 0.35.

(*d*)   Since the problem says "% of 1000," the base is 1000. The percentage is $2\frac{1}{2}\%$. From the formula:

$$\text{Part} = \frac{2\frac{1}{2}\%}{100\%} \times 1000 = \frac{5}{2} \times \frac{1}{100} \times 1000 = 25$$

Thus, $2\frac{1}{2}\%$ of 1000 is 25.

8.9   FINDING THE BASE GIVEN THE PERCENTAGE AND THE PART

When the percentage and part are given, to find the base use the formula:

$$\text{Base} = \frac{\text{part}}{\text{percentage}} \times 100\%$$

EXAMPLE 8.7   Find the base in each of the following problems:

(*a*)   16 is 20% of what number?

(*b*)   250% of what number is 300?

(*c*)   0.6% of what is equal to 42?

(*d*)   36 is equal to $3\frac{1}{3}\%$ of what number?

In each of these problems, the part and the percentage are known and the base is to be found.

(*a*)   Since the problem says, "% of what number," the base is unknown. The percentage is 20% and the part is 16. From the formula:

$$\text{Base} = \frac{16}{20\%} \times 100\% = \frac{16 \times 100}{20} = 80$$

Thus, 16 is 20% of 80.

(*b*)   The base is unknown. The percentage is 250% and the part is 300. From the formula:

$$\text{Base} = \frac{300}{250\%} \times 100\% = \frac{300 \times 100}{250} = 120$$

Thus, 250% of 120 is 300.

(c) The base is to be found. The percentage is 0.6% and the part is 42. From the formula:

$$\text{Base} = \frac{42}{0.6\%} \times 100\% = \frac{42 \times 100}{0.6} = \frac{4200}{0.6} = 7000$$

Thus, 42 is equal to 0.6% of 7000.

(d) Find the base. The percentage is $3\frac{1}{3}\%$ and the part is 36. From the formula:

$$\text{Base} = \frac{36}{3\frac{1}{3}\%} \times 100\% = \frac{36 \times 100}{3\frac{1}{3}} = 3600 \times \frac{3}{10} = 1080$$

Thus, $3\frac{1}{3}\%$ of 1080 is equal to 36.

8.10 PERCENTAGE STRENGTH OF SOLUTIONS

A solution consists of two parts mixed together: the *solute*, which is the substance that is dissolved or diluted, and a liquid that contains the solute. The solute can be either liquid or solid. When the solute is a liquid, it is said to be *diluted in a diluent*. For example, an alcohol solution consists of alcohol, a liquid, diluted in water as a diluent. When the solute is a solid (crystals or powders), it is said to be *dissolved in a solvent*. For example, a salt solution consists of solid crystals of salt dissolved in water as a solvent. The meaning of the percentage of a solution differs according to whether the solute is liquid or solid.

Liquid Solutes. For a solution that consists of a liquid solute in a liquid diluent, both solute and solution are measured in the same units of volume (for example, milliliters), and the *concentration* of a solution is the ratio of the volume of solute to the total volume of solution:

$$\text{Concentration} = \frac{\text{volume of solute}}{\text{total volume of solution}}$$

Since this is a ratio, it can also be expressed as a percentage:

Percentage concentration = the volume of solute contained in 100 mL volume of solution

See Fig. 8-1.

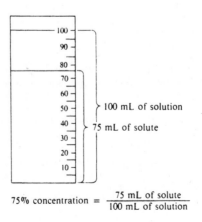

Fig. 8-1

EXAMPLE 8.8 7.5 mL of concentrated (i.e., full strength or undiluted) acetic acid is contained in 250 mL of solution. What is the percentage concentration of the solution?

Here, 7.5 mL of a liquid solute (the full-strength acetic acid) is contained in a total of 250 mL of solution. We must determine what percent of 250 mL is 7.5 mL. Since the part is 7.5 mL and the whole is 250 mL, the answer is:

$$\text{Percentage} = \frac{7.5 \text{ mL}}{250 \text{ mL}} \times 100\% = \frac{7.5 \times 100\%}{250} = 3\%$$

Thus, a concentration of 7.5 mL of solute in 250 mL of solution is a 3% concentration. This means that 3 mL of full-strength acetic acid is contained in 100 mL of solution.

EXAMPLE 8.9 How many milliliters of pure alcohol is contained in 750 mL of a 60% solution?

The problem here is to find 60% of 750 mL. That is, this is a problem in finding the part given the percent, 60%, and the whole, 750 mL.

$$\text{Part} = \frac{60\%}{100\%} \times 750 \text{ mL} = \frac{60 \times 750}{100} \text{ mL} = 450 \text{ mL}$$

Thus, there is 450 mL of pure alcohol in 750 mL of a 60% alcohol solution.

Solid Solutes. For solutions in which a solid is dissolved in solution, the percentage concentration gives the number of grams of solute per 100 mL of solution. For example, a 5% solution of glucose contains 5 g of glucose per 100 mL of solution. Thus, problems involving solutions containing a solid as a solute are conversion problems using the relationship given by the percentage. See Fig. 8-2.

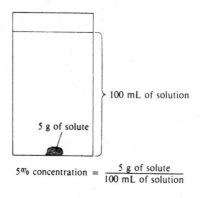

Fig. 8-2

EXAMPLE 8.10 How many grams of glucose is contained in 750 mL of a 5% glucose solution?

The percentage means that 100 mL of solution contains 5 g of glucose. The problem is to find how many grams of glucose is contained in 750 mL of solution.

The required conversion is: 750 mL → ? g (of glucose)

The relationship to use is: 100 mL = 5 g

Set up the calculation: $750 \text{ mL} \times \dfrac{5 \text{ g}}{100 \text{ mL}}$

Perform the calculation: $\dfrac{750 \times 5 \text{ g}}{100} = 37.5 \text{ g}$

Thus, 750 mL of a 5% glucose solution contains 37.5 g of glucose.

EXAMPLE 8.11 400 mL of solution contains 10 g of sodium bicarbonate. What is the percentage concentration of the solution?

Since a percentage concentration is the number of grams of solute contained in 100 mL of solution, we must calculate how many grams 100 mL of solution will contain if 400 mL contains 10 g.

The required conversion is: $100\,\text{mL} \rightarrow ?\,\text{g}$

The relationship to use is: $400\,\text{mL} = 10\,\text{g}$

Set up the calculation: $100\,\cancel{\text{mL}} \times \dfrac{10\,\text{g}}{400\,\cancel{\text{mL}}}$

Perform the calculation: $\dfrac{100 \times 10\,\text{g}}{400} = 2.5\,\text{g}$

100 mL of solution contains 2.5 g of sodium bicarbonate. Therefore, the percentage concentration is 2.5%.

EXAMPLE 8.12 How many milliliters of a 4% solution of boric acid can be made from 5 g of boric acid crystals?

Since the percentage concentration is 4%, 4 g of boric acid is contained in every 100 mL of solution. We must convert 5 g into the proper number of milliliters.

The required conversion is: $5\,\text{g} \rightarrow ?\,\text{mL}$

The relationship to use is: $4\,\text{g} = 100\,\text{mL}$

Set up the calculation: $5\,\cancel{\text{g}} \times \dfrac{100\,\text{mL}}{4\,\cancel{\text{g}}}$

Perform the calculation: $\dfrac{5 \times 100\,\text{mL}}{4} = 125\,\text{mL}$

Thus 5 g of boric acid crystals will make 125 mL of a 4% solution.

Solved Problems

8.1   Change each of the percentages to an equivalent simple fraction (or a whole or mixed number if the fraction is improper).

(a) 9%   (e) 175%   (i) $\dfrac{1}{4}\%$ (m) $67\dfrac{1}{2}\%$ (q) 12.5%

(b) 60%   (f) 100%   (j) $\dfrac{2}{3}\%$ (n) 0.8%   (r) 6.75%

(c) 45%   (g) 260%   (k) $\dfrac{1}{10}\%$ (o) 0.02%   (s) 99.9%

(d) 16%   (h) 300%   (l) $1\dfrac{1}{2}\%$ (p) 7.5%   (t) 0.004%

Solution

(a) $9\% = \dfrac{9}{100}$

(k) $\dfrac{1}{10}\% = \dfrac{\frac{1}{10}}{100} = \dfrac{1}{10} \times \dfrac{1}{100} = \dfrac{1}{1000}$

(b) $60\% = \dfrac{60}{100} = \dfrac{3}{5}$

(l) $1\dfrac{1}{2}\% = \dfrac{1\frac{1}{2}}{100} = \dfrac{3}{2} \times \dfrac{1}{100} = \dfrac{3}{200}$

(c) $45\% = \dfrac{45}{100} = \dfrac{9}{20}$

(m) $67\dfrac{1}{2}\% = \dfrac{67\frac{1}{2}}{100} = \dfrac{135}{2} \times \dfrac{1}{100} = \dfrac{27}{40}$

(d) $16\% = \dfrac{16}{100} = \dfrac{4}{25}$

(n) $0.8\% = \dfrac{0.8}{100} = \dfrac{8}{10} \times \dfrac{1}{100} = \dfrac{1}{125}$

(e) $175\% = \dfrac{175}{100} = \dfrac{7}{4} = 1\dfrac{3}{4}$

(o) $0.02\% = \dfrac{0.02}{100} = \dfrac{2}{100} \times \dfrac{1}{100} = \dfrac{1}{5000}$

(f) $100\% = \dfrac{100}{100} = 1$

(p) $7.5\% = \dfrac{7.5}{100} = \dfrac{7\frac{1}{2}}{100} = \dfrac{15}{2} \times \dfrac{1}{100} = \dfrac{3}{40}$

(g) $260\% = \dfrac{260}{100} = \dfrac{13}{5} = 2\dfrac{3}{5}$

(q) $12.5\% = \dfrac{12\frac{1}{2}}{100} = \dfrac{25}{2} \times \dfrac{1}{100} = \dfrac{1}{8}$

(h) $300\% = \dfrac{300}{100} = 3$

(r) $6.75\% = \dfrac{6\frac{3}{4}}{100} = \dfrac{27}{4} \times \dfrac{1}{100} = \dfrac{27}{400}$

(i) $\dfrac{1}{4}\% = \dfrac{\frac{1}{4}}{100} = \dfrac{1}{4} \times \dfrac{1}{100}$
$= \dfrac{1}{400}$

(s) $99.9\% = \dfrac{99\frac{9}{10}}{100} = \dfrac{999}{10} \times \dfrac{1}{100} = \dfrac{999}{1000}$

(j) $\dfrac{2}{3}\% = \dfrac{\frac{2}{3}}{100} = \dfrac{2}{3} \times \dfrac{1}{100}$
$= \dfrac{1}{150}$

(t) $0.004\% = \dfrac{\frac{4}{1000}}{100} = \dfrac{4}{1000} \times \dfrac{1}{100}$
$= \dfrac{1}{25,000}$

8.2 Write each percentage as an equivalent decimal numeral. Round the answer to the nearest thousandth if the decimal does not terminate.

(a) 112.5% (e) 9.2% (i) 130% (m) 0.25% (q) $133\dfrac{1}{3}\%$

(b) 38.0% (f) 75% (j) 200% (n) 0.01% (r) $\dfrac{1}{2}\%$

(c) 27.1% (g) 16% (k) 0.8% (o) $7\dfrac{1}{2}\%$ (s) $\dfrac{1}{10}\%$

(d) 4.0% (h) 2% (l) 0.30% (p) $66\dfrac{2}{3}\%$ (t) $\dfrac{2}{3}\%$

Solution

(a) $112.5\% \rightarrow 1.12.5 = 1.125$

(b) $38.0\% \rightarrow 0.38.0 = 0.38$

(c) $27.1\% \rightarrow 0.27.1 = 0.271$

(d) $4.0\% \rightarrow 0.04.0 = 0.04$

(e) $9.2\% \rightarrow 0.09.2 = 0.092$

(f) $75\% \rightarrow 0.75. = 0.75$

(g) $16\% \rightarrow 0.16. = 0.16$

(h) $2\% \rightarrow 0.02. = 0.02$

(i) $130\% \rightarrow 1.30. = 1.3$

(j) $200\% \rightarrow 2.00. = 2$

(k) $0.8\% \rightarrow 0.00.8 = 0.008$

(l) $0.30\% \rightarrow 0.00.30 = 0.003$

(m) $0.25\% \rightarrow 0.00.25 = 0.0025$

(n) $0.01\% \rightarrow 0.00.01 = 0.0001$

(o) $7\frac{1}{2}\% = 7.5\% \rightarrow 0.07.5 = 0.075$

(p) $66\frac{2}{3}\% \rightarrow 0.66.\frac{2}{3} = 0.667$

(q) $133\frac{1}{3}\% \rightarrow 1.33.\frac{1}{3} = 1.333$

(r) $\frac{1}{2}\% = 0.5\% \rightarrow 0.00.5 = 0.005$

(s) $\frac{1}{10}\% = 0.1\% \rightarrow 0.00.1 = 0.001$

(t) $\frac{2}{3}\% = 0.66\frac{2}{3}\% \rightarrow 0.00.66\frac{2}{3} = 0.007$

8.3 Write each decimal numeral as an equivalent percentage.

(a) 0.30 (e) 0.5625 (i) 0.0625 (m) 1.45 (q) 2.5

(b) 0.75 (f) 0.04 (j) 0.004 (n) 2.00 (r) 3

(c) 0.98 (g) 0.03 (k) 0.0058 (o) 2.623 (s) 12.1

(d) 0.341 (h) 0.027 (l) 0.0006 (p) 1.8 (t) 25

Solution

(a) $0.30 \rightarrow 0.30.\% = 30\%$

(b) $0.75 \rightarrow 0.75.\% = 75\%$

(c) $0.98 \rightarrow 0.98.\% = 98\%$

(d) $0.341 \rightarrow 0.34.1\% = 34.1\%$

(e) $0.5625 \rightarrow 0.56.25\% = 56.25\%$

(f) $0.04 \rightarrow 0.04.\% = 4\%$

(g) $0.03 \rightarrow 0.03.\% = 3\%$

(h) $0.027 \rightarrow 0.02.7\% = 2.7\%$

(i) $0.0625 \rightarrow 0.06.25\% = 6.25\%$

(j) $0.004 \rightarrow 0.00.4\% = 0.4\%$

(k) $0.0058 \rightarrow 0.00.58\% = 0.58\%$

(l) $0.0006 \rightarrow 0.00.06\% = 0.06\%$

(m) $1.45 \rightarrow 1.45.\% = 145\%$

(n) $2.00 \rightarrow 2.00.\% = 200\%$

(o) $2.623 \rightarrow 2.62.3\% = 262.3\%$

(p) $1.8 \rightarrow 1.80.\% = 180\%$

(q) $2.5 \rightarrow 2.50.\% = 250\%$

(r) $3 \rightarrow 3.00.\% = 300\%$

(s) $12.1 \rightarrow 12.10.\% = 1210\%$

(t) $25 \rightarrow 25.00.\% = 2500\%$

8.4 Express each fraction as an equivalent percentage.

(a) $\frac{1}{4}$ (e) $\frac{1}{100}$ (i) $1\frac{1}{2}$ (m) $3\frac{3}{4}$ (q) $\frac{1}{300}$

(b) $\frac{5}{8}$ (f) $\frac{5}{16}$ (j) 2 (n) $\frac{1}{3}$ (r) $1\frac{1}{3}$

(c) $\frac{1}{20}$ (g) $\frac{1}{250}$ (k) $2\frac{1}{4}$ (o) $\frac{1}{9}$ (s) $2\frac{3}{7}$

(d) $\frac{3}{10}$ (h) $\frac{7}{200}$ (l) $1\frac{3}{8}$ (p) $\frac{4}{15}$ (t) $1\frac{1}{30}$

Solution

(a) $\frac{1}{4} = 0.25 \to 0.25\, \% = 25\%$

(b) $\frac{5}{8} = 0.625 \to 0.62\,5\% = 62.5\%$

(c) $\frac{1}{20} = 0.05 \to 0.05\, \% = 5\%$

(d) $\frac{3}{10} = 0.3 \to 0.30\, \% = 30\%$

(e) $\frac{1}{100} = 0.01 \to 0.01\, \% = 1\%$

(f) $\frac{5}{16} = 0.3125 \to 0.31\,25\%$
$= 31.25\%$

(g) $\frac{1}{250} = 0.004 \to 0.00\,4\%$
$= 0.4\%$

(h) $\frac{7}{200} = 0.035 \to 0.03\,5\% = 3.5\%$

(i) $1\frac{1}{2} = 1.5 \to 1.50\, \% = 150\%$

(j) $2 \to 2.00\, \% = 200\%$

(k) $2\frac{1}{4} = 2.25 \to 2.25\, \% = 225\%$

(l) $1\frac{3}{8} = 1.375 \to 1.37\,5\% = 137.5\%$

(m) $3\frac{3}{4} = 3.75 \to 3.75\, \% = 375\%$

(n) $\frac{1}{3} = 0.33\frac{1}{3} \to 0.33\,\frac{1}{3}\% = 33\frac{1}{3}\%$

(o) $\frac{1}{9} = 0.11\frac{1}{9} \to 0.11\,\frac{1}{9}\% = 11\frac{1}{9}\%$

(p) $\frac{4}{15} = 0.26\frac{2}{3} \to 0.26\,\frac{2}{3}\% = 26\frac{2}{3}\%$

(q) $\frac{1}{300} = 0.003\frac{1}{3} \to 0.00\,3\frac{1}{3}\%$
$= 0.3\frac{1}{3}\%$

(r) $1\frac{1}{3} = 1.33\frac{1}{3} \to 1.33\,\frac{1}{3}\% = 133\frac{1}{3}\%$

(s) $2\frac{3}{7} = 2.42\frac{6}{7} \to 2.42\,\frac{6}{7}\% = 242\frac{6}{7}\%$

(t) $1\frac{1}{30} = 1.03\frac{1}{3} \to 1.03\,\frac{1}{3}\% = 103\frac{1}{3}\%$

8.5 Find the unknown quantity in each problem (percentage, part, or base).

(a) 30 is what percent of 60?

(b) What is 25% of 24?

(c) 25 is 50% of what number?

(d) What number is 4% of 75?

(e) What percent of 64 is 48?

(f) 9 is 60% of what number?

(g) What percent of 120 is 180?

(h) 100 is 80% of what number?

(i) What is 225% of 36?

(j) What percent of 75 is 25?

(k) 2 is what percent of 400?

(l) What is 0.6% of 40?

(m) What number is 2.5% of 180?

(n) 4.8 is what percent of 3.6?

(o) What percent of 2000 is 1?

(p) 27 is $1\frac{1}{2}\%$ of what number?

(q) What is 0.45% of 1200?

(r) What is $3\frac{1}{3}\%$ of 1500?

(s) What percent of 625 is 0.25?

(t) 200 is $66\frac{2}{3}\%$ of what number?

(u) What percent of 30 is $1\frac{1}{2}$?

(v) What percent of 75 is $2\frac{1}{2}$?

(w) $1\frac{1}{4}$ is $\frac{1}{2}\%$ of what number?

(x) What is 0.25% of 6.4?

Solution

(a) $$\frac{30}{60} \times 100\% = \frac{30 \times 100}{60}\% $$
$$= 50\%$$

(b) $$\frac{25\%}{100\%} \times 24 = \frac{25 \times 24}{100}$$
$$= 6$$

(c) $$\frac{25}{50\%} \times 100\% = \frac{25 \times 100}{50}$$
$$= 50$$

(d) $$\frac{4\%}{100\%} \times 75 = \frac{4 \times 75}{100}$$
$$= 3$$

(e) $$\frac{48}{64} \times 100\% = \frac{48 \times 100}{64}\%$$
$$= 75\%$$

(f) $$\frac{9}{60\%} \times 100\% = \frac{9 \times 100}{60}$$
$$= 15$$

(g) $$\frac{180}{120} \times 100\% = \frac{180 \times 100}{120}\%$$
$$= 150\%$$

(h) $$\frac{100}{80\%} \times 100\% = \frac{100 \times 100}{80}$$
$$= 125$$

(i) $$\frac{225\%}{100\%} \times 36 = \frac{225 \times 36}{100}$$
$$= 81$$

(j) $$\frac{25}{75} \times 100\% = \frac{25 \times 100}{75}$$
$$= 33\frac{1}{3}\%$$

(k) $$\frac{2}{400} \times 100\% = \frac{2 \times 100}{400}\%$$
$$= 0.5\%$$

(l) $$\frac{0.6\%}{100\%} \times 40 = \frac{0.6 \times 40}{100}$$
$$= 0.24$$

(m) $$\frac{2.5\%}{100\%} \times 180 = \frac{2.5 \times 180}{100}$$
$$= 4.5$$

(n) $$\frac{4.8}{3.6} \times 100\% = \frac{4.8 \times 100}{3.6}\%$$
$$= 133\frac{1}{3}\%$$

(o) $$\frac{1}{2000} \times 100\% = \frac{100}{2000}\%$$
$$= 0.05\%$$

(p) $$\frac{27}{1\frac{1}{2}\%} \times 100\% = \frac{27}{1} \times \frac{2}{3} \times 100$$
$$= 1800$$

(q) $$\frac{0.45\%}{100\%} \times 1200 = \frac{0.45 \times 1200}{100}$$
$$= 5.4$$

(r) $$\frac{3\frac{1}{3}\%}{100\%} \times 1500 = \frac{10}{3} \times \frac{1}{100} \times 1500$$
$$= 50$$

(s) $$\frac{0.25}{625} \times 100\% = \frac{0.25 \times 100}{625}\%$$
$$= 0.04\%$$

(t) $$\frac{200}{66\frac{2}{3}\%} \times 100\% = \frac{200}{\frac{200}{3}} \times 100$$
$$= 200 \times \frac{3}{200} \times 100 = 300$$

(u) $$\frac{1\frac{1}{2}}{30} \times 100\% = \frac{3}{2} \times \frac{1}{30} \times 100\%$$
$$= 5\%$$

(w) $$\frac{1\frac{1}{4}}{\frac{1}{2}\%} \times 100\% = \frac{5}{4} \times \frac{2}{1} \times 100$$
$$= 250$$

(v) $$\frac{2\frac{1}{2}}{75} \times 100\% = \frac{5}{2} \times \frac{1}{75} \times 100\%$$
$$= 3\frac{1}{3}\%$$

(x) $$\frac{0.25\%}{100\%} \times 6.4 = \frac{0.25 \times 6.4}{100}$$
$$= 0.016$$

PROBLEMS IN PERCENTAGE STRENGTH OF SOLUTIONS

8.6   What is the percentage strength of a solution that contains 75 mL of solute in 100 mL of solution?

Solution

   75 mL is what percent of 100 mL?

$$\frac{75 \text{ mL}}{100 \text{ mL}} \times 100\% = \frac{75 \times 100}{100}\% = 75\%$$

75 mL is 75% of 100 mL.

8.7   20 mL of concentrated hydrochloric acid is diluted with water to make 100 mL of solution. Calculate the percentage strength of the solution.

Solution

   20 mL is what percent of 100 mL?

$$\frac{20 \text{ mL}}{100 \text{ mL}} \times 100\% = \frac{20 \times 100}{100}\% = 20\%$$

20 mL is 20% of 100 mL.

8.8   How many milliliters of cresol are needed to make 1000 mL of a 2% cresol solution?

Solution

   What is 2% of 1000 mL?

$$\frac{2\%}{100\%} \times 1000 \text{ mL} = \frac{2 \times 1000 \text{ mL}}{100} = 20 \text{ mL}$$

20 mL is 2% of 1000 mL.

8.9   A solution of a drug contains 8 g dissolved in 100 mL of solution. What is the percentage concentration of the drug in the solution?

Solution

   8 g per 100 mL is an 8% concentration since the percentage concentration of a *solid* solute is equal to the *number of grams* in 100 mL.

8.10   How many grams of glucose are contained in 1500 mL of a 10% glucose solution?

Solution

   A 10% concentration means that the concentration is 10 g per 100 mL. Convert 1500 mL to grams using this concentration.

$$1500 \text{ mL} \times \frac{10 \text{ g}}{100 \text{ mL}} = \frac{1500 \times 10 \text{ g}}{100} = 150 \text{ g}$$

1500 mL of a 10% glucose solution contains 150 g of glucose.

8.11 How many liters of a 2% solution of potassium permanganate can be prepared from 5 g of crystals?

Solution

A 2% solution contains 2 g per 100 mL. Convert 5 g to liters.

$$5 \text{ g} \times \frac{100 \text{ mL}}{2 \text{ g}} \times \frac{1 \text{ L}}{1000 \text{ mL}} = \frac{5 \times 100 \text{ L}}{2 \times 1000} = 0.25 \text{ L}$$

5 g of potassium permanganate is dissolved in 0.25 L for a 2% solution.

8.12 How many grams of silver nitrate are contained in 500 mL of a 0.1% solution?

Solution

A percentage concentration of 0.1% means 0.1 g/100 mL. Convert 500 mL to grams.

$$500 \text{ mL} \times \frac{0.1 \text{ g}}{100 \text{ mL}} = \frac{500 \times 0.1 \text{ g}}{100} = 0.5 \text{ g}$$

0.5 g of silver nitrate is contained in 500 mL of a 0.1% solution.

8.13 How many milliliters of Lysol full strength are needed to prepare 0.5 L of a 0.5% solution?

Solution

First, note that 0.5 L = 500 mL. This is a liquid solute so we find 0.5% of 500 mL.

$$\frac{0.5\%}{100\%} \times 500 \text{ mL} = \frac{0.5 \times 500 \text{ mL}}{100} = 2.5 \text{ mL}$$

A 0.5% solution of Lysol contains 2.5 mL Lysol in 0.5 L of solution.

8.14 How many grams of sodium citrate are contained in a liter of a $2\frac{1}{2}\%$ solution?

Solution

A $2\frac{1}{2}\%$ concentration means 2.5 g/100 mL. Find the number of grams in 1 L.

$$1 \text{ L} \times \frac{1000 \text{ mL}}{1 \text{ L}} \times \frac{2.5 \text{ g}}{100 \text{ mL}} = \frac{1000 \times 2.5 \text{ g}}{100} = 25 \text{ g}$$

A liter of a $2\frac{1}{2}\%$ solution contains 25 g of sodium citrate.

8.15 In how many milliliters of solvent must 400 mg of Furacin be dissolved to prepare a 0.2% solution?

Solution

A concentration of 0.2% is 0.2 g per 100 mL. Find the number of milliliters containing 400 mg.

$$400 \text{ mg} \times \frac{1 \text{ g}}{1000 \text{ mg}} \times \frac{100 \text{ mL}}{0.2 \text{ g}} = \frac{400 \times 100 \text{ mL}}{1000 \times 0.2} = 200 \text{ mL}$$

400 mg dissolved in 200 mL will give a concentration of 0.2%.

Supplementary Problems

8.16 Change each percentage to an equivalent simple fraction (or a whole or mixed number if the fraction is improper).

(a) 21%   (e) 150%   (i) $\frac{1}{8}$%   (m) $37\frac{1}{2}$%   (q) 6.25%

(b) 30%   (f) 180%   (j) $\frac{1}{3}$%   (n) 0.6%   (r) 102.5%

(c) 65%   (g) 200%   (k) $\frac{1}{20}$%   (o) 0.25%   (s) 0.025%

(d) 24%   (h) 325%   (l) $2\frac{1}{4}$%   (p) 0.08%   (t) 0.005%

8.17 Write each percentage as an equivalent decimal numeral. Round answer to the nearest thousandth if the decimal does not terminate.

(a) 56.0%   (e) 4.5%   (i) 180%   (m) 0.45%   (q) $166\frac{2}{3}$%

(b) 120.0%   (f) 28%   (j) 300%   (n) 0.04%   (r) $\frac{1}{4}$%

(c) 38.7%   (g) 85%   (k) 0.9%   (o) $2\frac{1}{2}$%   (s) $\frac{3}{10}$%

(d) 7.0%   (h) 6%   (l) 0.70%   (p) $33\frac{1}{3}$% (t) $\frac{1}{3}$%

8.18 Write each decimal numeral as an equivalent percentage.

(a) 0.70   (e) 0.3106   (i) 0.0345   (m) 1.75   (q) 2.0
(b) 0.35   (f) 0.06   (j) 0.008   (n) 1.00   (r) 4
(c) 0.8   (g) 0.090   (k) 0.0095   (o) 2.105   (s) 10.2
(d) 0.0605   (h) 0.048   (l) 0.0004   (p) 2.2   (t) 15

8.19 Express each fraction as an equivalent percentage.

(a) $\frac{3}{4}$ (e) $\frac{1}{25}$ (i) $2\frac{1}{2}$ (m) $2\frac{5}{8}$ (q) $\frac{1}{60}$

(b) $\frac{3}{100}$ (f) $\frac{7}{16}$ (j) 1   (n) $\frac{2}{3}$ (r) $1\frac{7}{15}$

(c) $\frac{7}{10}$ (g) $\frac{1}{200}$ (k) $1\frac{3}{4}$ (o) $\frac{1}{12}$ (s) $\frac{1}{120}$

(d) $\frac{3}{8}$ (h) $\frac{3}{400}$ (l) $2\frac{1}{20}$ (p) $\frac{5}{9}$ (t) $\frac{1}{180}$

8.20 Find the unknown quantity in each problem (percentage, part, or base).

(a) What is 50% of 240?   (m) 12.5 is what percent of 7.5?

(b) 60 is what percent of 80?   (n) What is 4.5% of 250?

(c) 16 is 50% of what number?   (o) What percent of 4000 is 5?

(d) What percent of 125 is 75?   (p) 65 is $2\frac{1}{2}$% of what number?

(e) What number is 8% of 125?   (q) What is 0.9% of 1250?

(f) 56 is 80% of what number?   (r) What is $1\frac{1}{3}$% of 1200?

(g) 36 is 45% of what number?   (s) What percent of 300 is 0.75?

(h) What percent of 200 is 320?   (t) What percent of 40 is $\frac{1}{2}$?

(i) What is 175% of 16?   (u) 500 is $33\frac{1}{3}$% of what number?

(j) What percent of 60 is 20?   (v) What percent of 90 is $1\frac{1}{2}$?

(k) 3 is what percent of 750?   (w) $4\frac{1}{2}$ is $1\frac{1}{2}$% of what number?

(l) What is 1.8% of 120?   (x) What is 0.75% of 12.4?

PROBLEMS IN PERCENTAGE STRENGTH OF SOLUTIONS

8.21 How many milliliters of solute are contained in 200 mL of a 36% solution?

8.22 What is the percentage strength of a phenol solution that contains 30 mL of phenol in 3000 mL of solution?

8.23 A solution of a drug contains 80 mg dissolved in 120 mL of solution. What is the percentage concentration of the drug? Give answer to nearest hundredth.

8.24 How many grams of bicarbonate of soda are needed to prepare 500 mL of a 2% solution?

8.25 How many milliliters of cresol are contained in 250 mL of a 2% solution?

8.26 If 2 g of iodine crystals is dissolved in 500 mL of solvent, what is the percentage strength of the solution?

8.27 How many grams of magnesium sulfate are contained in 300 mL of a 25% solution?

8.28 How many grams of sodium chloride are contained in 1000 mL of a 0.45% solution?

8.29 A solution of mercuric chloride has a concentration of 0.5 g per 500 mL. What is the percentage concentration?

8.30   A solution of Merthiolate contains 0.4 g per 60 mL. Calculate the percentage strength of the solution, giving the answer to the nearest hundredth.

8.31   How many milliliters of Lysol full strength are needed to prepare 1.5 L of a 2.5% solution?

8.32   How many milligrams of solute are needed to make 250 mL of a 0.25% solution?

8.33   Choledyl pediatric syrup contains 50 mg of the drug per 5 mL of syrup. What is the percentage concentration of the drug?

8.34   A vial of Prostaphlin contains 250 mg per 1.5 mL. Calculate the percentage strength of the drug, giving the answer to the nearest whole.

8.35   How many milliliters of a 5% dextrose solution contain 5 g of dextrose?

8.36   A 15% solution of sodium bromide is to be prepared from 2.5 g of sodium bromide crystals. In how many milliliters should the crystals be dissolved? Give answer to the nearest tenth.

Answers to Supplementary Problems

8.16   (a) $\dfrac{21}{100}$ (e) $1\dfrac{1}{2}$ (i) $\dfrac{1}{800}$ (m) $\dfrac{3}{8}$ (q) $\dfrac{1}{16}$

(b) $\dfrac{3}{10}$ (f) $1\dfrac{4}{5}$ (j) $\dfrac{1}{300}$ (n) $\dfrac{3}{500}$ (r) $1\dfrac{1}{40}$

(c) $\dfrac{13}{20}$ (g) 2 (k) $\dfrac{1}{2000}$ (o) $\dfrac{1}{400}$ (s) $\dfrac{1}{4000}$

(d) $\dfrac{6}{25}$ (h) $3\dfrac{1}{4}$ (l) $\dfrac{9}{400}$ (p) $\dfrac{1}{1250}$ (t) $\dfrac{1}{20,000}$

8.17   (a) 0.56   (e) 0.045   (i) 1.8   (m) 0.0045   (q) 1.667
(b) 1.2   (f) 0.28   (j) 3   (n) 0.0004   (r) 0.0025
(c) 0.387   (g) 0.85   (k) 0.009   (o) 0.025   (s) 0.003
(d) 0.07   (h) 0.06   (l) 0.007   (p) 0.333   (t) 0.003

8.18   (a) 70%   (e) 31.06%   (i) 3.45%   (m) 175%   (q) 200%
(b) 35%   (f) 6%   (j) 0.8%   (n) 100%   (r) 400%
(c) 80%   (g) 9%   (k) 0.95%   (o) 210.5%   (s) 1020%
(d) 6.05%   (h) 4.8%   (l) 0.04%   (p) 220%   (t) 1500%

8.19 (a) 75%   (e) 4%   (i) 250%   (m) 262.5%   (q) $1\frac{2}{3}\%$

(b) 3%   (f) 43.75%   (j) 100%   (n) $66\frac{2}{3}\%$ (r) $146\frac{2}{3}\%$

(c) 70%   (g) 0.5%   (k) 175%   (o) $8\frac{1}{3}\%$ (s) $0.8\frac{1}{3}\%$

(d) 37.5%   (h) 0.75%   (l) 205%   (p) $55\frac{5}{9}\%$ (t) $0.5\frac{5}{9}\%$

8.20 (a) 120   (g) 80   (m) $166\frac{2}{3}\%$ (s) 0.25%

(b) 75%   (h) 160%   (n) 11.25   (t) 1.25%

(c) 32   (i) 28   (o) 0.125%   (u) 1500

(d) 60%   (j) $33\frac{1}{3}\%$ (p) 2600   (v) $1\frac{2}{3}\%$

(e) 10   (k) 0.4%   (q) 11.25   (w) 300

(f) 70   (l) 2.16   (r) 16   (x) 0.093

8.21 72 mL of solute in 200 mL of a 36% solution.

8.22 30 mL of phenol in 3000 mL of solution is a 1% concentration.

8.23 0.08 g of drug in 120 mL of solution is a 0.07% concentration (rounded to the nearest hundredth).

8.24 10 g of bicarbonate of soda in 500 mL yields a 2% solution.

8.25 5 mL of cresol is contained in 250 mL of a 2% solution.

8.26 2 g of iodine in 500 mL yields a 0.4% solution.

8.27 300 mL of a 25% solution of magnesium sulfate contains 75 g.

8.28 1000 mL of a 0.45% solution of sodium chloride contains 4.5 g.

8.29 0.5 g/500 mL is equivalent to a 0.1% concentration.

8.30 0.4 g/60 mL is equivalent to a concentration of 0.67% (rounded to the nearest hundredth).

8.31 37.5 mL of Lysol full strength will make 1.5 L of a 2.5% solution.

8.32 625 mg of solute will make 250 mL of a 0.25% solution.

8.33 50 mg per 5 mL is equivalent to a 1% concentration.

8.34 250 mg/1.5 mL is equivalent to a concentration of 17% (rounded to the nearest whole).

8.35 100 mL of a 5% dextrose solution will contain 5 g.

8.36 2 g dissolved in 16.7 mL will yield a 15% solution.

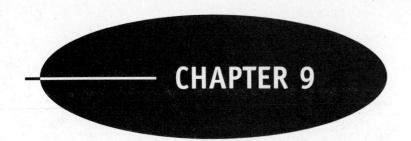

CHAPTER 9

Using the Electronic Calculator

9.1 CALCULATORS FOR NURSING

Only the simplest type of electronic calculator is necessary for nursing calculations. Such a calculator will perform the basic operations of addition, subtraction, multiplication, and division. It also has a percent key. A calculator of this kind looks basically like the illustration in Fig. 9-1.

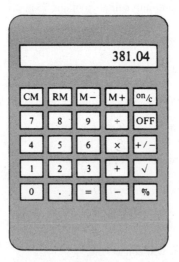

Fig. 9-1

The keys that will be of interest to us are:

1. The *numeric* keys ⓪ ① ② ③ ④ ⑤ ⑥ ⑦ ⑧ ⑨
2. The *decimal* key ⊡

3. The arithmetic *operation* keys
    $\boxed{+}$ addition
    $\boxed{-}$ subtraction
    $\boxed{\times}$ multiplication
    $\boxed{\div}$ division
4. The *equal* key $\boxed{=}$
5. The *percent* key $\boxed{\%}$
6. The on/clear key $\boxed{^{on}\!/_c}$ which turns the calculator on and also clears the calculator of all steps that have been performed previously. Whenever you start a calculation, be sure you clear the calculator first.
7. The $\boxed{\text{OFF}}$ key which turns the calculator off.

9.2   ELEMENTARY CALCULATIONS

Addition

EXAMPLE 9.1   Add $36.45 + 207.5$.

In the steps described below, Enter means to enter the indicated number, Press means to press the indicated key, and Display indicates what you will see on the display screen after that step has been performed.

	Enter	Press	Display
Step 1	36.45		36.45
Step 2		$\boxed{+}$	36.45
Step 3	207.5		207.5
Step 4		$\boxed{=}$	243.95

The answer is $36.45 + 207.5 = 243.95$. Note that the answer does not appear on the display until the equal key has been pressed.

Subtraction

EXAMPLE 9.2   Subtract $428.3 - 184.59$.

	Enter	Press	Display
Step 1	428.3		428.3
Step 2		$\boxed{-}$	428.3
Step 3	184.59		184.59
Step 4		$\boxed{=}$	243.71

The answer is $428.3 - 184.59 = 243.71$.

Multiplication

EXAMPLE 9.3   Multiply 26.87 × 0.073.

	Enter	Press	Display
Step 1	26.87		26.87
Step 2		⨯	26.87
Step 3	.073		0.073
Step 4		=	1.96151

The answer is 26.87 × 0.073 = 1.96151.

Division

EXAMPLE 9.4   Divide 4.28 ÷ 407.35.

	Enter	Press	Display
Step 1	4.28		4.28
Step 2		÷	4.28
Step 3	407.35		407.35
Step 4		=	0.0105069

The answer is 4.28 ÷ 407.35 = 0.0105069. The calculator gives answers to as many digits as will fit on the display. Usually you will not need all the digits and therefore will round the answer. In this case, the answer rounded to the nearest hundredth is 0.01.

9.3   EXTENDED CALCULATIONS

An extended sequence of calculations can be easily performed on the calculator as shown in the examples below.

EXAMPLE 9.5   Calculate 5.47 + 19.08 + 192.6.

	Enter	Press	Display
Step 1	5.47		5.47
Step 2		+	5.47
Step 3	19.08		19.08
Step 4		=	24.55
Step 5	192.6		192.6
Step 6		=	217.15

The answer is 5.47 + 19.08 + 192.6 = 217.15. Note that the number 24.55 displayed at Step 4 is the sum 5.47 + 19.08.

EXAMPLE 9.6   Calculate $192.6 + 74 - 45.93$.

	Enter	Press	Display
Step 1	192.6		192.6
Step 2		⊞	192.6
Step 3	74		74
Step 4		⊟	266.6
Step 5	45.93		45.93
Step 6		⊟	220.67

The answer is $192.6 + 74 - 45.93 = 220.67$.

EXAMPLE 9.7   Calculate $28.4 \times 0.24 \times 12$.

	Enter	Press	Display
Step 1	28.4		
Step 2		⊠	28.4
Step 3	.24		0.24
Step 4		⊠	6.816
Step 5	12		12
Step 6		⊟	81.792

The answer is $28.4 \times 0.24 \times 12 = 81.792$.

EXAMPLE 9.8   Calculate $630 \div 15.7 \times 0.65$.

	Enter	Press	Display
Step 1	630		630
Step 2		÷	630
Step 3	15.7		15.7
Step 4		⊠	40.127388
Step 5	.65		0.65
Step 6		⊟	26.082802

The answer is $630 \div 15.7 \times 0.67 = 26.082802$. Rounded to the nearest hundredth, this is 26.08.

9.4 WORKING WITH FRACTIONS ON THE CALCULATOR

Any arithmetic problem for which the answer is desired as a decimal numeral can be performed on the calculator. However, the calculator will not give answers in fractional form. For example, for a problem such as this,

$$\frac{1}{2} \times \frac{10}{3} = \frac{5}{3} = 1\frac{2}{3}$$

the calculator will give only the decimal approximation 1.6666666.

EXAMPLE 9.9   Change the fraction 2/3 into an equivalent decimal, rounded to the nearest hundredth. Since the fraction 2/3 means $2 \div 3$, this is performed on the calculator as follows:

	Enter	Press	Display
Step 1	2		2
Step 2		$\div$	2
Step 3	3		3
Step 4		$=$	0.6666666

The display shows 0.6666666, but we want to round the answer to the nearest hundredth. Thus, the answer is 0.67.

EXAMPLE 9.10   Calculate $250 \times \frac{3}{4} \times \frac{1}{60}$.

The problem can be written as $\frac{250 \times 3}{4 \times 60}$. Perform this calculation on the calculator by multiplying all the numbers *above* the line and dividing this product by all the numbers *below* the line.

	Enter	Press	Display
Step 1	250		250
Step 2		$\times$	250
Step 3	3		3
Step 4		$\div$	750
Step 5	4		4
Step 6		$\div$	187.5
Step 7	60		60
Step 8		$=$	3.125

The answer is 3.125.

EXAMPLE 9.11 Calculate $4.75 \times \dfrac{1}{1000} \times \dfrac{1}{\frac{1}{600}}$.

Write the problem as

$$4.75 \times \frac{1}{1000} \times \frac{600}{1} = \frac{4.75 \times 600}{1000}$$

On the calculator:

	Enter	Press	Display
Step 1	4.75		4.75
Step 2		$\times$	4.75
Step 3	600		600
Step 4		$\div$	2850
Step 5	1000		1000
Step 6		$=$	2.85

The answer is 2.85.

9.5 DOSAGE CALCULATIONS

The calculation of drug dosages using the calculator is especially easy when the technique of dimensional analysis is used to set up the problem. Some illustrations follow.

EXAMPLE 9.12 The doctor orders 40 mg of Prinivil. The label for the Prinivil available is shown in Fig. 9-2. How many tablets should you give?

Set up the calculation:
$$40 \text{ mg} \times \frac{1 \text{ tab}}{20 \text{ mg}}$$

Perform the calculation
on the calculator:
$$\frac{40}{20} \text{ tab} = 2 \text{ tab}$$

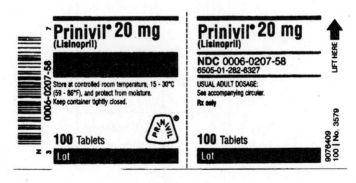

Fig. 9-2

EXAMPLE 9.13   The doctor orders 375 mg of a drug. On hand are tablets containing 125 mg each. How many tablets should you administer?

Set up the calculation:

$$375 \ \text{mg} \times \frac{1 \ \text{tab}}{125 \ \text{mg}}$$

Perform the calculation
on the calculator:

$$\frac{375}{125} \ \text{tab} = 3 \ \text{tab}$$

EXAMPLE 9.14   The order is for 0.6 g of a drug. The drug is available 450 mg per 5 mL. How many milliliters should you give?

Set up the calculation:

$$0.6 \ \text{g} \times \frac{1000 \ \text{mg}}{1 \ \text{g}} \times \frac{5 \ \text{mL}}{450 \ \text{mg}}$$

Perform the calculation
on the calculator:

$$\frac{0.6 \times 1000 \times 5}{450} \ \text{mL} = 6.7 \ \text{mL}$$

EXAMPLE 9.15   1000 mL of dextrose solution is to be infused over an 8-h period. The drop factor is 15. Calculate the drop rate.

Set up the calculation:

$$\frac{1000 \ \text{mL}}{8 \ \text{h}} \times \frac{1 \ \text{h}}{60 \ \text{min}} \times \frac{15 \ \text{gtt}}{1 \ \text{mL}}$$

Perform the calculation
on the calculator:

$$\frac{1000 \times 15}{8 \times 60} \ \text{gtt/min} = 31 \ \text{gtt/min}$$

9.6   THE PERCENT KEY

The percent key on most elementary calculators solves the three main types of percentage problems as follows.

Finding the Percentage.   Here, the part and the base are given. Divide the part by the base and change the answer to a percentage.

EXAMPLE 9.16   What percent of 360 is 24?

The part is 24 and the base is 360. Divide 24 by 360 and change the answer to a percentage. This is done on the calculator as follows:

	Enter	Press	Display
Step 1	24		24
Step 2		÷	
Step 3	360		360
Step 4		%	6.6666666

The answer (rounded) is 6.7%. Note that the equal key is *not* pressed.

Finding the Part.   Here, the base and the percentage are given. Multiply the base by the percentage.

EXAMPLE 9.17   What is 35% of 1250?
The base is 1250 and the percentage is 35%. Multiply 1250 by 35%. This is done on the calculator as follows:

	Enter	Press	Display
Step 1	1250		1250
Step 2		×	
Step 3	35		35
Step 4		%	437.5

The answer is 437.5. Again, it is not necessary to use the equal key.

Finding the Base.   Here, the part and the percentage are given. Divide the part by the percentage.

EXAMPLE 9.18   45 is 60% of what number?
The part is 45 and the percentage is 60%. Divide 45 by 60%. This is done on the calculator as follows:

	Enter	Press	Display
Step 1	45		45
Step 2		÷	45
Step 3	60		60
Step 4		%	75

The answer is 75. The equal key is not used.

EXAMPLE 9.19   25 g of a solute is dissolved in 1500 mL of water. What is the percentage concentration of the solution?
We must determine what percent of 1500 is 25. Divide 25 by 1500 and change the answer to a percent.

	Enter	Press	Display
Step 1	25		25
Step 2		÷	25
Step 3	1500		1500
Step 4		%	1.6666666

25 g/1500 mL is a 1.7% concentration (rounded to the nearest tenth).

EXAMPLE 9.20   How many grams of sodium chloride are dissolved in 2250 mL of a 0.9% solution? We must determine what is 0.9% of 2250. Multiply 2250 by 0.9%.

	Enter	Press	Display
Step 1	2250		2250
Step 2		×	2250
Step 3	.9		0.9
Step 4		%	20.25

2250 mL of a 0.9% solution contains 20.25 g of sodium chloride.

EXAMPLE 9.21   How many milliliters must be added to 50 mL of a full-strength solution to obtain a 5% solution?

The problem is to determine: 50 mL is 5% of what amount? Divide 50 mL by 5%. This gives the total amount of solution.

	Enter	Press	Display
Step 1	50		50
Step 2		÷	50
Step 3	5		5
Step 4		%	1000

50 mL is 5% of 1000 mL. Thus, you would add 950 mL to the 50 mL of full-strength solution to obtain 1000 mL of a 5% solution.

Solved Problems

9.1   Perform the following calculations on the calculator.

(a) $34 + 68 - 45$ (d) $24.56 \times 13.5 \times 0.35$

(b) $4.7 - 2.5 + 3.4$ (e) $6.78 \times 2.45 \div 4.20$

(c) $56 \times 23 \times 13$ (f) $456.8 \div 200 \times 2.5$

Solution

(a) 1. Enter 34   (b) 1. Enter 4.7
     2. Press +   2. Press −
     3. Enter 68   3. Enter 2.5
     4. Press −   4. Press +
     5. Enter 45   5. Enter 3.4
     6. Press =   6. Press =
         Answer is 57   Answer is 5.6

(c) 1. Enter 56
     2. Press ×
     3. Enter 23
     4. Press ×
     5. Enter 13
     6. Press =
         Answer is 16,744

(e) 1. Enter 6.78
     2. Press ×
     3. Enter 2.45
     4. Press ÷
     5. Enter 4.20
     6. Press =
         Answer is 3.955

(d) 1. Enter 24.56
     2. Press ×
     3. Enter 13.5
     4. Press ×
     5. Enter .35
     6. Press =
         Answer is 116.046

(f) 1. Enter 456.8
     2. Press ÷
     3. Enter 200
     4. Press ×
     5. Enter 2.5
     6. Press =
         Answer is 5.71

9.2 Perform the following calculations on the calculator.

(a) $\dfrac{3.8}{1.6}$

(d) $4 \times \dfrac{1}{200} \times 3.75$

(g) $0.65 \times \dfrac{1}{\frac{1}{30}} \times \dfrac{1}{1000}$

(b) $5 \times \dfrac{2}{3}$

(e) $12.5 \times \dfrac{3}{8} \times \dfrac{1}{30}$

(h) $\dfrac{1}{150} \times 125 \times \dfrac{1}{\frac{1}{120}}$

(c) $\dfrac{0.075}{\frac{1}{600}}$

(f) $66 \times \dfrac{1}{2.2} \times \dfrac{5}{125}$

(i) $0.0025 \times \dfrac{1}{200} \times \dfrac{1}{\frac{1}{250}}$

Solution

(a) $\dfrac{3.8}{1.6}$
     1. Enter 3.8
     2. Press ÷
     3. Enter 1.6
     4. Press =
         Answer is 2.375

(c) $\dfrac{0.075}{\frac{1}{600}} = 0.075 \times 600$
     1. Enter .075
     2. Press ×
     3. Enter 600
     4. Press =
         Answer is 45

(b) $5 \times \dfrac{2}{3} = \dfrac{5 \times 2}{3}$
     1. Enter 5
     2. Press ×
     3. Enter 2
     4. Press ÷
     5. Enter 3
     6. Press =
         Answer is 3.33 (rounded)

(d) $4 \times \dfrac{1}{200} \times 3.75 = \dfrac{4 \times 3.75}{200}$
     1. Enter 4
     2. Press ×
     3. Enter 3.75
     4. Press ÷
     5. Enter 200
     6. Press =
         Answer is 0.075

(e) $12.5 \times \dfrac{3}{8} \times \dfrac{1}{30} = \dfrac{12.5 \times 3}{8 \times 30}$

1. Enter 12.5
2. Press ×
3. Enter 3
4. Press ÷
5. Enter 8
6. Press ÷
7. Enter 30
8. Press =
    Answer is 0.15625

(h) $\dfrac{1}{150} \times 125 \times \dfrac{1}{\dfrac{1}{120}} = \dfrac{125 \times 120}{150}$

1. Enter 125
2. Press ×
3. Enter 120
4. Press ÷
5. Enter 150
6. Press =
    Answer is 100

(f) $66 \times \dfrac{1}{2.2} \times \dfrac{5}{125} = \dfrac{66 \times 5}{2.2 \times 125}$

1. Enter 66
2. Press ×
3. Enter 5
4. Press ÷
5. Enter 2.2
6. Press ÷
7. Enter 125
8. Press =
    Answer is 1.2

(i) $0.0025 \times \dfrac{1}{200} \times \dfrac{1}{\dfrac{1}{250}} = \dfrac{0.0025 \times 250}{200}$

1. Enter .0025
2. Press ×
3. Enter 250
4. Press ÷
5. Enter 200
6. Press =
    Answer is 0.003125

(g) $0.65 \times \dfrac{1}{\dfrac{1}{30}} \times \dfrac{1}{1000} = \dfrac{0.65 \times 30}{1000}$

1. Enter .65
2. Press ×
3. Enter 30
4. Press ÷
5. Enter 1000
6. Press =
    Answer is 0.0195

9.3 Set up the solution of each problem and perform the calculations on the calculator.

(a) You are to give 25 mg of Phenergan PO. The tablets available each contain 12.5 mg. How many tablets would you give?

(b) The order is for 250 mg of a drug. The drug label indicates a concentration of 60 mg/mL. How many milliliters should you administer?

(c) The patient is to receive 30 mEq of potassium chloride. On hand is a bottle labeled "potassium chloride 40 mEq/30 mL." How many milliliters will you give to the patient?

(d) A vial contains 1,000,000 U of penicillin G potassium as dry powder. The directions are to add 3.6 mL of diluent to obtain a concentration of 250,000 U/mL. How many milliliters of solution will contain 400,000 U?

(e) A bottle of digoxin elixir contains 50 μg/mL. How many milliliters contain 0.2 mg?

(f) Two grams of Amoxil PO is ordered for 1 h before a procedure. The label of the available Amoxil is shown in Fig. 9-3. How many of the chewable tables are to be given?

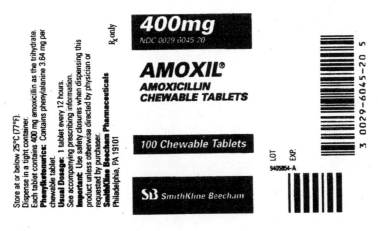

Fig. 9-3

(*g*)   An IV solution is being infused at the rate of 35 gtt/min. The drop factor is 10. Calculate the rate of infusion in mL/h.

(*h*)   1000 mL of a 5% glucose solution is to be administered IV over a period of 10 h. The drop factor is 20 gtt/mL. Calculate the drop rate.

(*i*)   A patient weighs 135 lb. The order is for 0.3 mg of a drug per kilogram of body weight. The drug label indicates a concentration of 5 mg/mL. How many milliliters should you give?

Solution

(*a*) $25 \text{ mg} \times \dfrac{1 \text{ tab}}{12.5 \text{ mg}} = \dfrac{25}{12.5} \text{ tab} = 2 \text{ tab}$

(*b*) $250 \text{ mg} \times \dfrac{1 \text{ mL}}{60 \text{ mg}} = \dfrac{250}{60} \text{ mL} = 4.2 \text{ mL}$

(*c*) $30 \text{ mEq} \times \dfrac{30 \text{ mL}}{40 \text{ mEq}} = \dfrac{30 \times 30}{40} \text{ mL} = 22.5 \text{ mL}$

(*d*) $400{,}000 \text{ U} \times \dfrac{1 \text{ mL}}{250{,}000 \text{ U}} = \dfrac{400{,}000}{250{,}000} \text{ mL} = 1.6 \text{ mL}$

(*e*) $0.2 \text{ mg} \times \dfrac{1000 \text{ } \mu g}{1 \text{ mg}} \times \dfrac{1 \text{ mL}}{50 \text{ } \mu g} = \dfrac{0.2 \times 1000}{50} \text{ mL} = 4 \text{ mL}$

(*f*) $2 \text{ g} \times \dfrac{1000 \text{ mg}}{1 \text{ g}} \times \dfrac{1 \text{ tab}}{400 \text{ mg}} = 5 \text{ tab}$

(*g*) $\dfrac{35 \text{ gtt}}{1 \text{ min}} \times \dfrac{60 \text{ min}}{1 \text{ h}} \times \dfrac{1 \text{ mL}}{10 \text{ gtt}} = \dfrac{35 \times 60}{10} \text{ mL/h} = 210 \text{ mL/h}$

(*h*) $\dfrac{1000 \text{ mL}}{10 \text{ h}} \times \dfrac{1 \text{ h}}{60 \text{ min}} \times \dfrac{20 \text{ gtt}}{1 \text{ mL}} = \dfrac{1000 \times 20}{10 \times 60} \text{ gtt/min} = 33 \text{ gtt/min}$

(*i*) $135 \text{ lb} \times \dfrac{1 \text{ kg}}{2.2 \text{ lb}} \times \dfrac{0.3 \text{ mg}}{1 \text{ kg}} \times \dfrac{1 \text{ mL}}{5 \text{ mg}} = \dfrac{135 \times 0.3}{2.2 \times 5} \text{ mL} = 3.7 \text{ mL}$

9.4   Solve the following percentage problems using the calculator.

   (*a*)   What percent of 120 is 90?   (*e*)   What is 0.4% of 1500?

   (*b*)   What is 35% of 180?   (*f*)   16 is 25% of what number?

   (*c*)   What is 120% of 75?   (*g*)   1250 is 250% of what number?

   (*d*)   What percent of 250 is 6?   (*h*)   0.8% of what number is 12?

Solution

(*a*) The base is 120 and the part is 90
   1. Enter 90
   2. Press ÷
   3. Enter 120
   4. Press %
       Answer is 75%

(*b*) The base is 180 and the percentage is 35%
   1. Enter 180
   2. Press ×
   3. Enter 35
   4. Press %
       Answer is 63

(*c*) The base is 75 and the percentage is 120%
   1. Enter 75
   2. Press ×
   3. Enter 120
   4. Press %
       Answer is 90

(*d*) The base is 250 and the part is 6
   1. Enter 6
   2. Press ÷
   3. Enter 250
   4. Press %
       Answer is 2.4%

(*e*) The base is 1500 and the percentage is 0.4%
   1. Enter 1500
   2. Press ×
   3. Enter .4
   4. Press %
       Answer is 6

(*f*) The part is 16 and the percentage is 25%
   1. Enter 16
   2. Press ÷
   3. Enter 25
   4. Press %
       Answer is 64

(*g*) The part is 1250 and the percentage is 250%
   1. Enter 1250
   2. Press ÷
   3. Enter 250
   4. Press %
       Answer is 500

(*h*) The part is 12 and the percentage is 0.8%
   1. Enter 12
   2. Press ÷
   3. Enter .8
   4. Press %
       Answer is 1500

9.5   Solve the following problems using the calculator.

(*a*) What is the percentage strength of a solution that contains 25 mL of solute in 150 mL of solution?

(*b*) What is the percentage concentration of a solution that contains 5 g of solute in 200 mL of solution?

(*c*) How many grams of dextrose are contained in 1200 mL of a 10% dextrose solution?

(*d*) How many grams of salt are contained in 1750 mL of a 0.9% saline solution?

(*e*) A 7.5% solution of sodium bromide is to be prepared from 15 g of sodium bromide crystals. In how many milliliters should the crystals be dissolved?

Solution

First determine the *type* of percentage problem each one is (finding the percentage, the part, or the base), then solve the problem using the calculator.

(*a*) We must calculate what percent of 150 is 25. The base is 150 and the part is 25.
   1. Enter 25
   2. Press ÷
   3. Enter 150
   4. Press %
       Answer is 16.7%

(*b*) We must calculate what percent of 200 is 5. The base is 200 and the part is 5.
   1. Enter 5
   2. Press ÷

3. Enter 200
4. Press %
    Answer is 2.5%

(c) We must calculate what is 10% of 1200. The base is 1200 and the percentage is 10%.
1. Enter 1200
2. Press ×
3. Enter 10
4. Press %
    Answer is 120 g

(d) We must calculate what is 0.9% of 1750. The base is 1750 and the percentage is 0.9%.
1. Enter 1750
2. Press ×
3. Enter .9
4. Press %
    Answer is 15.75 g

(e) We must determine: 7.5% of what amount is 50 mL? The part is 15 and the percentage is 7.5%.
1. Enter 15
2. Press ÷
3. Enter 7.5
4. Press %
    Answer is 200 mL

Supplementary Problems

9.6   Perform the following calculations on the calculator. Round your answers to the nearest tenth.

(a) $12 + 76 + 32$

(b) $6.7 + 0.9 + 3.5$

(c) $8.24 + 17.6 - 10.14$

(d) $156.2 - 35 - 79.13$

(e) $38 \times 20 \times 6$

(f) $76.2 \times 0.05 \times 30$

(g) $1500 \times 0.08 \div 25$

(h) $2.76 \div 4.5 \times 0.15$

(i) $2000 \div 240 \div 0.06$

(j) $0.0075 \div 15 \times 1250$

9.7   Perform the following calculations on the calculator. Round your answers to the nearest thousandth.

(a) $\dfrac{57.5}{25}$

(b) $\dfrac{0.6}{80}$

(c) $36 \times \dfrac{5}{9}$

(d) $\dfrac{1}{200} \times 240$

(e) $\dfrac{25}{\frac{1}{5}}$

(f) $\dfrac{0.0125}{\frac{1}{250}}$

(g) $\dfrac{3.6}{\frac{1}{150}}$

(h) $\dfrac{0.0024}{\frac{1}{600}}$

(i) $\dfrac{\frac{1}{6}}{\frac{1}{4}}$

(j) $\dfrac{\frac{1}{3}}{\frac{1}{300}}$

(k) $275 \times \dfrac{1}{300} \times 0.6$

(l) $0.64 \times \dfrac{1}{60} \times 2\dfrac{1}{2}$

(m) $0.005 \times \dfrac{1}{\frac{1}{60}} \times 2.75$

(n) $\dfrac{1.6}{\frac{1}{24}} \times 0.04 \times \dfrac{1}{30}$

(o) $0.01 \times \dfrac{1}{12} \times \dfrac{1}{\frac{1}{240}}$

9.8   Set up the solution of each problem and perform the calculations on the calculator.

(*a*)   You are to administer 750 mg of a drug from tablets which contain 375 mg each. How many tablets will you give?

(*b*)   The order is for 60 mg of Choledyl. The bottle of syrup on hand contains 50 mg per 5 mL. How many milliliters will you administer?

(*c*)   The directions on a vial containing 5 million U of penicillin G sodium are to add 3 mL of diluent to obtain a concentration of 1 million U/mL. How many milliliters are needed to give 2.5 million U?

(*d*)   The order is for 0.1 g of Talwin PO. The tablets available each contain 50 mg. How many tablets should you give?

(*e*)   A 1-mL dosette vial of scopolamine contains 400 μg of the drug. How many milliliters will contain 0.3 mg?

(*f*)   The order is for 1500 mg IM of a drug. The vial contains 2 g of the drug. The directions are to add 4.0 mL of sterile water to obtain a concentration of 1 g per 2.5 mL. How many milliliters will you administer?

(*g*)   The doctor orders 6 mg of morphine. The vial on hand contains 10 mg/mL. How many milliliters should you give?

(*h*)   The order is for 500 mg of a drug. The capsules on hand contain 0.25 g each. How many capsules will you administer?

(*i*)   500 mg of Flagyl is contained in 100 mL of lactated Ringer's injection, which is to be infused IV over 1 h. The drop factor is 20. What is the drop rate?

(*j*)   MVI (multivitamin infusion) 10 mL is contained in 1000 mL of normal saline for infusion over a period of 6 h. The drop factor is 15. Calculate the correct drop rate.

(*k*)   An IV solution is being infused at the rate of 40 gtt/min. The drop factor is 20. Calculate the rate of infusion in mL/h.

(*l*)   Using a tuberculin syringe, you are to give 75 U of insulin from a vial of U-100 insulin. How many milliliters will you give?

(*m*)   You are to give 36 U of U-100 insulin, using a tuberculin syringe. How many milliliters will you give?

(*n*)   You are to give 20 U of U-100 insulin by means of a 3/10-cc insulin syringe. How many units should you administer with the 3/10-cc syringe?

(*o*)   A 40-lb child is to receive 0.25 mL per kilogram of camphorated opium tincture tid. How many milliliters will the child be receiving daily?

(*p*)   Penicillin V potassium is ordered for a 60-lb child, at the rate of 15 mg per kilogram of body weight. On hand is oral solution containing 250 mg per 5 mL. How many milliliters should you give?

(*q*)   Aldomet (methyldopa) is to be given 10 mg per kilogram PO daily, in 3 equal doses, to a child who weighs 75 lb. The oral suspension contains 250 mg per 5 mL. How many milliliters should you give per dose?

(*r*)   Sulfadiazine is to be administered 4 g per square meter PO divided in 6 equal doses. The tablets contain 125 mg each. How many tablets per dose will you give to a child whose body surface area is 0.56 m^2?

(*s*)   Use Mosteller's formula to compute the surface area of a patient who is 5 ft tall and weighs 120 lb. A drug is to be administered 50 mg per square meter. Calculate the correct dosage for the patient.

(*t*)   Use Mosteller's formula to compute the surface area of a patient who is 122 cm tall and weighs 35 kg. A drug is to be administered 250 mg per square meter. Calculate the correct dosage for the patient.

9.9   Solve the following percentage problems using the calculator.

(*a*)   What percent of 75 is 6?   (*g*)   What is 120% of 4.5?

(*b*)   What is 18% of 200?   (*h*)   What percent of 1800 is 2?

(*c*)   What is 160% of 60?   (*i*)   35 is 20% of what number?

(*d*)   What percent of 300 is 75?   (*j*)   225 is 150% of what number?

(*e*)   What percent of 75 is 300?   (*k*)   0.8% of what number is 2?

(*f*)   What is 0.5% of 360?   (*l*)   24 is 0.05% of what number?

9.10   Solve the following problems using the calculator.

    (*a*)   What is the percentage strength of a solution that contains 6 g of solute in 250 mL of solution?

    (*b*)   What is the percentage concentration of a solution that contains 30 mL of solute in 360 mL of solution?

    (*c*)   Calculate the percentage strength of a solution that contains 250 mg of solute in 250 mL of solution.

    (*d*)   How many grams of solute are contained in 500 mL of a 20% solution?

    (*e*)   How many grams of sodium chloride are contained in 1750 mL of a half-normal (0.45%) saline solution?

    (*f*)   How many milliliters of pure alcohol are needed to prepare 1000 mL of a 15% alcohol solution?

    (*g*)   Calculate the number of milligrams of a pure drug needed to prepare 500 mL of a 0.06% solution.

    (*h*)   A solution of ampicillin contains 250 mg per 5 mL. Calculate the percentage strength of the solution.

    (*i*)   How many milliliters of full-strength acetic acid are needed to make 2000 mL of a 1.5% solution?

    (*j*)   How many milliliters of a 20% solution of hydrochloric acid can be prepared from 50 mL of concentrated hydrochloric acid?

    (*k*)   How many milliliters of a 2.5% solution of boric acid can be prepared from 20 g of boric acid crystals?

Answers to Supplementary Problems

9.6   (*a*) 120   (*c*) 15.7   (*e*) 4560   (*g*) 4.8   (*i*) 138.9
        (*b*) 11.1   (*d*) 42.1   (*f*) 114.3   (*h*) 0.1   (*j*) 0.6

9.7   (*a*) 2.3   (*d*) 1.2   (*g*) 540   (*j*) 100   (*m*) 0.825
        (*b*) 0.008   (*e*) 125   (*h*) 1.44   (*k*) 0.55   (*n*) 0.051
        (*c*) 20   (*f*) 3.125   (*i*) 0.667   (*l*) 0.027   (*o*) 0.2

9.8   (*a*) 2 tab   (*f*) 3.75 mL   (*k*) 120 mL/h   (*p*) 8.2 mL
        (*b*) 6 mL   (*g*) 0.6 mL   (*l*) 0.75 mL   (*q*) 2.3 mL
        (*c*) 2.5 mL   (*h*) 2 cap   (*m*) 0.36 mL   (*r*) 3 tab
        (*d*) 2 tab   (*i*) 33 gtt/min   (*n*) 20 U   (*s*) 1.52 m^2; 76 mg
        (*e*) 0.75 mL   (*j*) 42 gtt/min   (*o*) 13.6 mL   (*t*) 1.09 m^2; 272.5 mg

9.9   (*a*) 8%   (*d*) 25%   (*g*) 5.4   (*j*) 150
        (*b*) 36   (*e*) 400%   (*h*) 0.11%   (*k*) 250
        (*c*) 96   (*f*) 1.8   (*i*) 175   (*l*) 48,000

9.10   (*a*) 2.4%   (*d*) 100 g   (*g*) 300 mg   (*j*) 250 mL
        (*b*) 8.33%   (*e*) 7.9 g   (*h*) 5%   (*k*) 800 mL
        (*c*) 0.1%   (*f*) 150 mL   (*i*) 30 mL

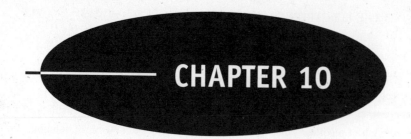

CHAPTER 10

Statistics for Nurses

10.1 STATISTICS FOR NURSING

Most undergraduate as well as graduate degree programs in nursing require a course in statistics. Nurses frequently encounter statistical measures in the material that accompanies drugs, in nursing magazines, in presentations sponsored by drug companies, and in other aspects of their profession. Nurses who are associated with medical research studies must be knowledgeable about statistics. This chapter discusses the most important statistical concepts that arise in nursing. In addition, you will be introduced to computer software that is used in statistics. Four important software packages are Microsoft Excel, Minitab, SAS, and SPSS. Statistical software has been around for about 25 years. Most users of statistics rely on some software package to perform their statistical analyses. Microsoft Excel is widely available on office computers as well as home computers. Many instructors of statistics, including this author, include Excel as an integral part of the statistics course that we teach to nurses. Excel can perform many of the statistical methods found in the course that nurses take. Excel also eliminates the need for all the tables found in statistics books. Areas under the normal curve, the student t curve, the chi-square curve, and others can be found using Excel. The examples and problems in this chapter that find areas under the normal curve use the functions NORMDIST and NORMINV in Excel.

10.2 BAR CHARTS AND PIE CHARTS FOR CATEGORICAL DATA

EXAMPLE 10.1 The number of emergency room visits to Metropolitan University Hospital for overdose of five legal drugs during the past year is given in Table 10-1.

Figure 10-1 shows the Microsoft Excel 2000 bar chart for the categorical data given in Table 10-1. The Chart Wizard in Excel is used to construct graphs and charts. In the bar chart, a box is constructed for each drug type, whose height is the frequency of occurrence for that drug. The tallest box corresponds to Tylenol because Tylenol has the

Table 10-1 Number of Emergency Room Visits for Five Legal Drugs

Drug	Emergency Room Visits
OxyContin	525
Valium	640
Aspirin	723
Advil	835
Tylenol	996

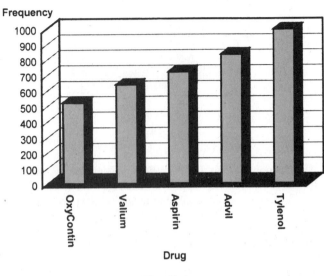

Fig. 10-1

highest frequency of occurrence. The shortest box corresponds to OxyContin because OxyContin has the lowest frequency of occurrence.

EXAMPLE 10.2   According to the Centers for Disease Control and Prevention, Americans made 724 million office visits to a physician during a recent year. Table 10-2 gives a breakdown of how much time was spent with the doctor during visits in a study conducted recently.

Table 10-2   Time Spent with Physicians

Time	Number of Patients
5 min or less	360
6–10 min	2180
11–15 min	3350
16–30 min	3270
31 min or more	840

Figure 10-2 gives the Microsoft Excel pie chart for the categorical data given in Table 10-2. The number of patients for each time category in Table 10-2 is converted to a percentage and then each slice of the pie has an angle equal to that percentage of 360°, since there are 360° in a circle. There were 10,000 patients in the study, and 2180 or 22% spent 6–10 min with the physician. The angle corresponding to the slice of the pie for 6–10 min is 22% of 360° or $360 \times 0.22 = 79.2°$. From Fig. 10-2 we see that the slice with the smallest angle corresponds to the category 5 min or less, and the slice with the largest angle corresponds to the category 11–15 min.

10.3 HISTOGRAMS AND DOT PLOTS FOR NUMERICAL DATA

When data are in the form of numbers rather than categories, bar and pie charts are not appropriate for displaying the data graphically. This section considers techniques for displaying such data.

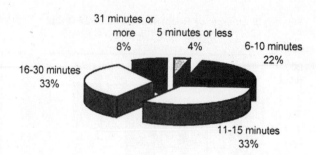

Fig. 10-2

EXAMPLE 10.3 Exercise is important in controlling as well as preventing many diseases such as diabetes and heart disease. Table 10-3 shows the number of minutes of planned exercise per week reported by 80 participants in a study. We shall consider two very useful techniques for displaying numerical data, the *histogram* and the *dot plot*.

Table 10-3   Minutes of Exercise Per Week Reported by Participants

180	840	180	750	150	840	840	750
240	250	150	250	180	240	250	250
150	250	750	750	250	480	250	0
180	250	840	60	750	250	180	150
250	250	750	750	250	840	750	250
250	750	150	250	750	0	180	150
180	240	750	150	750	750	250	150
250	840	250	240	750	150	150	250
180	60	750	250	240	150	840	250
150	250	60	480	480	750	250	750

Sorting data has a very simplifying effect and is often one of the first operations performed on a set of numerical data. Table 10-4 shows the data in Table 10-3 sorted from lowest to highest. We see that two individuals did not have any planned exercise time and seven had 840 min or 14 h per week planned.

Figure 10-3 is a Minitab-generated histogram for the exercise time data in Table 10-3. The histogram is composed of rectangles that have bases of width equal to 100 min. The height of the first rectangle is 5, since 5 of the times in Table 10-4 are between 0 and 100, and the height of the second rectangle is 20, since 20 of the times are between 100

Table 10-4   Minutes of Exercise Per Week Reported by Participants in Sorted Form

0	150	180	250	250	250	750	750
0	150	180	250	250	250	750	750
60	150	180	250	250	250	750	750
60	150	180	250	250	480	750	840
60	150	180	250	250	480	750	840
150	150	240	250	250	480	750	840
150	150	240	250	250	750	750	840
150	180	240	250	250	750	750	840
150	180	240	250	250	750	750	840
150	180	240	250	250	750	750	840

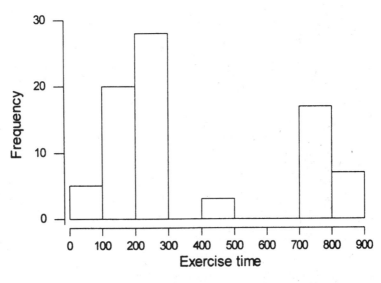

Fig. 10-3

and 200. The heights of rectangles 3 through 8 are 28, 0, 3, 0, 0, 17, and 7. Figure 10-4 is a Minitab-generated dot plot for the exercise time data. The exercise time line is scaled from 0 to 850. Two dots are above 0, three dots are above 60, twelve dots are above 150, and so forth.

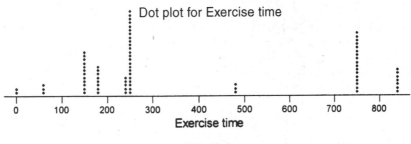

Fig. 10-4

10.4 NUMERICAL MEASURES FOR DESCRIBING NUMERICAL DATA

When we are faced with large sets of data it is difficult to determine the important characteristics of the data. A histogram or dot plot will tell us about the distribution of the data. That is, the histogram or dot plot will show how the data are spread out and what values occur frequently and what values occur rarely. The mean, median, and mode of a data set are numbers that in some sense represent the entire set of data. The standard deviation is a number that measures the dispersion or spread of the data.

EXAMPLE 10.4 Table 10-5 shows hemoglobin A1C values for a group of nondiabetic individuals as well as a group of diabetics.

The dot plots in Fig. 10-5 show that diabetics tend to have higher A1C values than nondiabetics, but there is an overlap of the two distributions. Also, there is more spread or dispersion of the diabetic values than the nondiabetic values. The statistical measures that help describe such situations are called *measures of central tendency* and *measures of dispersion*.

The Minitab descriptive statistics reproduced in Fig. 10-6 show two measures of central tendency. The *mean* is found by summing the A1C values and dividing by 45, the number of values. The *median* is the middle value. In this example, we would sort the 45 values and select the 23rd or middle one. On average, the diabetics' hemoglobin A1C values exceed the nondiabetics' hemoglobin A1C values by $2.278 = 7.540 - 5.262$ units if we use the mean as our

Table 10-5   Comparing Hemoglobin A1C Values for Diabetics and Nondiabetics

Nondiabetic Hemoglobin A1C Values					Diabetic Hemoglobin A1C Values				
4.2	7.1	5.1	6.4	5.1	6.8	7.0	6.2	6.5	4.2
4.0	4.4	4.9	5.6	4.0	8.6	8.8	11.5	5.3	6.3
4.9	7.9	4.1	4.5	6.0	9.8	12.0	6.5	5.1	5.8
4.5	4.7	5.1	6.1	6.2	4.6	11.6	8.2	8.0	8.5
6.7	4.1	3.6	5.1	6.6	7.0	7.9	6.7	9.3	10.1
2.9	4.1	5.2	6.3	5.7	7.4	7.8	5.9	8.5	7.2
5.2	5.4	8.3	4.6	5.7	8.1	5.8	6.6	11.3	6.6
4.9	7.1	4.5	4.2	5.0	4.3	7.3	7.5	8.1	12.4
7.0	5.3	4.6	3.9	6.0	3.6	8.1	5.9	8.9	5.7

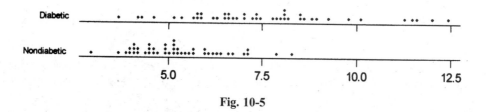

Fig. 10-5

measure of average, or 2.200 = 7.300 − 5.100 units if we use the median as our measure of average. The *mode* is the most frequently occurring value. Minitab does not give the mode, since often there is not a unique mode.

Three measures of dispersion can be obtained from Fig. 10-6. The simplest and easiest to compute is the *range*, defined as the maximum − minimum. For the diabetics the range = 12.4 − 3.6 = 8.8, and for the nondiabetics the range = 8.3 − 2.9 = 5.4. The *first quartile*, Q1, divides the lower 25% from the upper 75% of the data, and the *third quartile*, Q3, divides the lower 75% from the upper 25% of the data. A second measure of dispersion is the *interquartile range*, IQR, defined as IQR = Q3 − Q1. For the diabetics the IQR = 8.55 − 6.05 = 2.5, and for the nondiabetics, the IQR = 6.05 − 4.45 = 1.6. The IQR measures the spread of the middle 50% of the data. A third measure of dispersion is the *standard deviation*. The standard deviation of the diabetic values is 2.098, and the standard deviation of the nondiabetic values is 1.161. The standard deviation is represented by s and is found by either of the following equations:

$$ s = \sqrt{\frac{\sum(x - \bar{x})^2}{n - 1}} \quad \text{or} \quad \sqrt{\frac{\sum x^2 - (\sum x)^2/n}{n - 1}} $$

where $\bar{x}$ is the mean and n is the number of data values.

Descriptive Statistics: Nondiabetic, Diabetic

Variable	N	Mean	Median	TrMean	StDev	SE Mean
Nondiabetic	45	5.262	5.100	5.222	1.161	0.173
Diabetic	45	7.540	7.300	7.490	2.098	0.313

Variable	Minimum	Maximum	Q1	Q3
Nondiabetic	2.900	8.300	4.450	6.050
Diabetic	3.600	12.400	6.050	8.550

Fig. 10-6

The standard deviation is computed by most statistical software packages, including Microsoft Excel and Minitab.

EXAMPLE 10.5 To get a better understanding of the mean and standard deviation, consider a one-standard-deviation interval about the mean for the nondiabetic A1C values in Table 10-5. One standard deviation below the mean is $\bar{x} - s = 5.262 - 1.161 = 4.101$, and one standard deviation above the mean is $\bar{x} + s = 5.262 + 1.161 = 6.423$.

Table 10-6 gives the nondiabetic A1C values from Table 10-5 in ascending order. The 30 values shown in bold are between $\bar{x} - s$ and $\bar{x} + s$. Approximately 67% of the data are within one standard deviation of the mean. Forty-two of the A1C values are between $\bar{x} - 2s = 2.940$ and $\bar{x} + 2s = 7.584$. Approximately 93% of the data are within two standard deviations of the mean. All of the values are between $\bar{x} - 3s = 1.779$ and $\bar{x} + 3s = 8.745$; that is, 100% of the distribution is within three standard deviations of the mean.

Table 10-6 Nondiabetic Hemoglobin A1C Values

2.9	**4.2**	**4.9**	**5.3**	**6.3**
3.6	**4.4**	**4.9**	**5.4**	**6.4**
3.9	**4.5**	**5.0**	**5.6**	6.6
4.0	**4.5**	**5.1**	**5.7**	6.7
4.0	**4.5**	**5.1**	**5.7**	7.0
4.1	**4.6**	**5.1**	**6.0**	7.1
4.1	**4.6**	**5.1**	**6.0**	7.1
4.1	**4.7**	**5.2**	**6.1**	7.9
4.2	**4.9**	**5.2**	**6.2**	8.3

Two important results connecting the mean, standard deviation, and data distribution are Chebyshev's rule and the empirical rule. *Chebyshev's rule* applies to any set of data and assures us that:

1. At least 75% of any data set falls within two standard deviations of the mean.

2. At least 89% of any data set falls within three standard deviations of the mean.

3. Generally, at least $\left(1 - \dfrac{1}{k^2}\right) \times 100\%$ of any data set falls within k standard deviations of the mean.

The *empirical rule* applies to a bell-shaped set of data and assures us that:

1. Approximately 68% of a bell-shaped set of data falls within one standard deviation of the mean.

2. Approximately 95% of a bell-shaped set of data falls within two standard deviations of the mean.

3. Approximately 99.7% of a bell-shaped set of data falls within three standard deviations of the mean.

If a set of data has a dot plot or histogram with the general shape of Fig. 10-7, it is said to be *bell-shaped*.

10.5 PROPERTIES OF PROBABILITY AND THE BINOMIAL DISTRIBUTION

A few basic terms are needed to define probability. An *experiment* is defined as any procedure or operation whose outcomes cannot be predicted with certainty. The set of all possible outcomes for an experiment is called the *sample space* for the experiment. An *event* is a subset of the sample space. The definition of probability for experiments with equally likely outcomes is as follows. If an experiment has n equally likely outcomes and event A consists of k of those outcomes, then the probability of A, expressed as $P(A)$, is defined as the ratio of k divided by n. That is, we express the probability of A as $P(A) = \dfrac{k}{n}$.

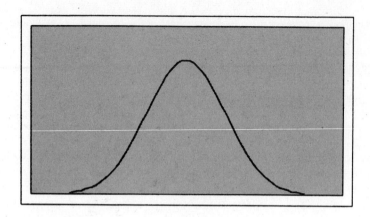

Fig. 10-7

EXAMPLE 10.6   A group of middle-aged men were classified according to whether they were overweight or not and as to whether they have hypertension or not. The results are shown in Table 10-7.

Table 10-7   **Hypertension/Weight Study**

	Hypertension	
Overweight	Yes	No
Yes	35	165
No	10	190

Suppose one of the 400 men in the study is randomly selected. Let A be the event that the man selected is overweight and let B be the event that the man selected has hypertension. Many of the properties of probability will now be developed in the context of this example, using the definition of probability given above. The probability of selecting an overweight man is represented as $P(A)$ and is equal $200/400 = 0.5 = 50\%$. Probabilities may be expressed as fractions, decimals, or percents. The probability of selecting a man who has hypertension is represented as $P(B)$ and is equal $45/400 = 0.1125 = 11.25\%$.

Operations such as *and*, *or*, and *not* are often performed on events. The probability that the selected man is overweight and has hypertension is represented as $P(A$ and $B)$ or $P(A \cap B)$. The event $A \cap B$ is read as A intersects B. Since there are 35 that are overweight and have hypertension, the probability is $P(A$ and $B) = 35/400 = 8.75\%$. That is, 8.75% in the study are both overweight and have hypertension.

The probability that the selected man is overweight or has hypertension is represented as $P(A$ or $B)$ or $P(A \cup B)$. The event $A \cup B$ is read as A union B. Note that there are $10 + 35 + 165 = 210$ men who are overweight or have hypertension. If we were to add those who were overweight to those who have hypertension, we would get $(35 + 165)$ and $(35 + 10)$, and 35 would be added twice and would need to be subtracted out. This is why the formula

$$P(A \text{ or } B) = P(A) + P(B) - P(A \text{ and } B)$$

is used to compute $P(A$ or $B)$. Therefore, $P(A$ or $B) = 50\% + 11.25\% - 8.75\% = 52.5\%$.

Since a man is either overweight or not, $P(A) + P(\text{not } A) = 100\%$. The event "not A" is called the *complement* of A and is represented by $\bar{A}$. We have the formula

$$P(A) + P(\bar{A}) = 100\%$$

Conditional probability $P(A|B)$ is read as the probability of event A given that event B is known to have occurred or to be true. We are asking what is the probability that the selected man is overweight if it is known that he has hypertension. Knowing that the selected man has hypertension reduces your space from 400 to 45. Of the 45 men with hypertension, 35 are overweight and therefore, $P(A|B) = 35/45 = 77.8\%$. Similarly, $P(B|A) = 35/200 = 17.5\%$. There is a formula that can be used to compute the conditional probabilities:

$$P(A|B) = \frac{P(A \cap B)}{P(B)} \quad \text{and} \quad P(B|A) = \frac{P(A \cap B)}{P(A)}$$

Recall that $P(A) = 50\%$, $P(B) = 11.25\%$, and $P(A \cap B) = 8.75\%$. Changing percents to decimals and using the formulas, $P(A|B) = \frac{0.0875}{0.1125} = 0.778$ or 77.8% and $P(B|A) = \frac{0.0875}{0.5} = 0.175$ or 17.5%. These results state that 77.8% of the hypertensive men are overweight and 17.5% of the overweight men have hypertension.

Finally, note that the conditional probability formulas may be also expressed as $P(A \cap B) = P(A|B)P(B) = P(B|A)P(A)$. If $P(A|B) = P(A)$ or $P(B|A) = P(B)$, events A and B are said to be *independent events*. For independent events, $P(A \cap B) = P(A)P(B)$.

A very important rule to remember from the discussion in Example 10.6 is that *when events are connected by OR you add probabilities and when events are connected by AND, you multiply probabilities.*

Example 10.7 illustrates how this AND/OR rule is used.

EXAMPLE 10.7 It was recently reported that 66% of adult males are overweight. If five adult males are randomly selected, find the probabilities that (*a*) all five are overweight, (*b*) exactly one of the five is overweight, and (*c*) none of the five is overweight.

To solve part (*a*), apply the AND rule as follows. All five are overweight if the first and second and third and fourth and fifth are overweight. The probability is $(.66)(.66)(.66)(.66)(.66) = (.66)^5 = 0.125$.

To solve part (*b*), apply both the OR and AND rules. Exactly one is overweight if the first is overweight and the other four are not; OR the first is not, the second is overweight, and the other three are not overweight; OR etc. This would be calculated as $(.66)(.34)(.34)(.34)(.34) + (.34)(.66)(.34)(.34)(.34) + (.34)(.34)(.66)(.34)(.34) + (.34)(.34)(.34)(.66)(.34) + (.34)(.34)(.34)(.34)(.66) = 5(.66)(.34)^4 = 0.044099$.

To solve part (*c*), apply the AND rule as follows. None of the five is overweight if the first and second and third and fourth and fifth are not overweight. The probability is $(0.34)(0.34)(0.34)(0.34)(0.34) = (0.34)^5 = 0.0045435$. The number overweight among the five men can be none, one, two, three, four, or five. The probabilities of each of the six outcomes can be generated using Microsoft Excel as follows. Enter the six numbers 0, 1, 2, 3, 4, and 5 in cells A1–A6 and then enter $=$BINOMDIST(A1,5,0.66,FALSE) in cell B1. Then, after obtaining the fill handle in cell B1, perform a click-and-drag from B1 to B6. Figure 10-8 shows the result. Compare the results for parts (*a*), (*b*), and (*c*) with the results for B6, B2, and B1, respectively.

If the word TRUE is used in place of FALSE, $=$BINOMDIST(A1,5,0.66,TRUE) will accumulate the probabilities from B1 to B6 rather than give them individually. The Excel function BINOMDIST calculates probabilities for the binomial distribution. The binomial distribution is applicable when there is a sequence of trials and each trial has only two possible outcomes. The trials are independent of one another. The two outcomes on

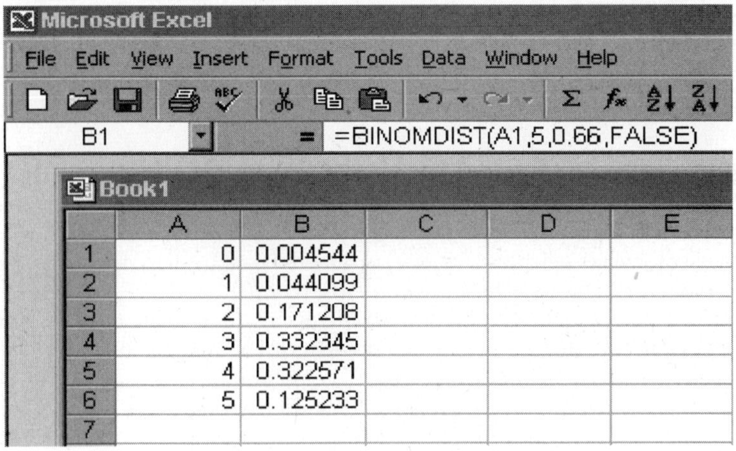

Fig. 10-8

each trial are usually referred to as *success* and *failure*. The probability of success and failure remains constant from trial to trial. In Example 10.7, the five selected males are the trials. The two possible outcomes on each trial are being overweight or not being overweight. On each trial, the probability of the selected male being overweight is 66% and the probability of the selected male not being overweight is 34%. The measure of interest, X, is the number of males among the five who are overweight. Figure 10-8 gives the possible values of X, namely, 0, 1, 2, 3, 4, and 5, in cells A1–A6 and the probabilities associated with these values in B1–B6. Note that four entities must be supplied to the function BINOMDIST. The first is the value of X for which the probability is to be computed, the second is the number of trials, the third is the probability of success on each trial, and the fourth is the word FALSE or TRUE. Individual probabilities will be computed if FALSE is used, and cumulative probabilities will be computed if TRUE is used.

10.6   THE NORMAL DISTRIBUTION

The *normal distribution curve*, often referred to as the *bell curve*, describes the distribution of many real-world phenomena. This curve is centered at the mean value of the characteristic being measured, and the total area under the curve is 1. Since the curve is symmetrical about the mean, the area to the left of the mean is 0.5 and so is the area to the right of the mean. Both Microsoft Excel and Minitab have built-in functions that find areas under the curve. The following example illustrates the usefulness of the distribution.

EXAMPLE 10.8   The heights of adult females are normally distributed with a mean value equal to 5 ft 6 in, or 66 in. The standard deviation of female heights is equal to 3 in. A graph of the normal distribution curve for female heights generated using Microsoft Excel is shown in Fig. 10-9.

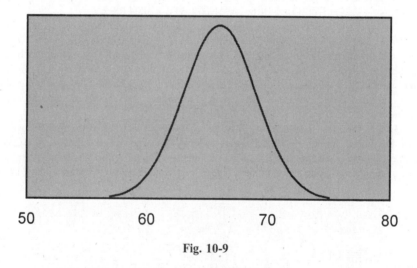

Fig. 10-9

The curve in Fig. 10-9 is centered at 66 in and is *asymptotic* to the horizontal axis. That is, the curve extends indefinitely to the right and to the left, approaching the horizontal axis but never touching it. From the empirical rule, we know that 99.7% of the area under the curve is between $66 - 3(3) = 57$ in and $66 + 3(3) = 75$ in. Suppose we wish to find the percentage of females taller than 70 in. This is represented by the shaded area shown in Fig. 10-11. It is the area under the curve to the right of 70 in.

This area may be found using the function NORMDIST in Excel. In any cell, enter $= 1$-NORMDIST(70,66,3, TRUE). The value 0.091211 in Fig. 10-10 is the area to the right of 70 on the normal curve in Fig. 10-11. That is, 9.12% of adult females are taller than 70 in.

The function NORMDIST returns the area to the left of 70 under a normal curve having a mean equal to 66 and a standard deviation equal to 3. The word TRUE indicates that we wish the cumulative area to the left of 70. Since the percentage of females taller than 70 in is the area to the right of 70, we have to subtract NORMDIST(70,66,3,TRUE) from 1 to find the shaded area. We subtract from 1 because the total area under the normal distribution curve is equal

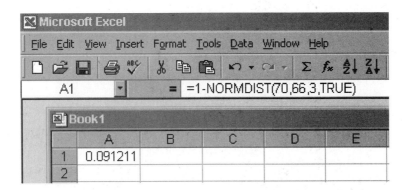

Fig. 10-10

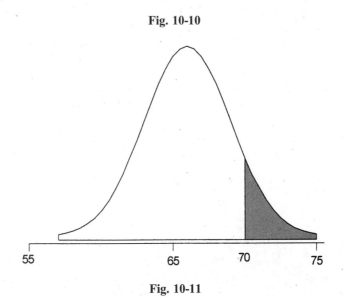

Fig. 10-11

to 1. In other words, we are using the property that $P(X \leq 70) + P(X \geq 70) = 1$. If we know an area under the normal curve, we can find the point on the horizontal axis that corresponds to this area. To do this we use the function NORMINV. If we wish to find the 90th percentile of female heights, then we need to find the point p90 shown in Fig. 10-12. The symbol p90 stands for the 90th percentile of female heights.

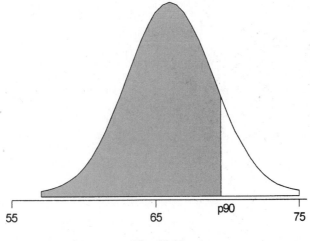

Fig. 10-12

The height p90 is found by using the Excel expression = NORMINV(0.90,66,3). The result is shown in Fig. 10-13.

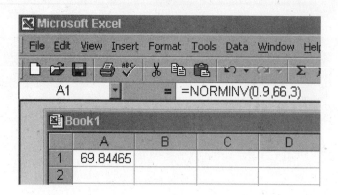

Fig. 10-13

The ninetieth percentile of female heights is 69.8 in. That is, 90% are shorter than 69.8 in and 10% are taller than 69.8 in. Note that the function NORMINV is the inverse of the function NORMDIST. For a given height, NORMDIST will find the percentage who are shorter than this height. For a given percentage, NORMINV will find the height so that the given percentage will be shorter than that height.

10.7 POPULATION AND SAMPLE

The concepts of sample and population are among the most important in statistics. The *population* is the collection of objects in which you are interested. For example, the population might be the nurses employed by Unified Health Care System. A *sample* is a subset of the population in which you are interested. A sample would be some of the nurses employed by Unified Health Care System. The sample is selected in such a way that it is representative of the population. A measure, such as the mean or median, on a sample is called a *statistic* and a measure on a population is called a *parameter*.

EXAMPLE 10.9 Unified Health Care System is interested in estimating patient satisfaction as well as other information for the nurse practitioners they employ. They decide to sample 10% of the patients seen by a nurse practitioner and to send the survey to the selected patients. Table 10-8 lists the patients whom Christine has seen in the past week.

Suppose the patients are numbered from 1 to 50 starting at the top of column 1 and proceeding down each column. Ten percent of 50 is 5, so a 10% sample would consist of 5 of the patients. Now Minitab or Excel can be used to select 5 random numbers between 1 and 50. Using Minitab, we obtained 3, 16, 19, 37, and 42. These random numbers selected the patients shown in bold in Table 10-8. For example, the third patient, J Murphy, is selected to be in the sample; the sixteenth patient, H Farhat is selected; the nineteenth patient, R Longmeyer, is selected; the thirty-seventh patient, P Ramos, is selected; and the forty-second patient, R Branca, is selected. This produces a *random sample*. In this case the population is the 50 patients and the random sample is the 5 shown in bold in Table 10-8. Many populations are more complex than this one, and the sampling technique is not applicable unless the items in the population can be enumerated in some manner. One parameter of interest is the average patient satisfaction of the 50 in Table 10-8. The average patient satisfaction of the 5 selected patients is a statistic that is an estimate of the average patient satisfaction of all 50 patients. Using a sample measurement to estimate the population parameter of interest saves time and money.

EXAMPLE 10.10 Length of patient stay in the hospital is of interest to hospital administrators. Table 10-9 gives the length of stay for 100 patients at Metropolitan Hospital. The mean length of stay for the data in Table 10-9 is 5.25 days, and the median is 5 days.

Table 10-8   Patients Seen by Christine in the Past Week

Konvalina, J	Soto, I	Aaron, H	Pete, C	Thompson, B
Shankle, C	Bush, G	Musial, S	Stengel, C	**Branca, R**
Murphy, J	Clinton, H	Tewilliger, W	Martin, B	Hazel, B
Scroggins, P	Grant, U	Limmer, L	Temple, J	Hoak, D
Kitchens, L	Madison, J	Jacobs, S	Skowron, B	Reno, J
Long, S	**Farhat, H**	Larson, D	Banks, E	Tuttle, B
Kidd, T	Kee, M	Gaedel, E	**Ramos, P**	Koufax, S
Liu, Y	Stafford, N	Kaline, A	Johnson, D	Miller, B
Maloney, J	**Longmeyer, R**	Feller, B	Rizzuto, P	Pickens, C
Carter, D	Armstrong, S	Trucks, V	Doby, L	Barlow, R

It is interesting to compare the mean and median of the table values with the mean and median of a sample of the table values. Suppose the cells in the table are numbered from 1 to 100 starting at the top of the first column and going down column by column from left to right. The following ten random numbers between 1 and 100 were selected by Minitab:

$$42 \quad 34 \quad 6 \quad 46 \quad 27 \quad 21 \quad 10 \quad 56 \quad 80 \quad 98$$

The 10 length-of-stay values determined by these random numbers are shown in bold in the table. The random number 42 determines length of stay, 7 days, the random number 34 determines length of stay, 4 days, etc. The ten sample values are: 5, 6, 4, 7, 4, 7, 3, 7, 2, and 4. The mean of this sample is 4.9 days and the median of this sample is 4.5 days.

Table 10-9   Length of Stay for 100 Patients at Metropolitan Hospital

6	1	**4**	2	5	**7**	6	5	7	7
4	5	9	6	**7**	3	8	7	4	6
4	7	4	2	8	4	3	5	7	6
2	4	5	**4**	3	2	5	2	8	3
3	8	6	3	7	3	2	3	5	4
5	1	5	8	**3**	7	4	11	12	6
2	3	**7**	3	7	6	10	3	10	6
5	8	10	7	5	6	1	3	3	**4**
2	3	6	4	9	11	3	9	6	7
6	5	5	6	4	4	10	**2**	5	6

To distinguish the population and sample means, statisticians use two different symbols. The Greek letter μ is used to represent the population mean and $\bar{X}$ is used to represent the sample mean. In this example, $\mu = 5.25$ days and $\bar{X} = 4.90$. If the sample mean is used to estimate the population mean, the absolute difference $|\bar{X} - \mu| = 0.35$ days is called the *error of estimation*. Usually μ is unknown and therefore when $\bar{X}$ is used to estimate μ, the error of estimation is unknown. As discussed in the next section, the margin of error is a computed quantity that gives us some idea concerning the error of estimation.

10.8 ESTIMATING POPULATION MEANS AND PERCENTAGES

Statistical techniques are often used to estimate the percentage of nurses who are satisfied with their job. Or the average number of overtime hours worked by nurses per year is often estimated. Because of the enormity of these projects if they were performed over the complete population of over 3 million nurses, statistical surveys and polls are used rather than a census of the population of nurses. A single number estimate called a *point estimate* along with a *margin of error* is given in such situations.

The sample mean, $\bar{X}$, is the point estimate of the population mean, μ. For samples greater than 30, the margin of error can be shown to equal $\pm z \dfrac{s}{\sqrt{n}}$, where s is the standard deviation of the sample, n is the sample size, and the value for z is determined using NORMINV in Excel. *Levels of confidence* are associated with different values of z. The most common level of confidence is 95% and the value of z is 1.96. Table 10-10 gives the values of z associated with the more common levels of confidence. This table will save you from using NORMINV to look these up.

Table 10-10 z Values for Different Levels of Confidence

Level of Confidence	z Value
80	1.282
90	1.645
95	1.960
99	2.575

EXAMPLE 10.11   The number of hours of overtime for the past year for 50 nurses in Midwestern City is given in Table 10-11. Estimate the average number of hours overtime for all nurses in Midwestern City for the past year and give a 95% margin of error for the estimate. Use Excel and Minitab to perform the computations.

The Excel output is shown in Fig. 10-14. The 50 overtime values are entered into A1–A50. The average is computed in cell C1, the standard deviation in C2, the margin of error in C3, the mean minus the margin of error in C4, and the mean plus the margin of error in C5. The interval that extends from 315.4073 to 323.9527 is called a *95% confidence interval* for the population mean.

Figure 10-15 gives the Minitab output for a 95% confidence interval for the population mean.

Because of the widespread availability of Microsoft Excel, the author recommends the use of the spreadsheet to compute the confidence interval for the population mean. Many universities and medical research hospitals also have Minitab, and it is also recommended when performing statistical estimation procedures. Both Excel and Minitab are user-friendly and save time and effort as compared to using a calculator to perform statistical computations.

When estimating the percentage in a population, p, who have a particular characteristic, a survey or poll of size n is taken and the percentage in the sample, $\bar{p}$, that has the characteristic is computed and is used as a point estimate of p. The margin of error can be shown to equal $\pm z \sqrt{\dfrac{\bar{p}(1 - \bar{p})}{n}}$.

EXAMPLE 10.12   A national survey of 1000 nurses was conducted and the question asked was, "Overall, are you satisfied with your job?" Six hundred and fifty answered yes. Estimate the percentage of all nurses who are satisfied with their job. Give a 95% confidence interval for the percentage of all nurses who are satisfied with their job. Use Excel and Minitab to perform the computations. The Excel computations are shown in Fig. 10-16. The

Table 10-11　Hours of Overtime for the Past Year

336	280	328	320	336
320	320	320	296	328
320	304	312	320	296
344	296	328	320	352
360	320	320	312	312
320	352	320	312	320
320	328	320	312	296
296	320	336	328	328
328	320	320	320	312
320	288	320	328	320

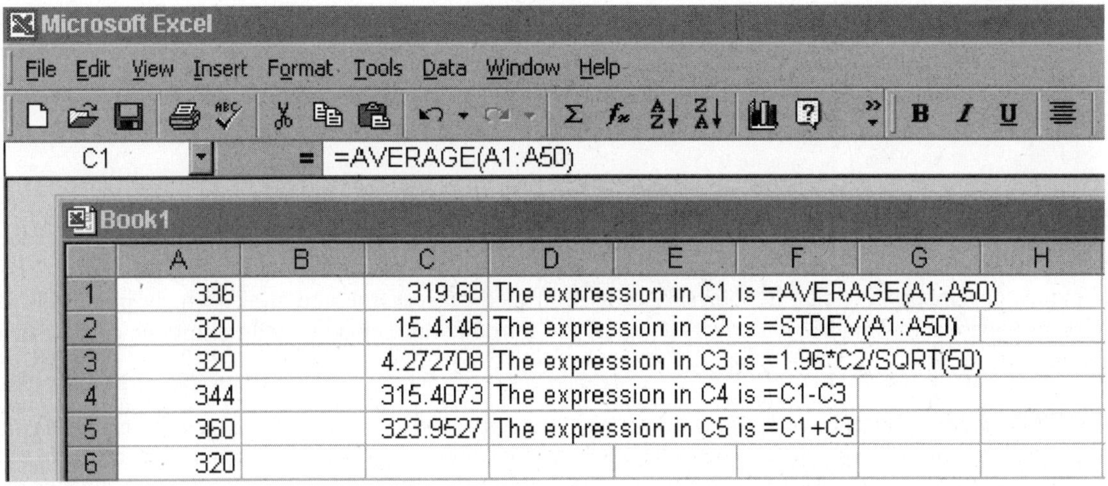

Microsoft Excel

File　Edit　View　Insert　Format　Tools　Data　Window　Help

C1　=　=AVERAGE(A1:A50)

Book1

	A	B	C	D	E	F	G	H
1	336		319.68	The expression in C1 is =AVERAGE(A1:A50)				
2	320		15.4146	The expression in C2 is =STDEV(A1:A50)				
3	320		4.272708	The expression in C3 is =1.96*C2/SQRT(50)				
4	344		315.4073	The expression in C4 is =C1-C3				
5	360		323.9527	The expression in C5 is =C1+C3				
6	320							

Fig. 10-14

Variable	N	Mean	StDev	SE Mean	95.0% CI
Hours	50	319.68	15.41	2.18	(315.41, 323.95)

Fig. 10-15

95% confidence interval for the percentage of nurses who are satisfied with their job extends from 62.04% to 67.95%.

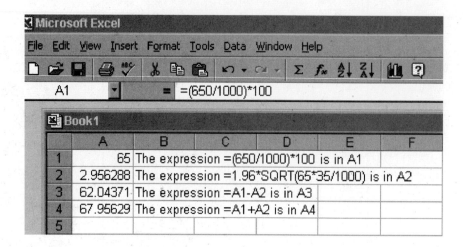

Fig. 10-16

The Minitab solution is shown in Fig. 10-17. The confidence interval is given for the proportion rather than the percentage in Fig. 10-17. To obtain percentages, simply multiply the results by 100.

```
Sample      X       N   Sample p         95.0% CI
1          650    1000   0.650000    (0.620438, 0.679562)
```

Fig. 10-17

10.9 TESTING HYPOTHESES ABOUT MEANS AND POPULATION PERCENTAGES

Statistical methods are used in making decisions. This use of statistics is called *testing hypotheses*. The techniques developed in testing hypotheses are used in medical research and are extremely important for nurses to understand. This section covers some of the introductory concepts and definitions of statistical hypothesis testing.

EXAMPLE 10.13 A study is conducted to determine if a zinc spray will shorten the duration of the common cold. Suppose the average duration of the common cold is 6 days. If μ represents the average duration of the common cold when the zinc spray is used, then the zinc spray is effective if $\mu < 6$. If there is no shortening of the cold's duration due to the zinc spray, then $\mu = 6$. The *research hypothesis* is that the zinc spray is effective in shortening the duration, and we state this as H_a: $\mu < 6$. The *null hypothesis* is that the duration is the same when the zinc spray is used, and we state this as H_0: $\mu = 6$. Table 10-12 gives the duration of colds for 50 patients with common colds who used the zinc spray.

The test of the hypothesis works as follows. The null hypothesis is assumed to be true and the following *test statistic* is computed:

$$z = \frac{\bar{x} - 6}{\frac{s}{\sqrt{50}}}$$

where $\bar{x}$ and s are computed from the data in Table 10-12. This test statistic follows a normal distribution that has mean 0 and standard deviation 1. A normal distribution having mean equal to 0 and standard deviation equal to 1 is

Table 10-12   Cold Duration Using Zinc Spray

4	4	5	4	4
4	4	3	7	4
5	4	4	2	4
6	5	5	2	7
3	4	4	4	4
4	5	6	3	4
5	5	3	4	3
3	3	3	5	4
4	4	3	4	3
5	5	5	4	2

called a *standard normal distribution*. Depending on where the computed test statistic falls on the standard normal curve, the null hypothesis is either rejected or not.

First the data are entered into the Excel worksheet in A1–A50 and the mean and standard deviation are computed. Then the test statistic is computed. These computations are shown in Fig. 10-18. The computed test statistic is $z = -12.2959$. The average duration of the cold for these 50 patients was 4.1 days. Since the sample mean centers on the population mean, $\mu < 6$ is much more reasonable than $\mu = 6$. Therefore, we reject the null hypothesis in favor of the research hypothesis. The probability of getting a value of z equal to -12.2959 or smaller is given by $= \text{NORMDIST}(B3,0,1,\text{TRUE})$, which for all practical purposes is 0. This computed probability is called the *p-value* for the test of hypothesis. The interpretation of the *p*-value is this: If the null hypothesis is true and the mean duration when using the zinc spray is 6 days, the probability of getting a sample with durations like those in Table 10-12 is practically zero. Because of these results, we will reject the null hypothesis and conclude that the zinc spray is effective in reducing the duration on the average.

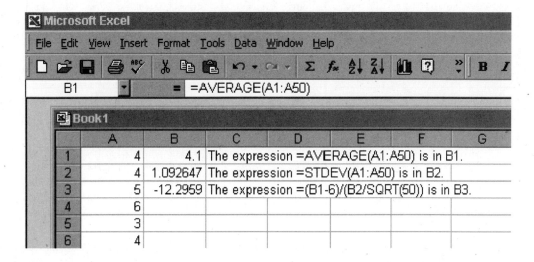

Fig. 10-18

The Minitab output for the same analysis is shown in Fig. 10-19. Because of the "less than" symbol ($<$) in the research hypothesis, and the fact that we used the lower tail of the standard normal distribution to compute the p value, this test is called a *lower-tail test*.

```
Test of mu = 6 vs mu < 6
The assumed sigma = 1.093

Variable            N       Mean     StDev    SE Mean
duration           50      4.100     1.093     0.155

Variable        95.0% Upper Bound        Z        P
duration                      4.354   -12.29    0.000
```

Fig. 10-19

EXAMPLE 10.14 Nationally, the average age of nurses is 45. Unified Health Care System employs thousands of nurses. Unified would like to know if the average age of their nurses is different from the national average. If μ represents the average age of Unified nurses, then the research hypothesis of interest is the following: $H_a: \mu \neq 45$. The null hypothesis is $H_0: \mu = 45$. The ages of a sample of 100 randomly selected nurses employed at Unified are shown in Table 10-13. The computations needed to test the hypothesis are shown in Fig. 10-20. The 100 ages are entered in A1–A100. The mean in B1 is 45.87 years. The computed test statistic in B3 is 1.663673. The computation of the p value in B4 determines the area to the right of 1.663673 and doubles it. The area is doubled because the research hypothesis contains the inequality symbol ($\neq$). Such a research hypothesis is called a *two-tailed test*.

Table 10-13   Ages of 100 Nurses Employed by Unified Health Care System

45	51	39	48	44	44	52	50	41	52
46	47	47	34	46	49	40	52	55	47
47	51	44	44	37	53	40	49	45	45
52	39	47	38	40	53	39	47	46	43
45	50	53	45	48	40	53	37	43	48
41	45	37	50	47	40	51	56	47	42
43	52	42	48	44	51	48	51	49	49
49	48	52	42	56	45	40	40	43	52
47	45	42	43	50	39	50	41	42	41
56	46	31	40	45	51	40	51	42	55

At the time the research hypothesis is formulated, *a level of significance* is stated. The value usually chosen for the level of significance is 0.05. The Greek letter α is used to represent the level of significance; that is, $\alpha = 0.05$. The null hypothesis is rejected and the research hypothesis is supported if the computed p value is less than the level of

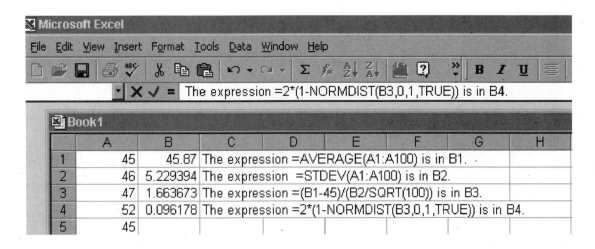

Fig. 10-20

significance. For the data in Table 10-13, the *p* value is 0.096178. Since the *p* value is not less than the level of significance, the data do not convince us that the mean age is different from the national average.

The Minitab output for the test is shown in Fig. 10-21.

```
Test of mu = 45 vs mu not = 45
The assumed sigma = 5.229

Variable            N        Mean      StDev    SE Mean
Age               100      45.870      5.229      0.523

Variable                  95.0% CI              Z       P
Age              (  44.845,   46.895)        1.66   0.096
```

Fig. 10-21

*In testing hypotheses, the null hypothesis is rejected and the research hypothesis is supported if the **p** value < α.*

EXAMPLE 10.15   A recent survey of 13,000 U.S. nurses found that only 33% said their unit had enough staff on hand to get the work done. Metropolitan Hospital conducted a survey to test the research hypothesis that a greater percentage of the nurses at Metropolitan would say that Metropolitan had enough staff on hand to get the work done. The hypothesis to be tested was H_0: $p = 33\%$ versus H_a: $p > 33\%$, and α was chosen to be 0.05. This research hypothesis is called an *upper-tail test* because of the "greater than" sign (>) in the research hypothesis. The test of the hypothesis works as follows. The null hypothesis is assumed to be true and the following *test statistic* is computed:

$$z = \frac{\bar{p} - 33\%}{\sqrt{\dfrac{(33\%)(67\%)}{n}}}$$

where *n* is the survey size and $\bar{p}$ is the percentage in the survey that has the characteristic of interest, which in this case is that the nurses believe there is enough staff on hand to get the work done. This test statistic follows a normal distribution that has mean 0 and standard deviation 1. The survey size at Metropolitan Hospital was 250, and 90 or 36% said that Metropolitan had enough staff on hand to get the work done.

Figure 10-22 gives the Excel computation of the percentage in the survey who said that Metropolitan had enough staff on hand to get the work done in A1, the computed test statistic in A2, and the computed *p* value in A3.

Figure 10-23 gives the Minitab computation for the test of hypothesis.

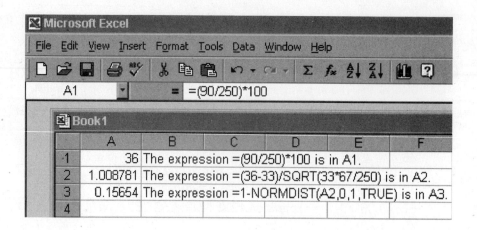

Fig. 10-22

```
Test of p = 0.33 vs p > 0.33

Sample      X      N  Sample p  95.0% Lower Bound  Z-Value  P-Value
1          90    250  0.360000            0.310066     1.01    0.157
```

Fig. 10-23

Because the p value $> \alpha$, the survey results do not support the research hypothesis. We cannot conclude that the percentage at Metropolitan Hospital exceeds the national percentage.

The hypothesis testing methods in this section have associated with them two types of errors that are very similar to two medical terms, namely, *false positives* and *false negatives*. If a lab test indicates that you have a disease when you do not, this is called a false positive; if a lab test indicates that you do not have a disease when you do, this is called a false negative. Table 10-14 summarizes the possible outcomes when testing these hypotheses.

Table 10-14   Type I and Type II Errors Defined

	Reject H_0	Do Not Reject H_0
H_0 is true	Type I error	Correct decision
H_a is true	Correct decision	Type II error

The probability of making a type I error is controlled by the level of significance that you set when performing a test of a hypothesis. When α is chosen to be 0.05, for example, and you reject the null hypothesis for p values $< \alpha$, you are actually controlling the probability of committing a type I error at 5%.

We close this section and chapter with a summary of the procedures for testing hypotheses about means and percentages. Microsoft Excel greatly facilitates the computation of test statistics and p values. Minitab actually performs all the computations for you.

Summary of Testing Hypotheses about a Mean and a Proportion
Lower-Tail Test of the Population Mean

First choose the level of significance at which the test is to be performed. That is, specify α.

For $H_0: \mu = \mu_0$ versus $H_a: \mu < \mu_0$, compute

$$z = \frac{\bar{x} - \mu_0}{\frac{s}{\sqrt{n}}}$$

The p value is the area under the standard normal curve to the left of the computed value of z. If the p value $< \alpha$, reject H_0. Otherwise, do not reject H_0.

Upper-Tail Test of the Population Mean

For $H_0: \mu = \mu_0$ versus $H_a: \mu > \mu_0$, compute

$$z = \frac{\bar{x} - \mu_0}{\frac{s}{\sqrt{n}}}$$

The p value is the area under the standard normal curve to the right of the computed value of z. If the p value $< \alpha$, reject H_0. Otherwise, do not reject H_0.

Two-Tail Test of the Population Mean

For $H_0: \mu = \mu_0$ versus $H_a: \mu \neq \mu_0$, compute

$$z = \frac{\bar{x} - \mu_0}{\frac{s}{\sqrt{n}}}$$

The p value is the area under the standard normal curve beyond the computed value of z, doubled. If the p value $< \alpha$, reject H_0. Otherwise, do not reject H_0.

Lower-Tail Test of the Population Percentage

For $H_0: p = p_0$ versus $H_a: p < p_0$, compute

$$z = \frac{\bar{p} - p_0}{\sqrt{\frac{p_0(1 - p_0)}{n}}}$$

The p value is the area under the standard normal curve to the left of the computed value of z. If the p-value $< \alpha$, reject H_0. Otherwise, do not reject H_0.

Upper-Tail Test of the Population Percentage

For $H_0: p = p_0$ versus $H_a: p > p_0$, compute

$$z = \frac{\bar{p} - p_0}{\sqrt{\frac{p_0(1 - p_0)}{n}}}$$

The p value is the area under the standard normal curve to the right of the computed value of z. If the p value $< \alpha$, reject H_0. Otherwise, do not reject H_0.

Two-Tail Test of the Population Percentage

For H_0: $p = p_0$ versus H_a: $p \neq p_0$, compute

$$z = \frac{\bar{p} - p_0}{\sqrt{\dfrac{p_0(1 - p_0)}{n}}}$$

The p value is the area under the standard normal curve beyond the computed value of z, doubled. If the p value $< \alpha$, reject H_0. Otherwise, do not reject H_0.

Solved Problems

10.1 A recent report by the Health Resources and Services Administration estimated the public health workforce to be 448,250. The Excel pie chart in Fig. 10-24 gives the percentages that are local, state, federal, and other.

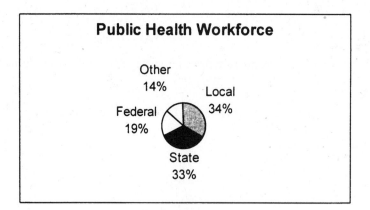

Fig. 10-24

(a) Give the number in each of the four groups.

(b) How many are state or federal?

(c) How many are local and state?

Solution

(a) Local: $.34 \times 448{,}250 = 152{,}405$; state: $.33 \times 448{,}250 = 147{,}923$; federal: $.19 \times 448{,}250 = 85{,}168$; other: $448{,}250 - 152{,}405 - 147{,}923 - 85{,}168 = 62{,}754$.

(b) $147{,}923 + 85{,}168 = 233{,}091$.

(c) 0, since the categories are mutually exclusive.

10.2 A recent survey of 10,000 nurses inquired about the stress that nurses faced on the job. The bar chart in Fig. 10-25 summarizes the results of the survey in percent. How many reported no or little stress associated with the job?

Job Stress in Nursing

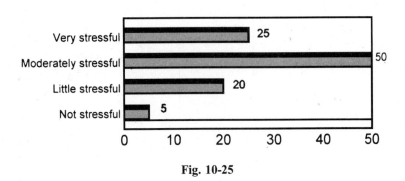

Fig. 10-25

Solution

The percentage is $20 + 5 = 25$, and $0.25 \times 10,000 = 2,500$.

10.3 The dot plot in Fig. 10-26 shows the systolic blood pressure readings for 50 individuals taken at a health fair.

Systolic Blood Pressures from Blood Pressure Screening

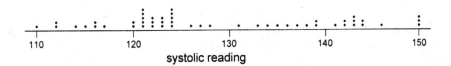

systolic reading

Fig. 10-26

(a) What percent are less than 120?

(b) What percent are between 120 and 140 (include 120 and 140)?

(c) What percent are more than 140?

Solution

(a) 8 out of 50 or 16%

(b) 30 out of 50 or 60%

(c) 12 out of 50 or 24%

10.4   The weights of 100 females are shown in Fig. 10-27.

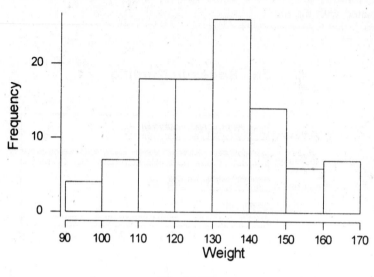

Fig. 10-27

(*a*)   What class has the smallest number of weights in it?

(*b*)   What class has the largest number of weights in it?

(*c*)   If you add the heights of the eight rectangles in the histogram, what do you obtain?

Solution

(*a*)   90 to 100   (*b*)   130 to 140   (*c*)   100

10.5   Fifty study participants with elevated cholesterol were divided into two groups. One group served as a control group and the other group served as the experimental group. The experimental group ate a fat-reduced diet and exercised 10 h per week. The cholesterol readings for the two groups after 6 months are given in Table 10-15. The output for the Descriptive statistics routine from the Data Analysis Add-in of Microsoft Excel is shown in Fig. 10-28. On average, how much lower are the cholesterol readings of the experimental group than of the control group?

Table 10-15   Cholesterol Readings for Control and Experimental Groups

Control Group Cholesterol Readings						Experimental Group Cholesterol Readings				
234	241	248	215	194		184	210	197	163	157
239	227	216	234	190		218	202	175	205	176
195	213	213	205	218		177	239	181	209	192
221	218	226	235	244		196	179	198	167	198
200	254	225	194	227		181	202	185	193	221

Solution

If the mean is used to compare the two groups, the experimental group is on average $221.04 - 192.2 = 28.84$ units lower than that of the control group. If the median is used to compare the two groups, the experimental

	A	B	C	D	E	F	G
1	Control	Experimental	*Control*		*Experimental*		
2	234	184					
3	239	218	Mean	221.04	Mean	192.2	
4	195	177	Standard Error	3.586307	Standard Error	3.831014	
5	221	196	Median	221	Median	193	
6	200	181	Mode	234	Mode	181	
7	241	210	Standard Deviation	17.93154	Standard Deviation	19.15507	
8	227	202	Sample Variance	321.54	Sample Variance	366.9167	
9	213	239	Kurtosis	-0.7867	Kurtosis	0.203229	
10	218	179	Skewness	-0.10256	Skewness	0.354939	
11	254	202	Range	64	Range	82	
12	248	197	Minimum	190	Minimum	157	
13	216	175	Maximum	254	Maximum	239	
14	213	181	Sum	5526	Sum	4805	
15	226	198	Count	25	Count	25	
16	225	185					

Fig. 10-28

group is $221 - 193 = 28$ units lower on average than that of the control group. If the cholesterol readings of the two groups were approximately the same at the beginning of the study, we might infer that the diet/exercise treatment reduced the cholesterol readings by 28 units on average.

10.6 Refer to the data in Table 10-15. Using the range as the measure of dispersion, which of the two groups has the greater dispersion? Using the standard deviation as the measure of dispersion, which of the two groups has the greater dispersion?

Solution

The range for the control group is 64 and the range for the experimental group is 82. Using the range, the experimental group has the greater dispersion. The standard deviation for the control group is 17.93154 and the standard deviation for the experimental group is 19.15507. Using the standard deviation, the experimental group has the greater dispersion.

10.7 For the experimental group cholesterol readings in Table 10-15, find the percentage of the data within one, two, and three standard deviations of the mean.

Solution

The experimental group data in sorted form is

157	163	167	175	176	177	179	181	181	184
185	192	193	196	197	198	198	202	202	205
209	210	218	221	239					

$\bar{x} - s = 192.2 - 19.16 = 173.04$ and $\bar{x} + s = 192.2 + 19.16 = 211.36$. Nineteen of the 25 readings, or 76%, are between the limits.
$\bar{x} - 2s = 192.2 - 38.32 = 153.88$ and $\bar{x} + 2s = 192.2 + 38.32 = 230.52$. Twenty-four of the 25 readings, or 96%, are between the limits.
$\bar{x} - 3s = 192.2 - 57.48 = 134.72$ and $\bar{x} + 3s = 192.2 + 57.48 = 249.68$. All readings, or 100%, are between these limits.

10.8   Study the Excel output in Fig. 10-28 and answer the following questions for the Control group.

(a)   What is the relationship between the mean, the sum, and the count?

(b)   What is the relationship between the standard deviation and the variance?

(c)   What is the relationship between the range, the minimum, and the maximum?

Solution

(a)   The mean equals the sum divided by the count or $221.04 = 5526/25$.

(b)   The variance equals the square of the standard deviation or $321.54 = (17.93154)^2$.

(c)   The range equals the maximum − the minimum or $64 = 254 - 190$.

10.9   Suppose a set of data has a mean equal to 75.5 and a standard deviation equal to 5.2. Use Chebyshev's rule to find an interval that will contain:

(a)   At least 75% of the values in the data set

(b)   At least 89% of the data

Solution

(a)   The interval from $\bar{x} - 2s = 75.5 - 2(5.2) = 65.1$ to $\bar{x} + 2s = 75.5 + 2(5.2) = 85.9$ will contain at least 75% of the data.

(b)   The interval from $\bar{x} - 3s = 75.5 - 3(5.2) = 59.9$ to $\bar{x} + 3s = 75.5 + 3(5.2) = 91.1$ will contain at least 89% of the data.

10.10   Refer to Problem 10.9 and assume the data distribution is known to be bell-shaped. Use the empirical rule to find an interval that will contain:

(a)   68% of the data

(b)   95% of the data

(c)   99.7% of the data

Solution

(a)   The interval from $\bar{x} - s = 75.5 - 5.2 = 70.3$ to $\bar{x} + s = 75.5 + 5.2 = 80.7$ will contain 68% of the data.

(b)   The interval from $\bar{x} - 2s = 75.5 - 2(5.2) = 65.1$ to $\bar{x} + 2s = 75.5 + 2(5.2) = 85.9$ will contain 95% of the data.

(c)   The interval from $\bar{x} - 3s = 75.5 - 3(5.2) = 59.9$ to $\bar{x} + 3s = 75.5 + 3(5.2) = 91.1$ will contain 99.7% of the data.

10.11   If no twins are born, the sex distribution of the babies born in a pediatric unit can be predicted using probability theory. On a day in which four babies are born in a pediatric unit and no twins are born, use the AND/OR rule to find the probabilities that none, one, two, three, or four girls are born.

Solution

The probability of no girls among the four is the same as the probability that a boy *and* a boy *and* a boy *and* a boy are born. Using the AND rule, this is $.5 \times .5 \times .5 \times .5 = (.5)^4 = 0.0625$.

The event that exactly one girl is born is: girl *and* boy *and* boy *and* boy *or* boy *and* girl *and* boy *and* boy *or* boy *and* boy *and* girl *and* boy *or* boy *and* boy *and* boy *and* girl. This could be written as GBBB or BGBB or BBGB or BBBG. Multiplying for *ands* and adding for *ors*, we add $.5 \times .5 \times .5 \times .5$ four times and obtain $4 \times (.5)^4 = 0.250$.

Exactly two girls are born if the sex orders are BGGB or BGBG or BBGG or GGBB or GBGB or GBBG. This results in $6 \times (.5)^4 = 0.375$.

Exactly three girls are born if the sex orders are BGGG or GBGG or GGBG or GGGB. This results in $4 \times (.5)^4 = 0.250$. If four girls are born, this is GGGG, and the probability of this is $.5 \times .5 \times .5 \times .5 = (.5)^4 = 0.0625$.

Summarizing, on days in which four babies are born, 6.25% of the time none of the four will be girls, 25% of the time exactly one will be a girl, 37.5% of the time two will be girls, 25% of the time three will be girls, and 6.25% all four will be girls.

The solution to this problem using the function BINOMDIST from Excel is shown in Fig. 10-29. The outcomes 0 through 4 are entered into A1–A5, =BINOMDIST(A1,4,0.5,FALSE) is entered into B1, and a click-and-drag is performed from B1 to B5.

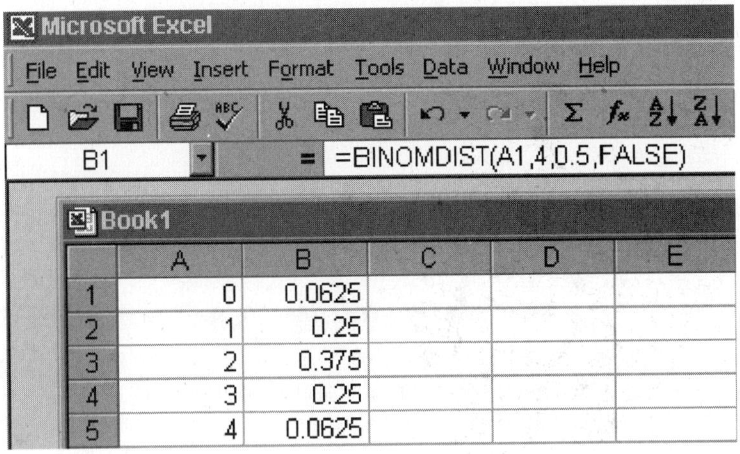

Fig. 10-29

10.12 This problem is a follow-up to Problem 10.11. It is assumed that you have worked that problem before this one. Figure 10-30 gives the probability distribution for the number of girls among 10 babies born one day in a pediatric unit. It is assumed that no twins were born in the unit on this day. Refer to Fig. 10-30 to answer the following questions.

(a) What percent of the time are all 10 girls?

(b) What percent of the time are at most four of the 10 girls?

(c) What percent of the time are eight or more girls?

(d) What are the most likely number of girls you would find among 10?

Solution

(a) $0.000977 \times 100 = 0.0977\%$, or about 1 day out of every 1000 will all 10 babies be girls.

(b) At most four of the 10 are girls means 0 or 1 or 2 or 3 or 4 of the 10 are girls. Because of the OR rule, we add the probabilities of 0, 1, 2, 3, and 4 to obtain the answer:

$$P(X \le 4) = 0.000977 + 0.009766 + 0.043945 + 0.117188 + 0.205078 = 0.376954$$

About 38% of the time, at most four of the 10 babies will be girls.

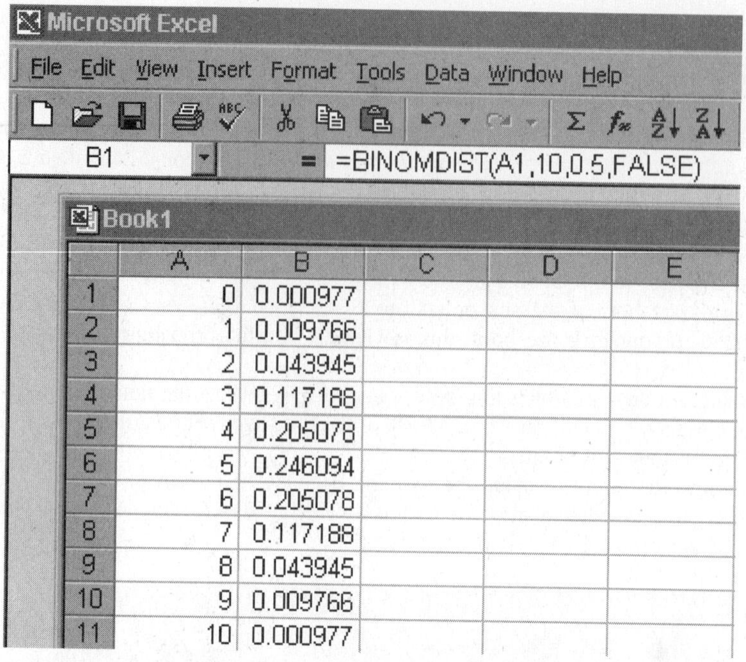
Microsoft Excel

File Edit View Insert Format Tools Data Window Help

B1 = =BINOMDIST(A1,10,0.5,FALSE)

Book1

	A	B	C	D	E
1	0	0.000977			
2	1	0.009766			
3	2	0.043945			
4	3	0.117188			
5	4	0.205078			
6	5	0.246094			
7	6	0.205078			
8	7	0.117188			
9	8	0.043945			
10	9	0.009766			
11	10	0.000977			

Fig. 10-30

(*c*) Eight or more girls means 8 or 9 or 10 of the 10 are girls. Because of the OR rule, we add probabilities to obtain

$$P(X \geq 8) = 0.043945 + 0.009766 + 0.000977 = 0.054688.$$

About 5.5% of the time, eight or more of the 10 babies will be girls.

(*d*) The most likely number of girl babies is five, because this number has the highest probability.

10.13 If male heights are normally distributed with mean equal to 70 in and standard deviation equal to 3 in, find the following:

(*a*) What percent are over 6 ft tall?

(*b*) What percent are shorter than 5 ft 5 in?

(*c*) What percent are between 5 ft 8 in and 5 ft 10 in?

(*d*) What is the third quartile (75th percentile) of male heights?

Solution

(*a*) The percent taller than 6 ft or 72 in is represented by the shaded area shown in Fig. 10-31. The Excel solution is shown in Fig. 10-32. The expression NORMDIST(72,70,3,TRUE) gives the area to the left of 72 in Fig. 10-31. Since the total area under the curve is 1, we subtract this from 1 to find the shaded area. Multiplying the area in cell A1 of Fig. 10-32 by 100, we see that a little over 25% are more than 6 ft tall.

(*b*) The percent shorter than 5 ft 5 in or 65 in is the area under the curve in Fig. 10-31 to the left of 65. The Excel solution to this is shown in Fig. 10-33. This figure shows that 4.8% are shorter than 5 ft 5 ins.

(*c*) Figure 10-34 shows that 24.8% have heights between 5 ft 8 in and 5 ft 10 in.

(*d*) From part (*a*), we know that about 25% of the heights exceed 72 in. This means that about 75% are less than 72 in tall. Therefore the 75th percentile or third quartile is 72 in or 6 ft.

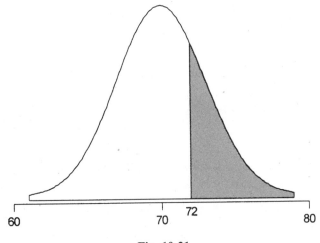

Fig. 10-31

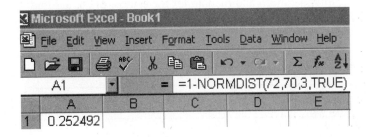

Fig. 10-32

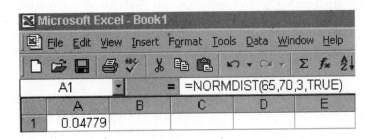

Fig. 10-33

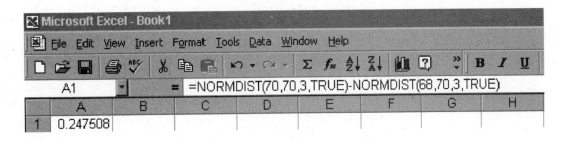

Fig. 10-34

10.14 Suppose you are to select a random sample of 5 from among the patients seen by Christine the past week as given in Table 10-8. Suppose Excel was used to select five random numbers between 1 and 50 and they were 7, 19, 28, 33, and 46. Who were the selected patients?

Solution

Assume the patients in Table 10-8 are numbered from 1 through 50 starting at the top of column 1 and proceeding down each column from left to right. The selected patients are Kidd, T, Longmeyer, R, Kaline, A, Martin, B, and Tuttle, B.

10.15 Table 10-9 shows lengths of hospital stays for 100 patients. The mean length of stay was 5.25 days and the median length of stay was 5 days for the 100 patients. Minitab was used to select 10 random numbers. The random numbers selected in order were

$$2 \quad 12 \quad 18 \quad 38 \quad 41 \quad 59 \quad 68 \quad 74 \quad 91 \quad 92$$

Suppose the cells in Table 10-9 are numbered from 1 to 100 starting at the top of the first column and going down column by column from left to right. Give the 10 lengths of stay determined by the random numbers. Find the mean and median for the sample of 10 and find the differences between the population and sample measurements.

Solution

Random number	2	12	18	38	41	59	68	74	91	92
Length of stay	4	5	8	7	5	11	1	2	7	6

The mean of the sample is 5.6 and the median is 5.5. The error of estimation for the mean is $|5.6 - 5.25| = 0.35$ days, and the error of estimation for the median is $|5.5 - 5| = 0.5$ days.

10.16 A survey of 100 nurses who work in intensive care units (ICUs) was taken, and the time from finishing nursing school until they began working in the ICU was determined for each. The mean was 30 months and the standard deviation was 5 months. Find a 95% confidence interval for the mean time from finishing nursing school until starting work in the ICU for all ICU nurses.

Solution

The point estimate for the mean is 30 months. The 95% margin of error is

$$\pm z \frac{s}{\sqrt{n}} = \pm 1.96 \frac{5}{\sqrt{100}} \qquad \text{or} \qquad \pm 1$$

The 95% confidence interval extends from $30 - 1 = 29$ months to $30 + 1 = 31$ months. Notice that in this problem, the mean and standard deviation was already given and we did not need to use Excel or Minitab to compute them.

10.17 A survey of 1000 nurses found that 68% of those surveyed performed duties other than nursing duties in addition to their nursing duties. Find a 99% confidence interval for the percent of all nurses who perform other than nursing duties.

Solution

The point estimate is $\bar{p} = 68\%$ and the margin of error is

$$\pm z \sqrt{\frac{\bar{p}(1 - \bar{p})}{n}} = \pm 2.575 \sqrt{\frac{68(32)}{1000}} \qquad \text{or} \qquad \pm 3.8\%$$

The 99% confidence interval for the percent of all nurses performing other duties extends from $68\% - 3.8\% = 64.2\%$ to $68\% + 3.8\% = 71.8\%$.

10.18 It is known that the mean response time for rats to a certain stimulus is 1.5 s. A researcher is interested in determining if drug A increases the mean response time to this stimulus. If μ is the mean response time of such rats when under the influence of drug A, then the hypotheses of interest are $H_0: \mu = 1.5$ and $H_a: \mu > 1.5$. The researcher determines the response times of 36 rats under the influence of drug A and finds that the mean response time is $\bar{x} = 2.1$ and the standard deviation is $s = 1.2$. If the level of significance $\alpha = 0.05$ is chosen by the researcher before the experiment is conducted, what conclusion does she reach?

Solution

The computed value of the test statistic is

$$z = \frac{\bar{x} - \mu_0}{\frac{s}{\sqrt{n}}} = \frac{2.1 - 1.5}{\frac{1.2}{\sqrt{36}}} = \frac{0.6}{0.2} = 3$$

Since this is an upper-tail test, the p value is the area to the right of 3 on the standard normal curve. The expression $= 1 - \text{NORMDIST}(3,0,1, \text{TRUE})$ is entered into any cell of the Excel worksheet and the value 0.00135 is returned. The p value $= 0.00135$ is less than $\alpha = 0.05$ and the null hypothesis is rejected. Our conclusion is that the drug increases the mean response time for rats of this type.

10.19 It is known that the mean response time for rats to a certain stimulus is 1.5 s A researcher is interested in determining if drug B decreases the mean response time to this stimulus. If μ is the mean response time of such rats when under the influence of drug B, then the hypotheses of interest are $H_0: \mu = 1.5$ and $H_a: \mu < 1.5$. The researcher determines the response times of 36 rats under the influence of drug B and finds that the mean response time is $\bar{x} = 1.3$ and the standard deviation is $s = 1.2$. If the level of significance $\alpha = 0.05$ is chosen by the researcher before the experiment is conducted, what conclusion does she reach?

Solution

The computed value of the test statistic is

$$z = \frac{\bar{x} - \mu_0}{\frac{s}{\sqrt{n}}} = \frac{1.3 - 1.5}{\frac{1.2}{\sqrt{36}}} = \frac{-0.2}{0.2} = -1$$

Since this is a lower-tail test, the p value is the area to the left of -1 on the standard normal curve. The expression $= \text{NORMDIST}(-1, 0,1,\text{TRUE})$ is entered into any cell of the Excel worksheet and the value 0.158655 is returned. The p value $= 0.158655$ is greater than $\alpha = 0.05$ and the null hypothesis is not rejected. We cannot conclude that the drug decreases response time.

10.20 It is known that the mean response time for rats to a certain stimulus is 1.5 s. A researcher is interested in determining if drug C changes the mean response time to this stimulus. If μ is the mean response time of such rats when under the influence of drug C, then the hypotheses of interest are $H_0: \mu = 1.5$ and $H_a: \mu \neq 1.5$. The researcher determines the response times of 36 rats under the influence of drug C and finds that the mean response time is $\bar{x} = 1.9$ and the standard deviation is $s = 1.2$. If the level of significance $\alpha = 0.05$ is chosen by the researcher before the experiment is conducted, what conclusion does she reach?

Solution

The computed value of the test statistic is

$$z = \frac{\bar{x} - \mu_0}{\frac{s}{\sqrt{n}}} = \frac{1.9 - 1.5}{\frac{1.2}{\sqrt{36}}} = \frac{0.4}{0.2} = 2$$

Since this is a two-tail test, the p value is the area to the right of 2 on the standard normal curve, doubled. The expression $= 2*(1 - \text{NORMDIST}(2,0,1,\text{TRUE}))$ is entered into any cell of the Excel worksheet and the value 0.0455 is returned. The p-value $= 0.0455$ is less than $\alpha = 0.05$ and the null hypothesis is rejected. We conclude that the drug changes the response time.

10.21 The most recent national C-section rate is reported as 22.6 per 100 births. A research study in Midwestern City randomly selected 10,000 birth records from the past year and used them to test the hypotheses: $H_0: p = 22.6\%$ versus $H_a: p \neq 22.6\%$, where p is the C-section rate in Midwestern City. In words, the study was trying to determine if the Midwestern City C-section rate was different from the national rate. If $\alpha = 0.01$ and $\bar{p} = 23.5\%$ of the 10,000 were C-sections, what conclusion would you draw?

Solution

The computed value of the test statistic is

$$z = \frac{\bar{p} - p_0}{\sqrt{\frac{p_0(1 - p_0)}{n}}} = \frac{23.5 - 22.6}{\sqrt{\frac{22.6(77.4)}{10,000}}} = 2.1519$$

Since this is a two-tail test, the p value is the area to the right of 2.1519 on the standard normal curve, doubled. The expression $= 2*(1 - \text{NORMDIST}(2.1519,0,1,\text{TRUE}))$ is entered into any cell of the Excel worksheet and the value 0.031 is returned. The p value $= 0.031$ is not less than $\alpha = 0.01$ and the null hypothesis is not rejected. We cannot conclude that the C-section rate in Midwestern City over the past year differs from the national rate.

10.22 The most recent national C-section rate is reported as 22.6 per 100 births. A research study in Northeastern City randomly selected 10,000 birth records from the past year and used them to test the hypotheses: $H_0: p = 22.6\%$ versus $H_a: p < 22.6\%$, where p is the C-section rate in Northeastern City. In words, the study was trying to determine if the Northeastern City C-section rate was less than the national rate. If $\alpha = 0.10$ and $\bar{p} = 16.3\%$ of the 10,000 were C-sections, what conclusion would you draw?

Solution

The computed value of the test statistic is

$$z = \frac{\bar{p} - p_0}{\sqrt{\frac{p_0(1 - p_0)}{n}}} = \frac{16.3 - 22.6}{\sqrt{\frac{22.6(77.4)}{10,000}}} = -15.06$$

Since this is a lower-tail test, the p value is the area to the left of -15.06 on the standard normal curve, doubled. The expression $= \text{NORMDIST}(-15.06,0,1,\text{TRUE})$ is entered into any cell of the Excel worksheet and the value 0 is returned. The p value $= 0$ is less than $\alpha = 0.1$ and the null hypothesis is rejected. We can conclude that the C-section rate in Northeastern City over the past year is less than the national average.

10.23 The most recent national C-section rate is reported as 22.6 per 100 births. A research study in Southwestern City randomly selected 10,000 birth records from the past year and used them to test the hypotheses: $H_0: p = 22.6\%$ versus $H_a: p > 22.6\%$, where p is the C-section rate in Southwestern City. In words, the study was trying to determine if the Southwestern City C-section rate was greater than the national rate. If $\alpha = 0.05$ and $\bar{p} = 23.2\%$ of the 10,000 were C-sections, what conclusion would you draw?

Solution

The computed value of the test statistic is

$$z = \frac{\bar{p} - p_0}{\sqrt{\dfrac{p_0(1 - p_0)}{n}}} = \frac{23.2 - 22.6}{\sqrt{\dfrac{22.6(77.4)}{10,000}}} = 1.43$$

Since this is an upper-tail test, the p value is the area to the right of 1.43 on the standard normal curve. The expression $= 1 - \text{NORMDIST}(1.43,0,1,\text{TRUE})$ is entered into any cell of the Excel worksheet and the value 0.076 is returned. The p value $= 0.076$ is not less than $\alpha = 0.05$ and the null hypothesis is not rejected. We cannot conclude that the C-section rate in Southwestern City over the past year is greater than the national average.

10.24 If a hypothesis test were conducted using $\alpha = 0.05$, for which of the following p values would the null hypothesis be rejected? (a) 0.06   (b) 0.11   (c) 0.02   (d) 0.003   (e) 0.249

Solution

In testing hypotheses, the null hypothesis is rejected and the research hypothesis is supported if the p value $< \alpha$. (a) Do not reject the null hypothesis. (b) Do not reject the null hypothesis. (c) Reject the null hypothesis. (d) Reject the null hypothesis. (e) Do not reject the null hypothesis.

10.25 For each α and p value, indicate whether the research hypothesis would be supported. (a) $\alpha = 0.05$ and p value $= 0.10$ (b) $\alpha = 0.05$ and p value $= 0.001$ (c) $\alpha = 0.01$ and p value $= 0.05$ (d) $\alpha = 0.01$ and p value $= 0.10$ (e) $\alpha = 0.01$ and p value $= 0.18$ (f) $\alpha = 0.10$ and p value $= 0.05$

Solution

(a) Research hypothesis not supported. (b) Research hypothesis supported. (c) Research hypothesis not supported. (d) Research hypothesis not supported. (e) Research hypothesis not supported. (f) Research hypothesis supported.

Supplementary Problems

10.26 The basic nursing education of the 2500 nurses at United Health Care System is given in Fig. 10-35. Give the number of nurses in each of the three education categories at Unified Health Care System.

10.27 Give the angles for each of the three pieces of the pie chart in Problem 10.26.

10.28 Suppose a bar chart was constructed using the three categories and their frequencies in Problem 10.26. Give the frequencies for each of the three categories.

10.29 For the bar chart discussed in Problem 10.28, which category has the tallest bar and which has the shortest bar?

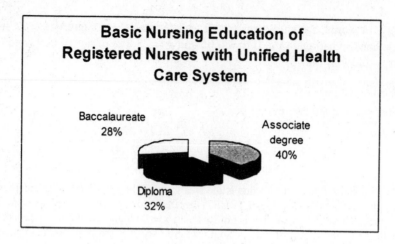

Fig. 10-35

10.30 Table 10-16 gives the resting pulse readings for 30 male and 30 female patients in a research study. A Minitab printout of the descriptive statistics for the data in Table 10-16 is given in Fig. 10-36. By how many beats per minute, on the average, do the female pulse readings exceed the male pulse readings?

Table 10-16   Resting Pulse Readings for Male and Female Patients

Male						Female				
69	71	77	73	68		80	87	74	82	70
69	80	66	71	61		69	73	72	69	86
61	72	71	60	66		72	68	82	77	86
77	73	64	60	60		89	81	74	90	65
70	67	61	73	76		86	65	67	65	85
64	76	65	77	69		77	82	68	87	83

```
Variable              N         Mean      Median      TrMean       StDev      SE Mean
Mpulse               30        68.90      69.00       68.85        5.89        1.07
Fepulse              30        77.03      77.00       77.00        8.12        1.48

Variable        Minimum      Maximum         Q1          Q3
Mpulse           60.00        80.00        64.00       73.00
Fepulse          65.00        90.00        69.00       85.25
```

Fig. 10-36

10.31 For the data in Problem 10.30, compare the variability of the male and female pulse readings by computing the range, interquartile range, and standard deviation for both males and females.

10.32 For the data in Problem 10.30, construct a dot plot for male and female pulse readings and comment on the relationship of the two dot plots.

10.33 For the male pulse readings in Problem 10.30, find the percentage of readings within one, two, and three standard deviations of the mean.

10.34 For the female pulse readings in Problem 10.30, find the percentage of readings within one, two, and three standard deviations of the mean.

10.35 Patients in a research study had a mean BMI (kilograms per square meter) equal to 25.7 and a standard deviation equal to 1.4. Nothing is known about the distribution of the BMI measurements. Apply Chebyshev's rule to find an interval that (*a*) contains at least 75% of the BMI measurements and (*b*) contains at least 89% of the BMI measurements.

10.36 Patients in a research study had a mean systolic blood pressure (mmHg) equal to 127 and a standard deviation equal to 13. Use Chebyshev's rule to answer the following.

(*a*) At least what percent of the systolic measurements were between 101 and 153?

(*b*) At least what percent of the systolic measurements were between 88 and 166?

10.37 Suppose that you know that the BMI measurements in Problem 10.35 have a bell-shaped distribution. Use the empirical rule to answer the following.

(*a*) What percent of the BMI measurements are between 24.3 and 27.1?

(*b*) What percent of the BMI measurements are between 22.9 and 28.5?

(*c*) What percent of the BMI measurements are between 21.5 and 29.9?

10.38 The hemoglobin A1C values for a group of insulin-dependent diabetics have a mean equal to 8.1% and a standard deviation equal to 1.8%. Suppose you know that the hemoglobin A1C values have a bell-shaped distribution. Use the empirical rule to answer the following.

(*a*) Find an interval in which approximately 68% of the hemoglobin A1C values lie.

(*b*) Find an interval in which approximately 95% of the hemoglobin A1C values lie.

(*c*) Find an interval in which approximately 99.7% of the hemoglobin A1C values lie.

10.39 An accident-avoidance study research coordinator is recruiting left-handed individuals to participate in the study. Approximately 15% of the population is left-handed. Use the AND/OR rules of probability to find the probabilities of the following events concerning the random selection of three individuals. Find the probability that of the three selected individuals:

(*a*) None of the three is left-handed.

(*b*) Exactly one of the three is left-handed.

(*c*) Exactly two of the three are left-handed.

(*d*) All three are left-handed.

10.40 Table 10-17 gives the blood type distribution for blacks and whites in the United States. Find the probability that among the next 10 white blood donors (assume they donate independently of one another):
(*a*) All will be type AB.   (*b*) None will be type AB.   (*c*) Half will be type AB.

Table 10-17   Blood Type Percent by Race

	Blood Type			
	O	A	B	AB
Black	49	27	20	4
White	45	40	11	4

10.41   Refer to Table 10-17. Find the probability that among the next 10 black blood donors (assume they donate independently of one another):

(*a*) All will be type B.   (*b*) None will be type B.   (*c*) Half will be type B.

10.42   Binomial probabilities may be found using the binomial probability formula. The binomial probability formula is

$$P(x) = \frac{n!}{x!(n-x)!}\, p^x (1-p)^{n-x}$$

Note: $2! = 2 \times 1$, $3! = 3 \times 2 \times 1$, and in general, $n! = n \times (n-1) \times (n-2) \times 1$. In Problem 10.41, let $n = 10$ and $p = 0.20$ and $x = 10$ for part (*a*), $x = 0$ for part (*b*), and $x = 5$ for part (*c*). Verify that using these values in the binomial probability formula will compute the same probabilities as were computed in Problem 10.41.

10.43   Refer to Problems 10.40 and 10.42 and then use the binomial probability formula to compute the probabilities in Problem 10.40.

10.44   If adult male weights are normally distributed with mean equal to 170 lb and standard deviation equal to 15 lb, use the function NORMDIST in Excel to find the following.

(*a*)   The percent who weigh over 200 lb

(*b*)   The percent who weigh between 150 and 200 lb

(*c*)   The percent who weigh less than 160 lb

10.45   For the male weights described in Problem 10.44, use the function NORMINV in Excel to find the following.

(*a*)   The first quartile of male weights

(*b*)   The third quartile of male weights

(*c*)   The 90th percentile of male weights

10.46   If adult female weights are normally distributed with mean equal to 135 lb and standard deviation equal to 19 lb, use the function NORMDIST in Excel to find the following.

(*a*)   The percent who weigh more than 175 lb

(*b*)   The percent who weigh between 100 and 150 lb

(*c*)   The percent who weigh less than 120 lb

10.47 For the female weights described in Problem 10.46, use the function NORMINV in Excel to find the following.

    (a)   The first quartile of female weights

    (b)   The third quartile of female weights

    (c)   The 90th percentile of female weights

10.48 Suppose you are to select a random sample of 5 from the patients seen by Christine the past week as given in Table 10-8. Suppose Excel was used to select five random numbers between 1 and 50 and they were 4, 17, 29, 36, and 43. Who were the selected patients?

10.49 Table 10-9 shows lengths of hospital stay for 100 patients. For these 100 patients, the mean length of stay was 5.25 days and the median length of stay was 5 days. Excel was used to select 10 random numbers. The random numbers selected in order were 3, 14, 19, 33, 47, 48, 59, 88, 93, and 99. Suppose the cells in Table 10-9 are numbered from 1 to 100 starting at the top of the first column and going down column by column from left to right. Give the 10 lengths of stay determined by the random numbers. Find the mean and median for the sample of 10 lengths of stay and find the differences between the population and sample measurements.

10.50 The mean total cholesterol (mmol/L) for 50 subjects in a research study was 4.0 and the standard deviation was 0.7. If 4.0 is used to estimate the population mean total cholesterol, find the following: (a) 80% margin of error; (b) 90% margin of error; (c) 95% margin of error; (d) 99% margin of error.

10.51 Use the results of Problem 10.50 to find an: (a) 80% confidence interval for μ; (b) 90% confidence interval for μ; (c) 95% confidence interval for μ; (d) 99% confidence interval for μ.

10.52 The mean triglycerides (mmol/L) for 50 subjects in a research study was 0.7 and the standard deviation was 0.2. If 0.7 is used to estimate the mean triglycerides for the population, find the following: (a) 80% margin of error; (b) 90% margin of error; (c) 95% margin of error; (d) 99% margin of error.

10.53 Use the results of Problem 10.52 to find an: (a) 80% confidence interval for μ; (b) 90% confidence interval for μ; (c) 95% confidence interval for μ; (d) 99% confidence interval for μ.

10.54 In a sample of 500 men over age 60, a total of 312 were found to have benign prostatic hyperplasia (BPH). (a) What is the point estimate of the percent of all men over age 60 who have BPH? (b) What is the 95% margin of error associated with this point estimate? (c) Give a 95% confidence interval for p.

10.55 In a sample of 900 women over age 60, a total of 715 were found to suffer from stress incontinence. (a) What is the point estimate of the percent of all women over age 60 who have stress incontinence? (b) What is the 95% margin of error associated with this point estimate? (c) Give a 95% confidence interval for p.

10.56 If a sample standard deviation, s, is known from a previous study, the sample size needed to obtain a 95% margin of error equal to E when estimating the population mean is given by the equation $n = \dfrac{1.96^2 s^2}{E^2}$.

A previous study of insulin-dependent diabetics found a mean BMI equal to $25.7 \,\mathrm{kg/m^2}$ with a standard deviation equal to 1.4. A new study is planned and a 95% margin of error equal to $0.25 \,\mathrm{kg/m^2}$ is required when estimating the population mean BMI. What sample size is required?

10.57 If a sample percent, $\bar{p}$, is known from a previous study, the sample size needed to estimate the population percent, p, with a 95% margin of error equal to E is given by the equation $n = \dfrac{1.96^2 \bar{p}(1 - \bar{p})}{E^2}$. A previous study of stress incontinence in women over age 60 found that 55% had stress incontinence. What sample size is required to estimate the population percent with a 95% margin of error equal to 3%?

10.58 If there is no previous study concerning a population percent, p, the sample size needed to estimate the population percent, p, with a 95% margin of error equal to E (expressed as a percent) is given by the equation $n = \dfrac{1.96^2 \times 2500}{E^2}$. No previous study of stress incontinence in women over age 60 has been conducted. What sample size is required to estimate the population percent that have stress incontinence with a 95% margin of error equal to 3%?

10.59 State whether you reject or do not reject the null hypothesis for the following cases: (a) $\alpha = 0.05$, p value $= 0.15$; (b) $\alpha = 0.01$, p value $= 0.003$; (c) $\alpha = 0.10$, p value $= 0.05$.

10.60 Classify each of the following research hypotheses as a lower-, upper-, or two-tailed test. (a) H_a: $\mu \neq 12$; (b) H_a: $\mu < 7$; (c) H_a: $p > 13.5$; (d) H_a: $p < 69$.

10.61 Calculate the value of the test statistic, z, for each of the following cases: (a) H_0: $\mu = 10$; $n = 35$, $\bar{x} = 11.5$, and $s = 2.3$; (b) H_0: $\mu = 120$; $n = 40$, $\bar{x} = 137.5$, and $s = 35.5$; (c) H_0: $p = 10\%$; $n = 350$, $\bar{p} = 11.5\%$; (d) H_0: $p = 70\%$; $n = 350$, $\bar{p} = 68.5\%$.

10.62 Calculate the p value for each of the following scenarios: (a) H_a: $\mu \neq 12$, $z = 1.78$; (b) H_a: $\mu < 75$, $z = -2.34$; (c) H_a: > 22, $z = 2.25$.

10.63 Calculate the p-value for each of the following scenarios: (a) H_a: $p \neq 25\%$, $z = 0.56$; (b) H_a: $p < 35\%$, $z = -2.77$; (c) H_a: $p > 45\%$, $z = 1.11$.

10.64 Table 10-18 gives the coronary flow reserve for 40 insulin-dependent diabetic patients. Test H_0: $\mu = 4.50$ versus H_a: $\mu < 4.50$ with $\alpha = 0.05$, where μ stands for the mean coronary flow reserve for insulin-dependent diabetics. Compute the test statistic and the p value, and give your conclusion.

Table 10-18   Coronary Flow Reserve Values

5.04	3.26	5.47	3.09	1.04
3.64	7.47	2.84	5.80	0.33
1.66	4.80	4.16	4.50	4.92
4.33	3.31	1.30	1.50	2.87
4.01	4.01	1.80	3.29	5.43
3.56	5.90	4.27	4.35	2.25
4.63	8.03	2.58	3.66	2.14
3.68	4.61	3.62	1.22	6.09

10.65   In order to test $H_0: p = 50\%$ versus $H_a: p > 50\%$ with $\alpha = 0.05$, where p is the percent of men over age 60 with benign prostatic hyperplasia (BPH), a random sample of 1500 men over age 60 was selected and 850 of the men had BPH. Compute the test statistic and the p value, and give your conclusion.

Answers to Supplementary Problems

10.26   Associate degree 1000   Diploma 800   Baccalaureate 700

10.27   Associate degree 144°   Diploma 115.2°   Baccalaureate 100.8°

10.28   Associate degree 1000   Diploma 800   Baccalaureate 700

10.29   Tallest bar is for Associate degree, shortest bar is for Baccalaureate

10.30   If the mean is used as the measure of average, female exceeds male by $77.03 - 68.90 = 8.13$ bpm.

10.31   Male: Range $= 20$, IQR $= 9$, $s = 5.89$ Female: Range $= 25$, IQR $= 16.25$, $s = 8.12$

10.32   The female dot plot is shifted to the right of the male dot plot. However, there is considerable overlap.

10.33   63.01 to 74.49, 60%   57.12 to 80.68, 100%   51.23 to 86.57, 100%

10.34   68.91 to 85.15, 56.7%   60.79 to 93.27, 100%   52.67 to 101.39, 100%

10.35   (*a*)   22.9 to 28.5   (*b*)   21.5 to 29.9

10.36   (*a*)   75%   (*b*)   89%

10.37   (*a*)   68%   (*b*)   95%   (*c*)   99.7%

10.38   (*a*)   6.3% to 9.9%   (*b*)   4.5% to 11.7%   (*c*)   2.7% to 13.5%

10.39   (*a*)   0.614125   (*b*)   0.325125   (*c*)   0.057375   (*d*)   0.003375

10.40   (*a*)   0.000000   (*b*)   0.664833   (*c*)   0.000021

10.41   (*a*)   0.000000   (*b*)   0.107374   (*c*)   0.026424

10.42   (*a*)   0.000000   (*b*)   0.107374   (*c*)   0.026424

10.43   (*a*)   0.000000   (*b*)   0.664833   (*c*)   0.000021

10.44   (*a*)   0.02275 or 2.275%   (*b*)   0.886039 or 88.6039%   (*c*)   0.252492 or 25.2492%

10.45   (*a*)   159.8826   (*b*)   180.1174   (*c*)   189.2233

10.46   (*a*)   0.017634 or 1.7634%   (*b*)   0.752353 or 75.2353%   (*c*)   0.214918 or 21.4918%

10.47   (*a*)   122.1847   (*b*)   147.8153   (*c*)   159.3495

10.48 Scroggins, P   Kee, M   Feller, B   Banks, E   Hazel, B

10.49 4, 4, 3, 2, 7, 5, 11, 3, 6, and 7,   sample mean = 5.2, population mean = 5.25, difference = 0.05
           sample median = 4.5, population median = 5, difference = 0.5

10.50 (a) $1.282 \times \dfrac{.7}{\sqrt{50}} = 1.282 \times 0.099 = 0.127$ (b) $1.645 \times 0.099 = 0.163$

      (c) $1.960 \times 0.099 = 0.194$ (d) $2.575 \times 0.099 = 0.255$

10.51 (a) 3.87 to 4.13   (b) 3.84 to 4.16   (c) 3.81 to 4.19   (d) 3.75 to 4.25

10.52 (a) $1.282 \times 0.028 = 0.036$ (b) $1.645 \times 0.028 = 0.046$
      (c) $1.960 \times 0.028 = 0.055$ (d) $2.575 \times 0.028 = 0.072$

10.53 (a) 0.664 to 0.736   (b) 0.654 to 0.746   (c) 0.645 to 0.755   (d) 0.628 to 0.772

10.54 (a) 62.4%   (b) 4.2%   (c) 58.2% to 66.6%

10.55 (a) 79.4%   (b) 2.6%   (c) 76.8% to 82.0%

10.56 120.4726, which we round up to 121

10.57 1056.44, which is rounded up to 1057

10.58 1067.11, which is rounded up to 1068

10.59 (a) Do not reject H_0 (b) Reject H_0 (c) Reject H_0

10.60 (a) Two-tail test   (b) Lower-tail test   (c) Upper-tail test   (d) Lower-tail test

10.61 (a) 3.858   (b) 3.118   (c) 0.935   (d) -0.612

10.62 (a) 0.075   (b) 0.00964   (c) 0.012

10.63 (a) 0.575   (b) 0.003   (c) 0.134

10.64 Test statistic $= -2.74$ p value $= 0.003$ Reject, since p value $< \alpha$

10.65 Test statistic $= 5.16$ p value $= 0.000$ Reject, since p value $< \alpha$

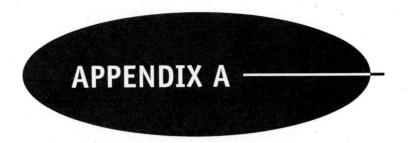

Temperature Conversions

The two temperature scales of importance in nursing are the *Celsius* scale and the *Fahrenheit* scale. Temperatures are measured on the Celsius scale in degrees Celsius (°C) and on the Fahrenheit scale in degrees Fahrenheit (°F). The Celsius scale divides the interval between the freezing point and the boiling point of water into 100 equal parts. The freezing point of water is set at 0°C, and the boiling point at 100°C. On the Fahrenheit scale, the freezing point of water is 32°F and the boiling point is 212°F (see Fig. A-1). The following formulas relate a temperature in one scale to a temperature in the other scale.

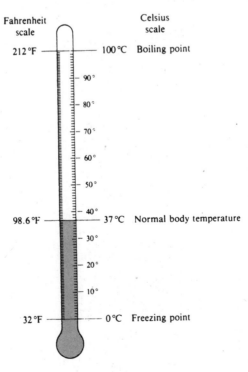

Fig. A-1

Conversion from degrees Celsius to degrees Fahrenheit:

$$F = \frac{9}{5}C + 32$$

Conversion from degrees Fahrenheit to degrees Celsius:

$$C = \frac{5}{9}(F - 32)$$

These formulas are equivalent to the following directions.
To convert from degrees Celsius to degrees Fahrenheit, start with the degrees Celsius and

1. Multiply by 9
2. Divide by 5
3. Add 32

To convert from degrees Fahrenheit to degrees Celsius, start with the degrees Fahrenheit and

1. Subtract 32
2. Multiply by 5
3. Divide by 9

Note that the steps followed in performing one conversion are just the opposite steps, taken in the reverse order, of the other conversion.

EXAMPLE 1 (*a*) Convert 20°C to degrees Fahrenheit. (*b*) Convert 68°F to degrees Celsius.

(*a*) Follow the steps for converting from degrees Celsius to degrees Fahrenheit.

1.   Multiply by 9: $20 \times 9 = 180$

2.   Divide by 5: $180 \div 5 = 36$

3.   Add 32: $36 + 32 = 68$

The answer is 68°F. You will see below that performing the *opposite* operations in the *reverse order* will lead back to the starting point.

(*b*) Follow the steps for converting from degrees Fahrenheit to degrees Celsius.

1.   Subtract 32: $68 - 32 = 36$

2.   Multiply by 5: $36 \times 5 = 180$

3.   Divide by 9: $180 \div 9 = 20$

The answer is 20°C as was expected.

Solved Problems

1.   Convert the following Celsius temperatures to Fahrenheit temperatures.

   (*a*)   37°C (normal body temperature)
   (*b*)   0°C (freezing point of water)
   (*c*)   100°C (boiling point of water)
   (*d*)   23.5°C

Solution

Follow the steps for converting from degrees Celsius to degrees Fahrenheit (multiply by 9, divide by 5, add 32).

(a)	(b)	(c)	(d)
37	0	100	23.5
×9	×9	×9	×9
5)333	5)0	5)900	5)211.5
66.6	0	180	42.3
+32	+32	+32	+32
98.6°F	32°F	212°F	74.3°F

2.   Convert the following Fahrenheit temperatures to Celsius temperatures.

(a)   98.6°F (normal body temperature)

(b)   32°F (freezing point of water)

(c)   212°F (boiling point of water)

(d)   104.2°F

Solution

Follow the steps for converting from degrees Fahrenheit to degrees Celsius (subtract 32, multiply by 5, divide by 9).

(a)	(b)	(c)	(d)
98.6	32	212	104.2
−32	−32	−32	−32
66.6	0	180	72.2
×5	×5	×5	×5
9)333	9)0	9)900	9)361
37°C	0°C	100°C	40.1°C

Supplementary Problems

3.   Convert each temperature from one scale to the other (Fahrenheit or Celsius).

(a)   38°C   (c)   110.5°F   (e)   99.4°F   (g)   36.8°C

(b)   72°F   (d)   39°C   (f)   29°C   (h)   102.8°F

Answers to Supplementary Problems

3.   (a)   100.4°F   (c)   43.6°C   (e)   37.4°C   (g)   98.2°F
          (b)   22.2°C   (d)   102.2°F   (f)   84.2°F   (h)   39.3°C

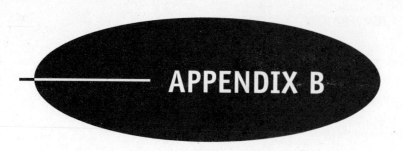

APPENDIX B

Some Commonly Used Medical Symbols and Abbreviations

Symbol	Meaning	Symbol	Meaning
a	before	mEq	milliequivalent
@	at	mg (mG)	milligram
a.a.	of each	mL (ml)	milliliter
ac	before meals	mm	millimeter
A.M.	morning (before noon)	m	minim
ad lib.	freely as desired	oz (℥)	ounce
aq	water	pc	after meals
bid	twice a day	per	by (for each)
c̄	with	P.M.	afternoon
caps	capsule	PO	by mouth
cc	cubic centimeter	prn	when necessary
cm	centimeter	pt	pint
cm³	cubic centimeter	qd	every day
°C	degrees Celsius	qh	every hour
dr (Ʒ)	dram	q2h	every 2 hours
°F	degrees Fahrenheit	q3h	every 3 hours
g (G, gm)	gram	q4h	every 4 hours
gr	grain	qid	four times a day
gtt	drop	qod	every other day
h (hr)	hour	qt	quart
hs	bedtime	s̄	without
IM	intramuscular	SC	subcutaneous
IU	international unit	s̄s̄	half (1/2)
IV	intravenous	stat.	immediately
IVPB	intravenous piggyback	T (tbs)	tablespoon
kg (kG)	kilogram	t (tsp)	teaspoon
L (l)	liter	tab	tablet
lb	pound	tid	three times a day
m	meter	U	Unit
m²	square meter	ut. dict.	as directed

INDEX